Movement Disorders

Unforgettable Cases and Lessons
From the Bedside

Movement Disorders

Unforgettable Cases and Lessons
From the Bedside

Edited By

HUBERT H. FERNANDEZ, MD
Professor of Medicine (Neurology)
Cleveland Clinic Lerner College of Medicine
and
Head of Movement Disorders
Center for Neurological Restoration, Cleveland Clinic
Cleveland, Ohio

MARCELO MERELLO, MD, PhD
Professor of Neurology and Director of Neuroscience Department
Raul Carrea Institute for Neurological Research (FLENI)
and
Clinical Researcher
Consejo Nacional de Investigaciones Científicas y Técnicas (CONICET)
Buenos Aires, Argentina

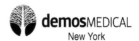

demosMEDICAL
New York

Visit our website at www.demosmedpub.com

ISBN: 9781936287284
e-book ISBN: 9781617050589

Acquisitions Editor: Beth Barry
Compositor: Newgen Imaging

Medicine is an ever-changing science. Research and clinical experience are continually expanding our knowledge, in particular our understanding of proper treatment and drug therapy. The authors, editors, and publisher have made every effort to ensure that all information in this book is in accordance with the state of knowledge at the time of production of the book. Nevertheless, the authors, editors, and publisher are not responsible for errors or omissions or for any consequences from application of the information in this book and make no warranty, express or implied, with respect to the contents of the publication. Every reader should examine carefully the package inserts accompanying each drug and should carefully check whether the dosage schedules mentioned therein or the contraindications stated by the manufacturer differ from the statements made in this book. Such examination is particularly important with drugs that are either rarely used or have been newly released on the market.

Library of Congress Cataloging-in-Publication Data

Movement disorders : unforgettable cases and lessons from the bedside / [edited by] Hubert H. Fernandez, Marcelo Merello.
     p. ; cm.
   Includes bibliographical references and index.
   ISBN 978-1-936287-28-4 — ISBN 978-1-61705-058-9 (e-book)
   1. Movement disorders—Case studies. I. Fernandez, Hubert H. II. Merello, Marcelo J., 1961-
   [DNLM: 1. Movement Disorders—Case Reports. 2. Movement Disorders—complications—Case Reports. WL 390]
   RC376.5.M692 2013
   616.8'3—dc23   2012013724

Printed in the United States of America by Gasch Printing.
12 13 14 15 / 5 4 3 2 1

We would like to dedicate this book
to all our patients, especially those who challenged us, kept us awake all night,
forced us to go back to our books, made us search the scientific literature, and call our
colleagues for advice. They have made us human, kept us humble, and most of all,
provided us our purpose on earth.

To each of our families, who understood our profession, along with its joys and
sacrifices. They have loved and supported us unconditionally, and sailed with us on our
life journey, faithfully, in calm or turbulent seas.

H.H.F.
M.M.

Contents

Contributors   *xiii*
Preface   *xxiii*
Acknowledgments   *xxvii*

I. Parkinson's Disease

1. Levodopa's Dark Side: The Remarkable Story of Dr B   *2*
   Howard I. Hurtig

2. Peanut Butter and Lottery: Two Impulse Control Disorders in an Elderly Parkinson Patient   *7*
   Hubert H. Fernandez

3. The Man Who Was Addicted to Levodopa: An Unforgettable Case Illustrating
   Dopamine Dysregulation Syndrome   *10*
   Mwiza Ushe and Joel Perlmutter

4. The Most Horrific Tactile Hallucination Described by a 78-Year-Old Colombian
   Man With Parkinson's Disease   *13*
   Oscar Bernal-Pacheco

5. Can a Research Subject Be Too Enthusiastic? An Important Lesson on Parkinson
   Trials From a 65-Year-Old Banker   *16*
   Richard M. Zweig

6. Parkinson's Disease Never Presents With Freezing—Except When It Does!   *18*
   Niall Quinn

7. From Hero to Villain: Walking the Tightrope in Impulse Control Disorders   *20*
   Junaid H. Siddiqui, Mayur Pandya, Anwar Ahmed, and Hubert H. Fernandez

8. Our Unforgettable Case of Malignant Motor Fluctuations in a Parkinson Patient   *24*
   Laura Silveira-Moriyama and Andrew J. Lees

9. Gaining Movement but Losing Speech: The Unexpected Side Effects of DBS Surgery   *27*
   Louis C.S. Tan and John Thomas

10. Strength (and Fun) in Numbers: Lessons From an "Extended Family" of Parkinson
    Patients and Their Spouses   *29*
    Ronald F. Pfeiffer

11. Help! My Spouse Is Out of Control! Three Cases of Dopamine Dysregulation
    in Parkinson's Disease   *31*
    Mayur Pandya and Ilia Itin

12. De Novo Parkinsonism Versus Depression: What to Treat First?   *33*
    Sergio E. Starkstein

13. How a Wife's Insomnia Led to Her Husband's Parkinson Diagnosis: The First
    Warning From REM Sleep Behavior Disorder   *35*
    Arturo Del Carmen Garay and Daniel P. Cardinali

II. *Other Parkinsonian Disorders*

14. Severe Hypophonia and Parkinsonism With Hepatitis C and Elevated
    Mn: Lessons From a Drug Abuser   *40*
    Anthony E. Lang

15. Ironing Out the Details: Two Sisters With Progressive Parkinsonism and Ataxia   *43*
    Matthew A. Bower and Paul J. Tute

16. Acute Onset of Akinetic Mutism With Rigidity in an Elderly Psychiatric
    Patient: A Reminder on Catatonia   *50*
    Joseph H. Friedman

17. Acute Onset Parkinsonism in a Middle-Aged Alcoholic: A "Great Case"   *54*
    Joseph H. Friedman

18. A 38-Year-Old Brazilian Woman Presenting With Reversible Parkinsonism
    Associated With Neurocysticercosis   *57*
    Hélio A.G. Teive

19. An Apparent Case of Early Onset Parkinsonism: A Lesson on Huntington's
    Disease From a Bus Driver in Italy   *60*
    Giovanni Abbruzzese, Monica Bandettini, Flavio Nobili, and Paola Mandich

20. A Vasculopathic Man With "Vascular Parkinsonism" Without Vasculopathy:
    My Humbling Case of Normal Pressure Hydrocephalus   *62*
    Alberto J. Espay

21. Too Young for Parkinson's Disease? Levodopa-Responsive Parkinsonism
    in an 8-Year-Old Boy   *66*
    Oscar S. Gershanik

22. The Misleading Phenotypes of PD and Parkinson-Plus Syndromes: Lessons I Learned
    From a 59-Year-Old Woman   *70*
    Oscar S. Gershanik

23. Atypical Parkinsonism With a Twist: My Memorable Case of an Indian Woman
    With Levodopa-Responsive Parkinsonism With Motor Fluctuations   *74*
    Kathleen M. Shannon

24. A Patient With Rapidly Progressive Dementia and Supranuclear Gaze Palsy: A Memorable
    Lesson on Prion Disorders   *77*
    Igor N. Petrovic, Laura Silveira-Moriyama, and Andrew J. Lees

25. A Lesson on Following One's Instincts: A Case of a Paraneoplastic Disorder Posing as PSP   *80*
    Chris Adams and Rajeev Kumar

26. A Sudden, Static, Supranuclear Syndrome After Surgical Repair of an Aortic Aneurysm in a
    Young Man From Thailand   *84*
    Roongroj Bhidayasiri and Duang Kawahara

27. Asymmetric Parkinsonism With Autonomic Dysfunction and Abnormal Sphincter EMG in a
    63-Year-Old English Woman: Why Not PSP?   *88*
    David R. Williams

28. Tremor Dominant Parkinsonism: Lesion or Deep Brain Stimulation?   *91*
Elisaveta Sokolov, Tipu Z. Aziz, Dipankar Nandi, and Peter G. Bain

29. The Miracle of Disappearance of Dyskinesias: The Case of an Elderly Italian
Woman Who Benefited From a Stroke   *95*
Giovanni Abbruzzese, Tiziano Tamburini, Laura Avanzino, and Roberta Marchese

30. Unforgettable Lessons From a Forgetful Museum Attendant With a Supranuclear Gaze Palsy   *98*
David J. Burn

31. Reversible Unilateral Parkinsonism Associated With Bipolar Affective Disorder in a
59-Year-Old Spanish Woman   *101*
Jaime Kulisevsky and Roser Ribosa Nogué

32. Sudden-Onset Mutism and Parkinsonism in a Psychiatric Patient: An Unusual Case of
"Central Pontine Myelinolysis"   *104*
Jaime Kulisevsky and Roser Ribosa Nogué

33. Acute Confusion and Rapidly Progressive Dementia in Diffuse Lewy Body Disease?   *107*
Eduardo Tolosa and Francesc Valldeoriola

34. Stereotypic Movements in a Nurse Referred for the Evaluation of Parkinson's Disease   *111*
Patrick Hickey and Mark Stacy

35. Familial Albers-Schonberg's Disease (Osteopetrosis) Complicated by Dystonia and
Dopa-Resistant Parkinsonism   *115*
Michelle Ferreira and Néstor Gálvez-Jiménez

III. Tremors

36. Not "X"-actly a Simple Tremor   *122*
Haitham M. Hussein, Matthew A. Bower, and Paul J. Tuite

37. The Tremulous Driver Who Could Not Find His Way Home   *127*
Ignacio Rubio-Agusti and Kailash Bhatia

38. The Shaky Professor: A Tale of Tremors   *131*
Amanda Jane Thompson

39. Early-Onset Hand Tremor and Later Adult Progression Without Speech Involvement:
An Unusual DYT6 Presentation   *134*
José C. Cabassa and Susan B. Bressman

40. Untwisting a Double-Twist: Severe Tremors in a Factory Worker With a Melanoma History   *137*
Thien Thien Lim, Ilia Itin, Stephen Hantus, and Hubert H. Fernandez

41. Disabling Postural and Resting Tremor: What Should One Aim to Treat?   *140*
Rafael Gonzalez-Redondo, Jorge Guridi, and José A. Obeso

42. Pseudopsychogenic Tremors and Parkinsonism: Two Presentations of Multiple
Sclerosis That Almost Fooled Us   *144*
Thien Thien Lim, Ilia Itin, and Hubert H. Fernandez

IV. Chorea

43. The Clumsy Piano Teacher Unable to Play the Organ in Church   *152*
Anthony E. Lang

44. Chorea in a Man With Peripheral Neuropathy and Hepatomegaly:
The Diagnosis Can Make a Difference!   *155*
Ruth H. Walker

45. When the HD Gene Test Is "Negative": Our Memorable Case of a Nursing Assistant
Fired From Her Job for Making Mistakes   *158*
Daniel Tarsy, Andrew V. Varga, and Penny Greenstein

46. Late-Onset Sydenham's Chorea in a Middle-Aged Brazilian Woman   *160*
Francisco Cardoso and Débora Maia

47. A Case of Calcium-Induced Marital Stress   *162*
Shawn F. Smyth, Liana Rosenthal, and Joseph M. Savitt

48. Discrepancy in CAG Repeat Lengths in a Case of Clinically Manifest Huntington's Disease:
The Pyschological Ordeal of My 24-Year-Old Patient   *165*
Juan Sanchez-Ramos

49. Evolving Movement Disorder in a 13-Year-Old Girl From the Philippines
Presenting Initially With Joint Pains   *168*
Lillian V. Lee, Rosalia A. Teleg, Jeannie Ahorro, Edwin Munoz, and Jose Robles

50. "Defiant and Rebellious" Behavior in a Canadian Teenager: Sarah's Difficult Journey   *172*
Marguerite Wieler and W.R. Wayne Martin

51. The Challenging Case of Progressive Cognitive Decline in a Student: History in the Making?   *175*
David J. Burn

52. Multiple Involuntary Movements in a Young Male Patient With Nephrocalcinosis: A
"Gold Medal" Story   *178*
Debabrata Ghosh

V. Dystonia

53. Seemingly "Progressive Postanoxic Dystonia" Finally Diagnosed 26 Years After Symptom Onset   *184*
Maja Kojovic and Kailash Bhatia

54. Dystonia, Ataxia, Dementia, and a Family History of "Huntington Disease"   *187*
Joseph Jankovic

55. Friedreich's Ataxia Presenting With Childhood Onset Progressive Dystonia and Spasticity   *191*
Joseph Jankovic

56. Dysarthria, Dystonia, and Cerebellar Ataxia: The Tale of Four Sisters   *194*
Marie Vidailhet, Mathieu Anheim, and Cécile Hubsch

57. Early-Onset Generalized Dystonia With Short Stature and Skeletal Dysplasia   *196*
Marie Vidailhet and Emmanuel Roze

58. The Highs and Lows of Deep Brain Stimulation in Dystonia: The Story of a Canadian Boy   *198*
W.R. Wayne Martin and Marguerite Wieler

59. The Opera Singer Who Cannot Hit the High Notes: Is It Always Spasmodic Dysphonia?   *201*
Ilia Itin and Hesham Abboud

60. An 18-Year-Old Woman Who Attacked a Policeman With a Knife: Our Memorable
Lesson on Treatable Causes of Dystonia   *204*
Shyamal H. Mehta and Kapil D. Sethi

61. Rapidly Progressive Dystonia in a 52-Year-Old Thai Woman With SCA Type 2   *207*
Roongroj Bhidayasiri, Wasan Akarathanawat, and Priya Jagota

62. A Young Girl With Presumed Cerebral Palsy and Her Grandfather With Depression,
Dystonia, and Daytime Sleepiness: As Always, Family Is the Clue   *211*
Mark S. LeDoux

63. I Cannot Eat, Even Though I Want To: An Illustrative Case From Mr A on the
Consequences of Dystonia   215
Mwiza Ushe and Joel Perlmutter

64. Painful Muscle Spasms, Twisting, and Loose Stools: What a Combination in an Adolescent Girl!   217
Raymond L. Rosales and Jacqueline E. Banzon

65. Why Did a Competitive Rower Lose His Skill? An Unusual Case of Task-Specific Action Dystonia   222
Jed Barash, Michael Ronthal, and Daniel Tarsy

66. "Tremors" and Gait Difficulties in an 18-Year-Old Hispanic Teenager: An Illustrative Case
on the Power of Levodopa   224
Daniel A. Roque and Carlos Singer

67. A Tendon Transfer That Could Have Been Avoided: My Memorable Case of a
College Student With Dopa-Responsive Dystonia   227
Robert L. Rodnitzky

68. The Serendipitous Discovery of the Beneficial Effect of Zolpidem on Dystonia   229
Virgilio Gerald H. Evidente

69. An Unusual Cause of Cervical Dystonia: Porencephalic Cyst, Putaminal, Pallidal, and
Cerebellar Atrophy, Aqueductal Stenosis, and Obstructive Hydrocephalus   232
Michelle Ferreira and Néstor Gálvez-Jiménez

VI. Ataxia

70. The ABC of Ataxia Should Also Include the E   238
Hasmet A. Hanagasi and Murat Emre

71. Speech and Gait Problems in a Patient Being Treated for Schizophrenia: A Lesson on
Psychiatric Comorbidity From an Afro-Caribbean Man   240
Ruth H. Walker

72. How Wiggling Movements in a 13-Year-Old Girl Helped Diagnose a Longstanding Ataxia   243
David Salat and Oksana Suchowersky

73. Acquired Cerebellar Ataxia Associated With Glutamic Acid Decarboxylase in a
52-Year-Old Brazilian Woman   247
Hélio A.G. Teive

74. Ataxia With Oculomotor Apraxia Type 2 in a 58-Year-Old Computer Programmer
Without Oculomotor Apraxia   249
Frances M. Velez-Lago and S.H. Subramony

75. A Patient With a Progressive Ataxia and Brain Iron Accumulation   252
Elisabeth Wolf and Werner Poewe

76. Evaluating Ataxia: The Eyes Have It—Or Do They?   255
Robert L. Rodnitzky

77. A Zebra Can Change Its Stripes: A Case of Inherited Ataxia   257
Liana S. Rosenthal, Shawn F. Smyth, and Joseph M. Savitt

78. Abrupt Onset "On Stage Ballerina-Like" Stair Descent in an Art Student   259
Marcelo Merello

VII. Tics and Stereotypies

79. Hereditary Syndrome With Multiple Tics: A Lesson on the Phenotypic
Variability of Huntington's Disease   264
Carlo Colosimo, Giovanni Fabbrini, and Alfredo Berardelli

80. Affective Changes and Involuntary Movements in a 29-Year-Old Man: Do Not Forget to Review the Medication List!   *266*
Kathleen M. Shannon

81. Hereditary Stereotypies From a Family in Canada   *268*
Justyna R. Sarna and Oksana Suchowersky

82. Tics From a Church Choir: A Unique Case Illustrating the Challenge of Distinguishing Organic From Psychogenic Tics   *272*
Nelson Hwynn, Genko Oyama, and Michael S. Okun

VIII. *Myoclonus and Startle Syndromes*

83. The Challenging Case of a Man With Paroxysmal Irregular Jerking of the Right Arm   *276*
A. Zangerle, J. Willeit, and W. Poewe

84. A Stiff and Jerky Person: How Useful Is a DAT Scan in the Differential Diagnosis?   *279*
Nicola Modugno, Giovanni Fabbrini, Carlo Colosimo, and Alfredo Berardelli

85. The Torture of Tortuosity: Lessons From a 45-Year-Old Woman With Myoclonus, Dystonia, Chorea, and Ataxia   *281*
Bart P.C. van de Warrenburg and Bastiaan R. Bloem

86. On the Priority of Clinical Diagnosis: A Complex Case With Myoclonus   *285*
Franziska Hopfner and Günther Deuschl

IX. *Psychogenic Movement Disorder Presentations*

87. Walking Out of the Psychogenic "Bizarre-Gait" Pigeonhole: A Lesson From the Psychiatry Ward   *290*
Alberto J. Espay

88. My Unforgettable Parkinson Patient With Psychogenic Tremors   *292*
Kelvin L. Chou

89. Bizarre "Exorcist-Like" Movements and Behavioral Change in an Adolescent Filipino: A Mystery Case   *295*
Lillian V. Lee, Ma. Lourdes Ebero, Nelma Magpusao, and Jose Robles

90. Intermittent Tunnel Vision in a Patient With Multiple Drug Abuse History   *298*
Katrin Bürk, Adam Strelczyk, and Wolfgang H. Oertel

91. "Psychogenic Tremor" in a 32-Year-Old Factory Worker: The Eyes Do Not Lie!   *300*
Richard M. Zweig

About the Editors   *303*
Index   *305*

Contributors

Hesham Abboud, MD
Center for Neurological Restoration
Cleveland Clinic
Cleveland, Ohio

Department of Neurology
University of Alexandria
Alexandria, Egypt

Giovanni Abbruzzese, MD
Department of Neurosciences, Ophthalmology
  and Genetics
University of Genova
Genoa, Italy

Chris Adams, MS
Movement Disorders Center
Colorado Neurological Institute
Englewood, Colorado

Anwar Ahmed, MD
Center for Neurological Restoration
Cleveland Clinic
Cleveland, Ohio

Jeannie Ahorro, MD
Calamba Doctors' Hospital
Calamba, Philippines

Wasan Akarathanawat, MD
Department of Neurology
Chulalongkorn Center of Excellence on
  Parkinson's Disease and Related Disorders
Chulalongkorn University Hospital
Bangkok, Thailand

Department of Medicine
Chulalongkorn University and King
  Chulalongkorn Memorial Hospital
Bangkok, Thailand

Mathieu Anheim, MD
Department of Neurogenetics
CRICM UPMC/INSERM UMR-S 975 CNRS
  UMR7225
Pierre Marie Curie Paris 6 University
Salpêtrière Hospital
Paris, France

Laura Avanzino, MD, PhD
Department of Neurosciences, Ophthalmology
  and Genetics
University of Genova
Genoa, Italy

Tipu Z. Aziz, MD, FRCS(SN) DMedSci
Nuffield Department of Surgery
University of Oxford
Oxford, UK

Peter G. Bain, MA, MD, FRCP
Department of Neurosciences
Imperial College London
London, UK

Monica Bandettini, MD
Department of Neuroscience
University of Genova
Genoa, Italy

Jacqueline E. Banzon, MD
Department of Neurology and Psychiatry
University of Santo Tomas Hospital
Manila, Philippines

Jed Barash, MD
Department of Medicine
Yale University School of Medicine
New Haven, Connecticut

Alfredo Berardelli, MD
Department of Neurology and Psychiatry
Neuromed Institute
Sapienza University of Rome
Rome, Italy

Oscar Bernal-Pacheco, MD
Movement Disorders Clinic
Hospital Militar Central–Clínica Nueva
Universidad Militar Nueva Granada
Bogota, Colombia

Kailash Bhatia, MD, FRCP
Sobell Department of Motor Neuroscience and
   Movement Disorders
UCL Institute of Neurology
London, UK

Roongroj Bhidayasiri, MD, FRCP, FRCPI
Chulalongkorn Center of Excellence for
   Parkinson's Disease and Related Disorders
Chulalongkorn University Hospital
Bangkok, Thailand

Department of Medicine
Chulalongkorn University and King
   Chulalongkorn Memorial Hospital
Bangkok, Thailand

Department of Neurology
Geffen School of Medicine at UCLA
Los Angeles, California

Bastiaan R. Bloem, MD, PhD
Department of Neurology
Donders Centre for Neuroscience
Radboud University Nijmegen Medical Centre
Nijmegen, The Netherlands

Matthew A. Bower, MS, CGC
Institute of Human Genetics
University of Minnesota Medical Center
Minneapolis, Minnesota

Susan B. Bressman, MD
Department of Neurology
Center for Movement Disorders
Philips Ambulatory Care Center
Beth Israel Medical Center
New York, New York

Katrin Bürk, MD
Department of Neurology
University of Marburg
Marburg, Germany

David J. Burn, FRCP, MD, MA
Institute for Ageing and Health
Clinical Ageing Research Unit
Newcastle University
Newcastle upon Tyne, UK

José C. Cabassa, MD
Center for Movement Disorders
Philips Ambulatory Care Center
Beth Israel Medical Center
New York, New York

Daniel P. Cardinali, MD, PhD
Departamento de Docencia e Investigación
Pontificia Universidad Católica Argentina
Buenos Aires, Argentina

Francisco Cardoso, MD, PhD
Departamento de Clínica Médica
Universidade Federal de Minas Gerais
Belo Horizonte, Brazil

Kelvin L. Chou, MD
Department of Neurology
University of Michigan
Ann Arbor, Michigan

Carlo Colosimo, MD
Department of Neurology and Psychiatry
Neuromed Institute
Sapienza University of Rome
Rome, Italy

Arturo del Carmen Garay, MD, PhD
Medicina del Sueño
Unidad de Neurociencias
Centro de Educación Médica e Investigaciones
   Clínicas "Norberto Quirno"
Buenos Aires, Argentina

Günther Deuschl, MD
Department of Neurology
University of Kiel
University-Hospital-Schleswig-Holstein
Kiel, Germany

Ma. Lourdes Ebero, MD
Child Neuroscience Center
Philippine Children's Medical Center
Quezon City, Philippines

Murat Emre, MD, DMsc
Department of Neurology
Behavioral Neurology and Movement
Disorders Unit
Istanbul University
Istanbul, Turkey

Alberto J. Espay, MD, MSc
Gardner Family Center for Parkinson's Disease
and Movement Disorders
University of Cincinnati Academic
Health Center
Department of Neurology
University of Cincinnati
Cincinnati, Ohio

Virgilio Gerald H. Evidente, MD
Department of Neurology
Mayo Clinic Arizona
Scottsdale, Arizona

Giovanni Fabbrini, MD
Department of Neurology and Psychiatry
and
Neuromed Institute
Sapienza University of Rome
Rome, Italy

Hubert H. Fernandez, MD
Department of Neurology
Cleveland Clinic Lerner College of Medicine
Cleveland, Ohio

Center for Neurological Restoration
Cleveland Clinic
Cleveland, Ohio

Michelle Ferreira, DO
Department of Neurology
Cleveland Clinic Florida
Weston, Florida

Joseph H. Friedman, MD
Department of Clinical Neurosciences
Brown University
Providence, Rhode Island

**Néstor Gálvez-Jiménez, MD, MSc,
MHA, FACP**
Department of Neurology
Cleveland Clinic Florida
Weston, Florida

Oscar S. Gershanik, MD
Movement Disorders Unit
Institute of Neuroscience
Favaloro Foundation University Hospital
Buenos Aires, Argentina

Debabrata Ghosh, MD, DM
Child Neurology Center
Movement Disorders and Spasticity Program
Neurological Institute
Cleveland Clinic
Cleveland, Ohio

Rafael Gonzalez-Redondo, MD
Department of Neurosciences
Center for Applied Medical Research CIMA
Pamplona, Spain
Department of Neurology and Neurosurgery
Clínica Universidad de Navarra
Pamplona, Spain

Centro de Investigación Biomédica en Red
sobre Enfermedades Neurodegenerativas
CIBERNED
Instituto Carlos III
Ministerio de Investigación y Ciencias
Madrid, Spain

Penny Greenstein, MD
Department of Neurology
Beth Israel Deaconess Medical Center
Boston, Massachusetts

Jorge Guridi, MD
Center for Applied Medical Research CIMA
University of Navarra
Pamplona, Spain

Department of Neurology and Neurosurgery
Medical School
Clínica Universidad de Navarra
Pamplona, Spain

Hasmet A. Hanagasi, MD
Department of Neurology
Behavioral Neurology and Movement
Disorders Unit
Istanbul University
Istanbul, Turkey

Stephen Hantus, MD
Epilepsy Center
Center for Neurological Restoration
Cleveland Clinic
Cleveland, Ohio

Patrick Hickey, DO
Division of Neurology
Duke University Medical Center
Durham, North Carolina

Franziska Hopfner, MD
Department of Neurology
University of Kiel
University-Hospital-Schleswig-Holstein
Kiel, Germany

Cécile Hubsch, MD
Department of Neurology
CRICM UPMC/INSERM UMR-S 975
   CNRS UMR7225
Pierre Marie Curie Paris 6 University
Salpêtrière Hospital
Paris, France

Howard I. Hurtig, MD
Department of Neurology
Pennsylvania Hospital
Philadelphia, Pennsylvania

Haitham M. Hussein, MD, MSc
Department of Neurology
University of Minnesota
Minneapolis, Minnesota

Nelson Hwynn, DO
Division of Neurology
Scripps Clinic
La Jolla, California

Ilia Itin, MD
Center for Neurological Restoration
Cleveland Clinic
Cleveland, Ohio

Priya Jagota, MD
Department of Neurology
Chulalongkorn Center of Excellence on
   Parkinson's Disease and Related Disorders
Chulalongkorn University Hospital
Bangkok, Thailand

Department of Medicine
Chulalongkorn University and King
   Chulalongkorn Memorial Hospital
Bangkok, Thailand

Joseph Jankovic, MD
Department of Neurology
Movement Disorders
Parkinson's Disease Center and Movement
   Disorders Clinic
Baylor College of Medicine
Houston, Texas

Duang Kawahara, MD
Nopparat Rachatanee Hospital
Bangkok, Thailand

Maja Kojovic, MD
Sobell Department of Motor Neuroscience and
   Movement Disorders
UCL Institute of Neurology
London, UK

Jaime Kulisevsky, MD
Movement Disorders Unit
Hospital de la Santa Creu i Sant Pau
Barcelona, Spain

Rajeev Kumar, MD
Movement Disorders Center
Colorado Neurological Institute
Englewood, Colorado

Anthony E. Lang, MD, FRCPC
University of Toronto
Toronto Western Hospital
Movement Disorders Clinic
Toronto, Canada

Mark S. LeDoux, MD, PhD
Department of Neurology
University of Tennessee Health Science Center
Memphis, Tennessee

Lillian V. Lee, MD, FPNA, FCNSP, MHSA
Child Neuroscience Center
Philippine Children's Medical Center
Quezon City, Philippines

Andrew J. Lees, MD, FRCP
Department of Neurology
Reta Lila Weston Institute
UCL Institute of Neurology
London, UK

Nelma Magpusao, MD
Child Neuroscience Center
Philippine Children's Medical Center
Quezon City, Philippines

Débora Maia, MD
Departamento de Clínica Médica
Universidade Federal de Minas Gerais
Belo Horizonte, Brazil

Paola Mandich, MD
Department of Neurosciences, Ophthalmology
and Genetics
University of Genova
Genoa, Italy

Unit of Medical Genetics
Azienda Ospedaliera Universitaria
San Martino of Genova
Genoa, Italy

Roberta Marchese, MD
Department of Neurosciences,
Ophthalmology and Genetics
University of Genova
Genoa, Italy

Shyamal H. Mehta, MD, PhD
Movement Disorders Program
Georgia Health Sciences University
Augusta, Georgia

Marcelo Merello, MD, PhD
Neuroscience Department
Institute for Neurological Research
Raul Carrea (FLENI)
Buenos Aires, Argentina

Nicola Modugno, MD, PhD
Department of Neurology and Psychiatry
Neuromed Institute
Sapienza University of Rome
Rome, Italy

Edwin Munoz, MD
Department of Pathology
Philippine Children's Medical Center
Quezon City, Philippines

Dipankar Nandi, FRCS(SN), DPhil
Department of Neurosciences
Imperial College London
London, UK

Flavio Nobili, MD
Department of Neurosciences,
Ophthalmology and Genetics
Clinical Neurophysiology Unit
University of Genova
Genoa, Italy

José A. Obeso, MD
Department of Neurology and Neurosurgery
Medical School
Clínica Universidad de Navarra
Pamplona, Spain

Center for Applied Medical Research CIMA
University of Navarra
Pamplona, Spain

Wolfgang H. Oertel, MD
Department of Neurology
University of Marburg
Marburg, Germany

Michael S. Okun, MD
Department of Neurology
Movement Disorders Center
McKnight Brain Institute
University of Florida
College of Medicine
Gainesville, Florida

Genko Oyama, MD, PhD
Department of Neurology
Movement Disorders Center
McKnight Brain Institute
University of Florida
College of Medicine
Gainesville, Florida

Mayur Pandya, DO
Cleveland Clinic Lerner College of Medicine
Cleveland, Ohio
Center for Neurological Restoration
Cleveland Clinic
Cleveland, Ohio

Joel Perlmutter, MD
Department of Neurology
Department of Anatomy and Neurobiology
Program in Physical Therapy
Program in Occupational Therapy
Mallinckrodt Institute of Radiology
Washington University School of Medicine
St Louis, Missouri

Igor N. Petrovic, MD
Neurology Clinic
Clinical Center of Serbia
Belgrade, Serbia

Ronald F. Pfeiffer, MD
Division of Neurodegenerative Diseases
Department of Neurology
University of Tennessee Health Science Center
Memphis, Tennessee

Werner Poewe, MD
Department of Neurology
Medical University Innsbruck
Innsbruck, Austria

Niall Quinn, MA, MD, FRCP, FAAN
Department of Clinical Neurology
Sobell Department of Motor Neuroscience and
    Movement Disorders
UCL Institute of Neurology
London, UK
National Hospital for Neurology and
    Neurosurgery
London, UK

Roser Ribosa Nogué
Movement Disorders Unit
Hospital de la Santa Creu i Sant Pau
Barcelona, Spain

Jose Robles, MD, FPNA, FCNSP
Philippine Movement Disorder Surgery Center
Cardinal Santos Medical Center
Metro Manila, Philippines

Child Neuroscience Center
Philippine Children's Medical Center
Quezon City, Philippines

Robert L. Rodnitzky, MD
Department of Neurology
University of Iowa Roy J. and Lucille A. Carver
    College of Medicine
Iowa City, Iowa

Michael Ronthal, MbBCh, FRCP
Department of Neurology
Harvard Medical School
Beth Israel Deaconess Medical Center
Boston, Massachusetts

Daniel A. Roque, MD
Department of Neurology
University of Miami
Miami, Florida

Raymond L. Rosales, MD
Department of Neurology and Neurosciences
University of Santo Tomas Hospital
Manila, Philippines

Liana S. Rosenthal, MD
Department of Neurology
Johns Hopkins School of Medicine
Baltimore, Maryland

Emmanuel Roze, MD, PhD
Department of Neurology
and
CRICM UPMC/INSERM UMR-S 975
    CNRS UMR7225
Pierre Marie Curie Paris 6 University
Salpêtrière Hospital
Paris, France

Ignacio Rubio-Agusti, MD
Sobell Department of Motor Neuroscience and
    Movement Disorders
UCL Institute of Neurology
London, UK

Neurology Department
Hospital Universitari La Fe
Valencia, Spain

David Salat, MD
Department of Clinical Neurosciences
University of Calgary
Calgary, Canada

Juan Sanchez-Ramos, PhD, MD
Department of Neurology
HDSA Center of Excellence
University of South Florida College of Medicine
Tampa, Florida

Justyna R. Sarna, MD, PhD, FRCPC
Health Sciences Centre
Department of Clinical Neurosciences
University of Calgary
Calgary, Canada

Joseph M. Savitt, MD, PhD
Institute for Cell Engineering
Parkinson Disease and Movement Disorders
    Center of Maryland
Elkridge, Maryland

Department of Neurology
Johns Hopkins University
Elkridge, Maryland

Kapil D. Sethi, MD, FRCP(UK)
Movement Disorders Program
Georgia Health Sciences University
Augusta, Georgia

Kathleen M. Shannon, MD
Department of Neurological Sciences
Rush University Medical Center
Chicago, Illinois

Junaid H. Siddiqui, MD
Center for Neurological Restoration
Cleveland Clinic
Cleveland, Ohio

Laura Silveira-Moriyama, MD, PhD
Reta Lila Weston Institute
UCL Institute of Neurology
London, UK

Department of Neurology
University of Campinas
Campinas, Brazil

Carlos Singer, MD
Department of Neurology
Movement Disorders Division
University of Miami
Miami, Florida

Shawn F. Smyth, MD
Department of Neurology
Johns Hopkins School of Medicine
Baltimore, Maryland

Elisaveta Sokolov, MSc
Department of Neurosciences
Imperial College London
London, UK

Mark Stacy, MD
Division of Neurology
Duke University Medical Center
Durham, North Carolina

Sergio E. Starkstein, MD, PhD
Fremantle Hospital
University of Western Australia
Perth, Australia

Adam Strelczyk, MD
Department of Neurology
University of Marburg
Marburg, Germany

S.H. Subramony, MD
Department of Neurology
Movement Disorders Center
McKnight Brain Institute
University of Florida
Gainesville, Florida

Oksana Suchowersky, MD, MSc,
    FRCPC, FCCMG
Department of Medicine & Medical Genetics
University of Alberta Hospital
Edmonton, Canada

Tiziano Tamburini, MD
Department of Neurosciences, Ophthalmology
    and Genetics
University of Genova
Genoa, Italy

Louis C.S. Tan, FRCP
Department of Neurology
Parkinson's Disease and Movement Disorder Centre
National Neuroscience Institute
Singapore, Singapore

Daniel Tarsy, MD
Department of Neurology
Harvard Medical School
Parkinson's Disease and Movement Disorders
    Center
Beth Israel Deaconess Medical Center
Boston, Massachusetts

Hélio A.G. Teive, MD, PhD
Movement Disorders Unit
Neurology Service
Hospital de Clínicas
Federal University of Paraná
Curitiba, Brazil

Rosalia A. Teleg, MD, FPNA
Child Neuroscience Center
Philippine Children's Medical Center
Quezon City, Philippines

Philippine Movement Disorder Surgery Center
Cardinal Santos Medical Center
Metro Manila, Philippines

Thien Thien Lim, MD
Center for Neurological Restoration
Cleveland Clinic
Cleveland, Ohio

John Thomas, FRCS
Department of Neurosurgery
Parkinson's Disease and Movement Disorder Centre
National Neuroscience Institute
Singapore, Singapore

Amanda Jane Thompson, MD
Department of Neurology
University of Florida
Movement Disorders Center
McKnight Brain Institute
Gainesville, Florida

Eduardo Tolosa, MD
Movement Disorders Unit
Neurology Service
Institut Clínic de Neurociències
Hospital Clínic de Barcelona
Barcelona, Spain

Centro de Investigación Biomédica en Red sobre
    Enfermedades Neurodegenerativas
Hospital Clínic Universitari
Universitat de Barcelona
Barcelona, Spain

Paul J. Tuite, MD
Movement Disorders Center
Department of Neurology
University of Minnesota
Minneapolis, Minnesota

Mwiza Ushe, MD
Department of Neurology
Washington University School of Medicine
St. Louis, Missouri

Francesc Valldeoriola, MD
Movement Disorders Unit
Neurology Service
Institut Clínic de Neurociències
Hospital Clínic de Barcelona
Barcelona, Spain

Centro de Investigación Biomédica en Red sobre
    Enfermedades Neurodegenerativas
Hospital Clínic Universitari
Universitat de Barcelona
Barcelona, Spain

Bart P.C. van de Warrenburg, MD, PhD
Department of Neurology
Donders Centre for Neuroscience
Radboud University Nijmegen Medical Centre
Nijmegen, The Netherlands

Andrew V. Varga, MD, PhD
Department of Neurology
Beth Israel Deaconess Medical Center
Boston, Massachusetts

Frances M. Velez-Lago, MD
Department of Neurology
Movement Disorders Center
McKnight Brain Institute
University of Florida
Gainesville, Florida

Marie Vidailhet, MD
Department of Neurology
and
CRICM UPMC/INSERM UMR-S 975 CNRS
    UMR7225
Pierre Marie Curie Paris 6 University
Salpêtrière Hospital
Paris, France

Ruth H. Walker, MB, ChB, PhD
Department of Neurology
James J. Peters Veterans Affairs Medical Center
Bronx, New York

W.R. Wayne Martin, MD, FRCPC
Movement Disorders Program
University of Alberta
Edmonton, Canada

Movement Disorders Clinic
Glenrose Rehabilitation Hospital
Edmonton, Canada

Marguerite Wieler, BScPT, MSc
Movement Disorders Program
University of Alberta
Edmonton, Canada

Glenrose Rehabilitation Hospital
Movement Disorders Clinic
Edmonton, Canada

J. Willeit, MD
Department of Neurology
Medical University Innsbruck
Innsbruck, Austria

David R. Williams, MBBS, PhD, FRACP
Movement Disorders Program
Faculty of Medicine
Van Cleef Roet Centre for Neurological Diseases
Monash University
Alfred Hospital
Melbourne, Australia

Elisabeth Wolf, MD
Department of Neurology
Medical University Innsbruck
Insbruck, Austria

A. Zangerle, MD
Department of Neurology
Medical University Innsbruck
Innsbruck, Austria

Richard M. Zweig, MD
Department of Neurology
LSU Health Sciences Center in Shreveport
Shreveport, Louisiana

Preface

The Hippocratic Oath, originally written in Ionic Greek in the late 5th Century, is an oath historically taken by physicians swearing to practice medicine ethically. It is a rite of passage for practitioners of medicine from the ancient civilizations to today's modern world.

I swear by Apollo the Physician and Asclepius and Hygieia and Panaceia and all the gods, and goddesses, making them my witnesses, that I will fulfill according to my ability and judgment this oath and this covenant:

To hold him who has taught me this art as equal to my parents and to live my life in partnership with him, and if he is in need of money to give him a share of mine, and to regard his offspring as equal to my brothers in male lineage and to teach them this art – if they desire to learn it – without fee and covenant; to give a share of precepts and oral instruction and all the other learning to my sons and to the sons of him who has instructed me and to pupils who have signed the covenant and have taken the oath according to medical law, but to no one else.

I will apply dietic measures for the benefit of the sick according to my ability and judgment; I will keep them from harm and injustice.

I will neither give a deadly drug to anybody if asked for it, nor will I make a suggestion to this effect. In purity and holiness I will guard my life and my art.

I will not use the knife, not even on sufferers from stone, but will withdraw in favor of such men as are engaged in this work.

Whatever houses I may visit, I will come for the benefit of the sick, remaining free of all intentional injustice, of all mischief and in particular of sexual relations with both female and male persons, be they free or slaves.

What I may see or hear in the course of treatment or even outside of the treatment in regard to the life of men, which on no account one must spread abroad, I will keep myself holding such things shameful to be spoken about.

If I fulfill this oath and do not violate it, may it be granted to me to enjoy life and art, being honoured with fame among all men for all time to come; if I transgress it and swear falsely, may the opposite of all this be my lot.

Although a modernized version of this text is used nowadays, the principles of medicine, as an art and a science, and as a gift and a responsibility, have remained unchanged for centuries. It is what makes our profession noble, timeless, and universal.

It is also, perhaps, the most rapidly growing and evolving discipline in the modern world—with its body of knowledge now expanding at its most rapid pace. The effective and continued learning of concepts in medicine, both basic and complex, established and evolving, is therefore critical, more than ever, for the just and meaningful practice of medicine. Various learning methods have now been introduced, using technology such as the Internet and computerized simulations, robotic models, small group sessions, evidence-based curricula, audience-response system, and multimedia education. Multimedia uses a combination of different content forms, including text, audio, still images, animation, video, and other interactive mediums. Multimedia has now taken its rightful place as a standard approach in education, including medicine, and most especially in movement disorders where videotapes of patients have now started to replace the careful and vivid description of cases in textbooks, journals and specialty board examinations.

We both believe in progressive education! In fact, as the current comedical editors of the *Movement Disorders Society* website, we both have made the utilization and optimization of multimedia technology as the single greatest vehicle in enhancing education and communication in our international society. Nonetheless, despite all the technological advancements, we believe that there are some things that will never change. Frank Smith, a contemporary British psycholinguist, recognized for his contributions in linguistics and cognitive psychology captured perfectly, why we, co-medical editors who have championed and continue to champion the use of technology, decided to "go back to the basics" in this special project.

>...I do not agree with the view that writing will become redundant in our own culture because other technologies are taking its place. I cannot imagine any technology making writing obsolete, in the sense of providing a complete alternative to writing. Technologies may sometimes offer acceptable substitutes-they may occasionally be more efficient than writing, occasionally less-but they are not the same; they do not do what writing does in the way writing does it. Therefore they cannot wholly take the place of writing, any more than photography can take the place of the painter's art (though photography introduces new possibilities for art). Consider the technological alternatives that are commonly proposed for writing, the telephone or radio and television, and their more permanent forms, recording and film...Recordings can only overcome constraints of time in a limited way, taking a spoken language event out of one particular moment of time, the moment it is produced, so that it can be heard and repeated at other times. But listeners to a recording do not have the power to manipulate time that readers have: they cannot skip, hurry ahead, or go back and review, at least not with the facility of a reader. You could not ask me to repeat a sentence I produced five minutes ago if you were listening to me talk, nor could you so easily find that sentence on a tape recording or even a computer disk. Certainly you could not ask me to tell you in advance the sentence I might produce five minutes from now, although you can easily look forward in a letter or a book. Nor could you attend to either of those sentences at your own pace, as slowly or as rapidly as you might wish...

Indeed, the pen remains mightier than the screen!

Moreover, from the traditional classroom learning, we will always remember the most intimidating professor, the funniest professor, or the one with the most unusual style. Who will forget the professor who made us tremble? The one who challenged us the most? Or the one who inspired us to pursue the profession of healing? However, by now, while their image sticks to our memories, we have probably forgotten the actual content of their lectures! To this date, the most enduring lessons we never forget are those taught to us by our patients. Patients remain, universally, our best teachers and the ones that provide us with the most memorable lessons.

Therefore, with this time-tested learning methodology in medicine in mind, we have assembled the most memorable cases in Movement Disorders, in written form, from some of the most respected clinicians around the globe. As you read through each case, you will realize that our primary goal was not to simply assemble rare cases, but rather to capture the scientific and human challenges and create a truly special collection of memorable teaching patient encounters. The lessons learned need not be all scientific, such as describing the first case on a new genetic disorder. More often, the lessons are that about human frailty, medical intuition, a caregiver's strength, a doctor's uncertainty, or a patient's determination and will to survive. This book and its collection of cases, is as much about the art and the compassion, as it is about the science of our profession. Each case will invoke a lesson on persistence or practicality, thoroughness or focused observation, objectivity or intuition, and professionalism or empathy. It is our hope that the cases will inspire us, and once again remind all of us of the main reason why we chose our life-long profession.

H.H.F.
M.M.

Acknowledgments

We would like to thank our friends and colleagues from around the globe for sharing with us their most memorable cases for all of us to learn from.

Our deepest gratitude goes to Ms. Christine Moore, our Editorial Assistant, who was instrumental in organizing this amazing project—for connecting with all our contributors, editing the chapters to the publisher's specifications, and keeping us all on track and on time, with grace and efficiency.

Movement Disorders

Unforgettable Cases and Lessons
From the Bedside

I

Parkinson's Disease

1

Levodopa's Dark Side: The Remarkable Story of Dr B

HOWARD I. HURTIG

THE CASE

I can remember the phone call in the fall of 1983 as though it happened yesterday. Dr B, a 49-year-old Philadelphia rheumatologist, somehow found out that I was using the experimental dopamine agonist pergolide mesylate (Eli Lilly) for compassionate use in patients with advanced Parkinson's disease (PD). In a controlled, soft voice, he briefly told me the following story of his illness.

It began at the age of 42 with stiffness of the left hand. PD was diagnosed and he responded well to carbidopa/levodopa (Sinemet). However, within 3 years, his illness had rapidly progressed to a nightmarish state of severe parkinsonism and unmodulated motor fluctuations, called by Dr B his "double dystonia." This term characterized a daily harrowing and rigidly timed biphasic sequence of events that initially came close to destroying his will to live, but he realized he had no choice but to devise a strategy of survival under terrible circumstances. His response to levodopa was eventually made tolerable after a lot of meticulous tinkering with doses of Sinemet and other modifiable factors such as diet, sleep, and exercise. Thus, his daily routine evolved into a stereotyped daily sequence of events: (1) on arising at 7 a.m., he was severely bradykinetic and immediately took the first daily dose of Sinemet (750 mg); (2) 15–20 minutes later, a rapid crescendo of wrenching dystonic spasms of the face and upper body occurred, during which time he became intensely sweaty and felt an intense restlessness and need to walk, even run around until the dystonia subsided about 15 minutes later; (3) after recovering from postdystonic exhaustion, he was able to function well enough to see patients in the morning and spend the afternoon relaxing with reasonably good "on" time as long as he took a dose of Sinemet 25/250 mg every 2 to 3 hours; (4) each evening, he and his wife, a nurse, prepared for the onslaught of severe, unrelenting generalized dystonia that occurred about 2 hours after he took the last dose of Sinemet, usually around 9 p.m., and lasted 45 to 90 minutes. They coped with this agonizing evening ordeal by having him lie down on a special mattress with padded side rails on the floor of the bedroom, where he writhed continually until the dystonia subsided. Moderately severe generalized bradykinesia ensued, but he was able to get to bed with his wife's assistance before starting the entire arduous cycle again the next day and the day after that and every day without apparent end.

Sometime after the onset of double dystonia, Dr B and his wife found and sought the help of Dr Manfred Muenter, a movement disorders specialist at the Mayo Clinic in Rochester, MN. In 1977, Dr Muenter authored an important paper (1), in which he reported the results of a clinical and pharmacokinetic study of 39 mostly young patients with PD who had developed motor fluctuations in response to the chronic use of levodopa. Five of these, all under 50 years of age, had the very same pattern of double dystonia or "dystonia-improvement-dystonia (DID)" that Dr B had been experiencing. In the paper, Muenter and coworkers documented the classic "on" and "off" responses to a dose of levodopa, termed the "short-duration response," and correlated the clinical phenomenology with rising and falling blood levels of levodopa in two distinct patterns: improvement-dystonia-improvement (IDI) and DID. According to their findings, the episode of morning dystonia occurs in DID when the concentration of dopa in plasma rises in the blood through a critical but relatively low zone of vulnerability (the "dystonia" zone) following ingestion of the first dose of the day, resolving without recurrence as long as the plasma concentration of dopa is kept above a critical threshold by frequent dosing of levodopa throughout the day. Dystonia occurring after the last dose of levodopa at the end of the day lasts considerably longer and is less modifiable than the morning episode, as the plasma level of dopa slowly descends through the dystonia zone. The authors hypothesized that in IDI, dystonia occurred as the result of overstimulation of dopamine or other receptors as the brain level of dopa increased, whereas in DID, the physiologic response was somehow inverted, with overstimulation occurring as the level rose and depolarizing blockade occurring (to abolish the dystonia) as the dopa level passed through and rose above the dystonia zone.

In the early days, Dr B refused to be defeated by the terrible hand he had been dealt, so he resolved to make the best of a bad situation. He learned several lessons by trial and error. First, he was unable to take levodopa around the clock because the dystonia eventually broke through the high plasma levodopa "shield" and was more severe than when he stopped taking levodopa in the early evening. Second, he found that he could ameliorate the severe post dystonia "off" period in the evening sufficiently to get a decent night's sleep by taking amantadine 100 mg every 2 hours until bedtime, when a dose of diphenhydramine gave him additional relaxation. Because of the intense suffering that accompanied the two episodes of dystonia each day, Dr B continued to seek help from the local community of neurologists, hoping that he could find someone who had the knowledge, imagination, and commitment to discover an innovative new therapy that would restore a modicum of quality to his life.

In 1981, Dr B consulted a neurologist who advised him to taper and stop Sinemet in favor of starting the potentially more effective and better tolerated antiparkinson drug bromocriptine, which had recently been marketed as a safer upgrade over levodopa and the first of its class of synthetic dopamine agonists. The experiment was a disaster. On the third day after rapid withdrawal of Sinemet, he began to shake violently and became so rigid that he could not breathe. His nurse wife, recognizing that his life was in danger, calmly and decisively had him transported by ambulance to the nearest hospital, where he was intubated and mistakenly treated for status epilepticus. Ignoring the insistent pleas of Ms B that Dr B had PD and desperately needed to resume taking Sinemet, the treating doctors continued to administer antiepileptic drugs while maintaining ventilator support. Ms B, realizing she needed to intervene more aggressively, contacted Dr Muenter and had Dr B air evacuated to one of the Mayo hospitals in Rochester, MN, whereupon Sinemet was immediately resumed and within 3 days, he had returned to the livable baseline of levodopa-controlled parkinsonism with double dystonia.

At Mayo, attempts to adjust the dosing schedule of Sinemet to his advantage were unsuccessful. On lower doses, he was severely dystonic (as small as 1/2 tablet of the 10/100 formulation) and had barely any "on" time. Therefore, he was forced to default to the prior regimen that at least allowed him to function independently for 6–8 hours a day between the daily bookends of morning and evening dystonia. Additional trials of available drugs led to slight improvement in "off" comfort by an evening combination of amantadine and benztropine, an anticholinergic given into muscle or intravenously.

He was able to return home, but, with the passage of time, everything gradually grew worse, especially the evening dystonia. These wildly writhing, thrashing involuntary movements became so violent that he dislocated a shoulder on two occasions, and he developed a considerable bald spot on the back of his head where continuous rubbing of his scalp against the mattress each evening as a result of dystonic retrocollis caused permanent damage to hair follicles.

When I first met Dr B for an evaluation on an afternoon in late 1983, he was "on" with only a mildly parkinsonian appearance. His voice was soft, speech slightly muffled but understandable, and cognitive function was normal. There was a definite steely resolve emanating from his persona. He had no tremor, dystonia, or other involuntary movement. He was slow to get out of a chair but could do so without assistance and stood with a mildly stooped posture. His gait was shuffling and he hesitated on turns. He retropulsed moderately when the pull test was administered.

THE APPROACH

I started him on a low dose of pergolide mesylate and gradually ramped it up to a moderate level of 0.7 mg three times a day. As the dose incremented, he was gratified that the morning dystonia shrank from 15 to 5 minutes, and the evening dystonia was much less severe but just as drawn out at 45 minutes. Functional "on" time during the day increased from 8 to 12 hours. He was happy and optimistic that pergolide was truly a remedy worth praising. However, as if to forecast future developments, the improvement was only temporary. After a few weeks on the combination of frequent doses of Sinemet and pergolide three times a day, he began to notice, for the first time, typical dopaminergic choreiform dyskinesia, which abated when he lowered the dose of pergolide, at which point the dystonia reemerged with its previous ferocity. During the ensuing months, the favorable, delicate balance that he had achieved early on slowly eroded, and he was faced with worsening dystonia, increasing amounts of superadded choreiform dyskinesia, and a shrinking window of functional "on" time. Valiant efforts to regain the earlier good balance between Sinemet and pergolide failed and were complicated by extreme breakthrough dystonia/chorea and two additional admissions to a hospital intensive care unit (ICU) with acute renal failure from severe rigidity and rhabdomyolysis on one occasion and respiratory arrest on another.

Dr B kept trying to modify the medication schedule and was able to find periods of relative calm between drug-induced crises that were caused by unexplained, random spikes in life threatening dystonia and necessary visits to his local hospital's ICU for intensive management. Overall, the combination of frequent large doses of Sinemet and a modest amount of pergolide two to three times a day improved the pattern of drug response enough for him to be ever so slightly more comfortable. However, the relentless march of the underlying degenerative process slowly undermined whatever temporary progress he had made with the latest pharmacologic manipulations. It was the story of Sisyphus and the stone writ large in neurologic imagery.

Dr B was clearly losing ground at an accelerated pace. The drugs in whatever combination he tried were increasingly ineffective. Despite doing his best to work effectively in his office, he was forced to retire. Driving became out of the question. The quality of the "on" time for performing basic activities of daily living began to hover on the brink of dependency. Episodes of loss of balance and falling, initially rare, were becoming more frequent. Evening dystonia was once again severe, but he had discovered that the intensity could be mitigated by taking several doses of lorazepam. Lorazepam given intravenously was more effective and lasting, so an indwelling portacath was installed, notwithstanding the reluctance of his treating doctors to expose him to a constant risk of bloodstream infection.

During the years 1986 and 1987, management of Dr B's illness became more of a high wire act than ever before. He was hospitalized twice for sepsis related to the indwelling portacath and four times for severe dystonia. Somehow, he summoned the moxie to recover from each of these. He was using lorazepam more frequently, but it was becoming less effective. The morning dose of Sinemet had increased to 1,000 mg, the amount now required to push the blood dopa level rapidly through the dystonia zone and above the levodopa response threshold. But dystonia-free time after the morning ritual was becoming erratic and punctuated by short breakthrough periods of relatively minor dystonic spasms during the day. Evening dystonia began to appear earlier than before, changing from onset typically at 8 or 9 p.m. to 5 or 6 p.m., and was just as severe as ever. Speech had deteriorated to a whisper, and he could no longer stand or walk without maximal assistance. Swallowing was becoming precarious and he was losing weight.

In August 1987, Dr B was hospitalized proactively under my care for a comprehensive review of any additional therapeutic options that might have the potential to offer even a small degree of benefit. New trials of bromocriptine, high-dose intravenous benztropine, and an intraduodenal infusion of an acidic solution of levodopa through a nasogastric tube failed or were counterproductive. A swallowing evaluation showed typical cricopharyngeal incoordination and silent aspiration. A percutaneous gastrostomy was recommended and reluctantly accepted. Throughout this latest iteration of his Job-like marathon, Dr B remained stoic, determined, and focused. He was not ready to give up the fight.

In April 1987, the *New England Journal of Medicine* published a report of two patients with advanced, young-onset PD who had responded dramatically and rapidly to treatment with an adrenal medulla to caudate autograft. The effect on the global neurologic community was electrifying, and others quickly fell into line, often carelessly, to duplicate the results but without doing a randomized trial. When Dr B learned of this potentially game changing development, he insisted that he was ready to take the chance that this radical new treatment just might return him to independent living. From his vantage, there was little to lose and little time to waste, especially in light of the failure of the August hospitalization to improve his condition. Therefore, in late September 1987, he traveled to New York City and had the procedure done by a well-known and experienced neurosurgeon. The operation was done according to plan and without immediate problems. I was present in the operating room as an observer and recalled a subdued feeling of excitement that Dr B, at last, would get lucky.

Unfortunately, fate had a different script for Dr B. The outcome of surgery was disappointing, even catastrophic. The postoperative course was complicated by more severe parkinsonism and a resurgence of severe dystonia. Aspiration pneumonia and another bout of sepsis attributable to the indwelling portacath were major setbacks, but each responded to intravenous antibiotics. After 2 months of hospitalization and modified rehabilitation, he was able to return home but in a much diminished state of health than before the surgery. He had lost more weight, looked cachectic, and was totally dependent for all activities of daily living. He was unable to tolerate even small doses of oral Sinemet because of an unaccountably lowered threshold for the dystonia. A glimmer of hope penetrated the gloom when a homemade solution of carbidopa/levodopa given as an infusion through a jejunal extension of the gastrostomy tube enabled him to become somewhat stable, but he still had frequent severe dystonia, was unable to walk without help, and relied totally on others for carrying out basic functions. Surprisingly, cognitive function remained relatively preserved and his mood, although depressed, showed flashes of his strong and determined core personality.

In January 1988, Dr B complained of pain in the neck, and he developed a fever. His wife took him to a local hospital's emergency department (ED), where an evaluation documented the fever and disclosed a high white blood count. The presumptive diagnosis was aspiration pneumonia. He was started on an antibiotic and sent home. On a Saturday evening 48 hours later, he abruptly noticed numbness from the middle of his chest down to his toes. Within the next few hours, weakness appeared in the legs and left arm and he was brought urgently late that evening to the University Hospital where I work. One of my partners was on duty and responded immediately to the call from the ED that Dr B was there in serious trouble. The neurologic exam showed triplegia (legs and left arm) and severe weakness of the right hand. A cervical myelogram showed a complete block at C6 from a mass lesion originating from the left side. An immediate cervical laminectomy revealed a large epidural abscess, which was drained. Blood cultures were positive for *Staphylococcus aureus*.

The postoperative course was yet one more tragic chapter in the narrative of Dr B's life with PD. He was kept intubated and supported, but he showed no improvement after the laminectomy and, in fact, became quadriplegic with preserved function above the neck. He was fully aware of the recent chain of events, and, despite ventilator dependency and loss of his voice to intubation, he let everyone around him know how despondent he was. The levodopa and other infusions were stopped, the portacath removed, and the cruel irony of his liberation from the daily agony of dystonia—not lost on him or others around him—was the only absurdly positive result of his new neurologic predicament.

Dr B's paralysis and ventilator dependence persisted unchanged. On the 10th hospital day, knowing that he was hopelessly and permanently disabled, he communicated clearly that he had finally suffered enough and wanted us to let him die. With full concurrence from every member of his family, all members of the health care team, hospital administration, and legal advisors, an infusion of morphine induced a state of unconsciousness and he was disconnected from the ventilator. Thus ended the life of the most courageous human being I had and still have ever met (3).

THE LESSON

Many are the lessons that I drew and still ponder from my intense involvement with Dr B, his illness, and his devoted family. The war against PD has a way of burrowing deeply into your mind and the marrow of your bones. I often think about the enormity of Dr B's suffering and how furiously he struggled to find comfort and dignity as his disease slowly ravaged and eventually overwhelmed him. His case was unique in my 40 years of caring for patients with PD, so it is impossible to generalize lessons on management from Dr B to others. Yet, there are a few universal constants that typify the way most patients learn to live with their disease, the most important of which is the will to go on and the hope for a stable future—not necessarily a cure, although that four letter word receives a lot of lip service—but faith in those of us in the helping professions to care, to listen, to be available, to apply our knowledge to devise the best and most creative treatments, and to stay for the long haul. Patients' hopeful expectations are usually sustaining, but fear of an unpredictable future is an opposing undercurrent for many, offset to some extent by the more immediate demands and challenges of everyday living. I am forever amazed at how most people develop their own highly individual and ultimately successful methodology for coping. These resilient people are my personal heroes, fighting off desperation, soldiering on, making me proud and privileged that I have chosen a career that allows me to serve my fellow human beings. The life of a physician in the trenches is exhilarating and exhausting. We cannot afford to be sissies because there are too many out there counting on us to make a permanent difference. Maybe someday we will.

REFERENCES

1. Muenter M, Sharpless N, Tyce GM, et al. Patterns of dystonia ("I-D-I" and "D-I-D") in response to L-dopa therapy for Parkinson's disease. *Mayo Clin Proc.* 1977;52:163–174.
2. Madrazo I, Drucker-Colin R, Diaz V, et al. Open microsurgical autograft of adrenal medulla to right caudate nucleus in two patients with intractable Parkinson's disease. *NEJM.* 1987;316:831–834.
3. Hurtig H, Joyce J, Sladek J, Trojanowski JQ. Post mortem analysis of an adrenal medulla to caudate autograft in a patient with Parkinson's disease. *Ann Neurol.* 1989;25:607–614.

2

Peanut Butter and Lottery: Two Impulse Control Disorders in an Elderly Parkinson Patient

HUBERT H. FERNANDEZ

THE CASE

I was just a first year neurology resident and this patient was one of the first Parkinson patients I had ever seen. He was an 81-year-old man who first noted the onset of mild tremor and bradykinesia over 20 years ago. His past medical history was significant for heavy alcohol abuse and a family history of psychiatric disease (two siblings were mentally retarded and one daughter had schizophrenia). He initially responded well to levodopa although increasing disability resulted in early retirement at the age of 63. When he was first seen at my training institution at age 79, he was on carbidopa/levodopa 25/250 mg three times per day with significant "wearing off" symptoms. A regimen of carbidopa/levodopa, 25/100 mg, two tablets four times per day and the addition of pergolide 0.25 mg (which was still available at that time), three tablets four times per day was reached in 6 months, which significantly lessened his fluctuations. However, within 3 months, his family noted that he had become more impulsive over the past several months and had been obsessed with lottery tickets. His son told us that his father would frequent multiple stores within a day spending up to $200 on lottery tickets in each store. His life savings quickly dwindled from $9,000 to $50 within a span of a couple of months.

On further questioning about other behaviors during that outpatient visit, his son also told us that he caught his father several times engaged in sexual contact with the family dog. Specifically, he was caught placing peanut butter on his penis and then allowing the family dog to lick it. Although he confessed guilt and dismay, this occurred with increasing frequency over the ensuing months despite angry condemnations from the son and threats that he would be placed in a nursing home. Prior to this occurrence, his son was unaware of any similar aberrant behavior or intense sexual urges practiced by his father.

THE APPROACH

We admitted the patient directly from clinic. On admission, he complained of frequent mood swings and intermittent hallucinations but denied aberrant sexual behavior even when confronted with this history from the son. He was an alert and fully oriented elderly man. His speech was hypophonic but fluent. His writing was micrographic. He had mild to moderate bradykinesia with trace cogwheeling, but he did not exhibit tremors or dyskinesias. He had some difficulty arising but was able to do so unassisted. His gait showed flexion posturing of the head and trunk, and reduced stride with some hesitation when approaching a narrow space. His cranial nerves, reflexes, sensory, and cerebellar examinations were unremarkable. Complete blood count (CBC) and blood chemistries were within normal. We started him on clozapine 12.5 mg by mouth every night without any adjustment to his antiparkinsonian medication. While in the hospital, we never witnessed any hypersexual behavior; however, he had intermittent hallucinations requiring increasing doses of clozapine. He was discharged on 50 mg of clozapine every night. I followed him, along with my former mentor for over 2 years, in the outpatient clinic. He would always be accompanied by a family member, usually his son, who attested that there had been no recurrence of impulsivity or hypersexuality, but that his hallucinations had diminished but did not totally resolve.

THE LESSON

I never thought that one of my first patients during training would be the one to introduce me to the multifaceted and colorful world of Parkinson's disease (PD). This case fascinated me, so I wrote it up (1), but more than that, it inspired me and intrigued me, and made me pursue fellowship training in movement disorders. Since then I have become interested in psychosis, antipsychotic drugs, and nonmotor complications of PD.

Impulse control disorders (ICDs) are increasingly reported in PD. Examples of these iatrogenic behaviors seen in PD include binge eating, excessive spending, compulsive shopping, pathological gambling, and hypersexuality (2–6). Hypersexuality in particular is a psychiatric issue that patients are often reluctant to discuss. Voon et al. (2) found the lifetime prevalence of pathologic hypersexuality in PD to be 2.4%. While no direct cause has been identified, Voon et al. (2) found hypersexuality to be significantly associated with male sex and an earlier age of PD onset. Treatment with dopamine agonist therapy and a history of ICDs has also been proposed as possible risk factors (3).

This is a case of zoophilia (in which animals are preferentially incorporated into the arousal fantasies and sexual activities) in a PD patient that appears to have arisen de novo in a setting of increasing dopaminergic medication. This behavior was successfully treated with clozapine. Since a concurrent reduction of medication was not required, the patient was able to maintain adequate antiparkinsonian response. The true incidence of paraphilia (i.e., disorders of specialized sexual fantasies, intense sexual urges, and practices that are repetitive and distressing to the affected individual) in PD patients receiving dopaminergic therapy is difficult to assess. Due to social repercussions, patients and their families may not volunteer such information. My patient's behavior, for example, would not have been volunteered by his son, if not for the accompanying pathological gambling that dwindled his father's savings.

In hindsight, this single case experience, purely from an anecdotal basis, gave me several insights that were confirmed using more rigorous methodology many years later:

1. While all PD medications were capable of inducing ICDs, dopamine agonists put patients at higher risk than other classes of drugs (3).
2. Clozapine was truly an atypical antipsychotic that allowed control of behavior without sacrificing motor control (7–9).
3. It was not uncommon that ICDs occurred together, and more often from patients with previous behavioral or psychiatric history (3,10,11).
4. The true incidence of ICDs would be difficult to ascertain and that it would need a standardized, rigorous, and prospective method to get a truly good handle on this fascinating phenomenon (3).
5. Hallucinations in PD were a unique phenomenon that, most of the time, can be controlled, but cannot be completely eradicated, even by the best antipsychotic medications (12,13).

REFERENCES

1. Fernandez HH, Durso R. Clozapine for dopaminergic-induced paraphilias in Parkinson's disease. *Mov Disord.* 1998;13(3):597–598.
2. Voon V, Hassan K, Zurowki M, et al. Prevalence of repetitive and reward-seeking behaviors in Parkinson disease. *Neurology.* 2006;67:1254–1257.
3. Weintraub D, Siderowf AD, Potenza MN, et al. Association of dopamine agonist use with impulse control disorders in Parkinson disease. *Arch Neurol.* 2006;63:969–973.
4. Nguyen FN, Chang Y-L, Okun MS, et al. Prevalence and characteristics of punding and repetitive behavior among Parkinson patients in North Central Florida. *Int J Geriatr Psych.* 2010;25(5):540–541.

5. Cooper CA, Jadidian A, Paggi M, et al. Prevalence of hypersexual behavior in Parkinson disease patients: non-restricted to males and dopamine agonist use. *Int J Gen Med*. 2009;2:51–61.
6. Shapiro MA, Okun, MS, Chang YL, et al. The 4 "A"s associated with pathological Parkinson gamblers: anxiety, anger, age and agonists. *Neuropsych Dis Treat*. 2007;3(2):1–7.
7. Fernandez HH, Friedman JH. The role of atypical antipsychotics in the treatment of movement disorders. *CNS Drugs*. 1999;11(6):467–483.
8. Friedman JH, Fernandez HH. Atypical antipsychotics in Parkinson sensitive populations. *J Geriatr Psych Neurol*. 2002;15(3):156–170.
9. Zahodne LB, Fernandez HH. Pakinson's psychosis. *Curr Treat Option Neurol*. 2010;12(3):200–211.
10. Zahodne LB, Susatia F, Ong TL, et al. Binge eating in PD: prevalance, correlates and the contribution of deep brain stimulation. *J Neuropsych Clin Neurosci*. 2011 Fall;23(1):56–62.
11. Voon V, Fox SH. Medication-related impulse control and repetitive behaviors in Parkinson disease. *Arch Neurol*. 2007;64(8):1089–1096.
12. Forsaa EB, Larsen JP, Wentzel-Larsen T, et al. A 12-year population-based study of psychosis in PD. *Arch Neurol*. 2010;67(8):996–1001.
13. Factor SA, Fuestel PJ, Friedman JH, et al. Parkinson Study Group. Longitudinal outcome of Parkinson's disease patients with psychosis. *Neurology*. 2003;60(11):1756–1761.

3

The Man Who Was Addicted to Levadopa: An Unforgettable Case Illustrating Dopamine Dysregulation Syndrome

Mwiza Ushe and Joel Perlmutter

THE CASE

Mr A is a 48-year-old right-handed man with a chief complaint of shaking. Four years ago, he first noticed shaking of his right hand and leg on one particular occasion as he was screwing in a lightbulb. He then began to shake during particularly tense moments. Over the next few months, he became slower doing his usual activities and his arms became stiffer. About a year after the onset of the shaking, he started to shuffle his feet when walking. He continued to work managing apartments he owned. About a year later, he developed more difficulty managing the repairs at the apartments. Handwriting became smaller and voice softer. Six months prior to his first evaluation, he was catching his foot when walking, but did not fall. He complained of anxiety and low mood with crying spells but denied visual or auditory hallucinations and delusions.

About 2 years ago, his primary physician initiated dopaminergic therapy with reduction of tremor and stiffness with improved movement. Medications were titrated to carbidopa/levodopa/entacapone 37.5/150/200 mg every 4 hours as well as carbidopa/levodopa 25/100 mg 1.5 tablets at 6 and 10 a.m., rasagiline 1 mg daily, and ropinirole 4 mg three times a day. He developed wearing off about 30 minutes prior to each dose and the next dose would take 60 to 75 minutes to provide benefit. He had mild peak dose dyskinesias and when "off," he had dystonia in the right foot. When "on," anxiety diminished and mood improved. Other side effects included increased daytime sleepiness, vivid dreaming, and increased libido.

No etiologic risks for parkinsonism were identified in his history including relevant medication exposure, encephalitis, brain injury, or environmental exposure. He was taking no other medications and had no allergies. His past medical history was significant for infrequent migraine for the last 25 years and required no preventive medication. He had no other medical problems. He continued to work as a real estate manager for apartments, which he owned and lived in with his family.

We examined Mr A in the "on" state 2 hours after medication administration. He had a normal general medical examination without orthostasis. Mental status was normal with no signs of hallucinations or delusions. Language was normal. His cranial nerves, gross motor, sensory, coordination, and reflex examinations were normal. He did not have dystonia. His Unified Parkinson Disease Rating Scale subscale III score was 15/108. His major parkinsonian signs were bradykinesia and rigidity, which were worse on the left side.

He had mild stage 2 parkinsonism likely due to idiopathic Parkinson's disease (PD). His major complaints were latency to drug effect and wearing off of doses especially in the late afternoon and evening. He also had peak dose dyskinesias that were not bothersome and excessive daytime sleepiness. As a first step, we decided to reduce wearing off by adding a levodopa dose at 6 p.m., with the goal of eventually simplifying the regimen and changing from the long-acting preparation of levodopa to the regular levodopa (to reduce the delay in onset of benefit).

Over the course of the next month, he continued to have wearing off at least 30 minutes prior to the next dose and complained of severe anxiety during these "off" times. He was also very anxious about tapering ropinirole (which was likely contributing to excessive daytime sleepiness). At this point, levodopa was increased to 2 tablets three times a day. After stopping ropinirole, he noticed that his morning dose did not improve symptoms. The carbidopa/levodopa/entacopone combination was discontinued and tolcapone was added to improve the duration of levodopa effect. However, he continued to complain that the medication benefits did not last for more than 2 hours. He also began complaining of depressive symptoms including low mood, guilt, anhedonia, poor concentration, and increased sleep. Mirtazapine was prescribed by a psychiatrist for depression. Depression continued to worsen and duloxetine was added.

Over the next 3 months, he continued to have wearing off associated with increased tremor and increased anxiety. He began adding additional tablets of levodopa each time he began to wear off. He described wearing off as a feeling of unease and anxiety. He noticed these symptoms more than any motor symptoms, although he did have a return of his resting tremor during these states (but at times this was a sense of an internal tremor rather than one visible to others). He continued to increase the daily amount of levodopa intake until he reached about 21 pills (2,100 mg) per day. Although when he was at the peak effect of the levodopa he had reduced anxiety, overall he had worsening anxiety, mood, and sleep. Then Mr A began calling our office more frequently seeking more medication. He also began to complain of feeling air in his body that was building a pressure sensation inside his chest and abdomen and was escaping from different orifices. He was afraid that the pressure would be sufficiently severe that he would not be able to breathe and would kill him. This sensation was sufficiently frightening that he asked his wife to jump up and down on his chest to push the air out of his body. He had insight that he was taking too much medication that may have contributed to his delusions, but he could not stop himself from continuing to take more medicine at the hint of wearing off.

He finally presented to the emergency department (ED) due to sense of impending doom and severe anxiety related to the sensation of air building inside his body. General medical examination was normal. Motor examination revealed dyskinesia but was otherwise unchanged from his last clinic examination. He had substantial thought disorder with delusions and suicidal ideation. He was oriented to person, place, and time and had insight into his situation. He had no alteration of consciousness.

THE APPROACH

Mr A is a 48-year-old man with 4 year history of parkinsonism diagnosed as idiopathic PD. His motor manifestations are dopamine responsive, but his care was complicated by somatic delusions, depression, and anxiety. He presented acutely to the ED with severe anxiety and delusions. Laboratory evaluations were normal including blood count, chemistry, thyroid stimulating hormone and T4, urinalysis, and urine drug screen. Differential diagnosis included drug-induced psychosis due to multiple dopaminergic medications, major depressive episode with psychotic features, and delirium. Delirium seemed unlikely due to his intact level of arousal. Although he had a history of major depressive disorder, he did not endorse acute worsening of depressive symptoms. In the ED, psychotic symptoms seemed to improve at the end of his levodopa dose and worsen at the peak motor effect although he had only modest motor wearing off. We diagnosed dopamine dysregulation syndrome (DDS) and discontinued amantadine and mirtazapine, tapering levodopa to his previous therapeutic dose. Psychotic symptoms gradually improved and he returned home. His wife now controls administration of his dopaminergic medication.

THE LESSON

DDS is a dopamine replacement therapy (DRT) abuse disorder that complicates the long-term management of PD, affecting about 3% to 5% of patients with PD (3). Related and concurrent disorders include punding in PD and impulse control disorders such as hypersexuality and pathological gambling (1). Like Mr A, patients with DDS often exhibit disabling nonmotor fluctuations including dysphoria, anhedonia, fatigue, anxiety, and panic during the "off" state (1). These may be replaced by euphoria, hypomania, and hyperactivity in the "on" state. This cycle of fluctuations may lead to a psychological and physiological dependence on DRT. In fact, it seems that the nonmotor fluctuations are more likely to drive the behavior of taking more medication than the motor fluctuations (2). As in our memorable case, patients often report the onset of anhedonia and dysphoria prior to motor symptoms. These nonmotor symptoms are so disabling that patients continue to take large amounts of DRTs to avoid them. These patients often have continuous dyskinesias while complaining that the medication is ineffective in controlling symptoms. Patients with DDS exhibit many of the same drug seeking behaviors seen in patients addicted to other drugs such as narcotics and cocaine. These patients will request early refill of medications, often complain of early wearing off symptoms, or report that medications are ineffective and require larger and larger doses of DRTs. DDS patients may also have complex dosing schedules crafted to avoid the negative effects of the "off" period (1,2). PD patients with DDS may report a "high" from peak effects of DRT. The treatment of DDS requires cessation of dopamine agonists as well as other drugs likely to contribute to psychosis like amantadine or anticholinergics and then gradual decrement of dopaminergic therapy to a point that controls motor symptoms without significant untoward side effects. This may be difficult as the anxiety and depression may temporarily worsen during this time. Psychiatric admission may be necessary to treat the depression with medication and cognitive behavioral therapy. In the case of Mr A, his presentation to the ED was the one that led to the correct diagnosis and the subsequent implementation of his treatment plan. There are currently little data regarding further options for treatment in this disorder. However, the treatment of PD patients with DDS requires a coordinated team approach to avoid relapse. The neurologist, primary medical doctor, caregiver, and family should be involved in producing a fixed dosage schedule and monitoring of medications (1). Data are also currently limited regarding risk factors for the development of DDS in PD.

REFERENCES

1. O'Sullivan SS, Evans AH, Lees AJ. Dopamine dysregulation syndrome: an overview of its epidemiology, mechanisms and management. *CNS Drugs.* 2009;23(2):157–170.
2. Evans AH, Lawrence AD, Cresswell SA, et al. Compulsive use of dopaminergic therapy in Parkinson's disease: reward and anti-reward. *Mov Disord.* 2010;25(7):867–875.
3. Evans AH, Lees AJ. Dopamine dysregulation syndrome in Parkinson's disease. *Curr Opin Neurol.* 2004;17(4):393–398.

4

The Most Horrific Tactile Hallucination Described by a 78-Year-Old Colombian Man With Parkinson's Disease

OSCAR BERNAL-PACHECO

THE CASE

The incredible variability in the phenomenology of motor and nonmotor symptoms in patients with Parkinson's disease (PD) makes this disorder unique in every patient. Sometimes symptoms can be extreme and almost unimaginable. This is one such case.

A 78-year-old Colombian man, who first noticed tremor, rigidity, and bradykinesia 18 years ago, initially received treatment with levodopa with good control of movements. Complications such as dyskinesia and dystonic posture were noticed after 7 years of treatment. The patient then developed nonmotor symptoms such as depression, anxiety, and REM sleep behavior disorders. During his first visit with me, he was taking levodopa/carbidopa/entacapone 200/50/200 mg at 7 a.m., 3 p.m., and 8 p.m., carbidopa/levodopa 25/250 at 11 a.m., pramipexole 0.5 mg at 7 a.m., 3 p.m., and 9 p.m., and amantadine 100 mg at 8 a.m. and 2 p.m.

He volunteered to have good control of motor and nonmotor symptoms including tremor, bradykinesia, and rigidity, although dyskinesias were present more than 50% of the day. When he was asked about nonmotor symptoms, he denied significant cognitive dysfunction, depression, anxiety, or insomnia. However, when I asked about hallucinations, psychosis, and other related symptoms, the patient seemed embarrassed. He initially denied symptoms of impulsive or compulsive behaviors and dopamine dysregulation syndrome. However, his daughter, accompanying him during his visit, described that she has been noticing her father frequently touching his penis. After several minutes, the patient eventually opened up to me and his daughter and started describing the unusual experiences throughout the day that persisted at night and during his sleep to try to explain why he was frequently caught touching his penis.

The "episodes" were clear, occurring any time of the day, but more frequently in the mornings when he entered the bathroom, and during sleep. Embarrassingly and awkwardly, he described hearing four men talking to him, with one of them saying, "We are going to rape you." Although he does not see them, he then feels the first man grabbing hold of him followed by a violent penetration in his anus with something that feels like an erect penis; then he feels the second man biting his penis while the other two men touched him on his other body parts. He described the sensations as painful and with great discomfort. Although he has generally retained his insight and knew that these were probably hallucinations, he often tried to fight against these four men because the hallucinations were so vivid and uncomfortable. He said that the rape continued at night and even while sleeping, such that he was not always sure whether they occurred in his dreams or when he was still awake. His daughter, surprised about all these, then described that although she did not know about the hallucinations, she indeed had noticed that he fought, talked, and even screamed during his sleep and sometimes when he was awake.

Furthermore, when I asked about any other hallucinations that he might be experiencing, he volunteered that sometimes, the tip of the zipper turned into a worm that crawled over his legs, and then dug deep into his skin and caused numbness in his legs and pain in his heels.

The patient admitted that he was ashamed because of the bizarre nature of these hallucinations, and most especially because his daughter was always with him during his doctor's visits.

THE APPROACH

It is important to notice that there were no cognitive issues. He scored a 30/30 on the mini-mental state examination, and his daughter denied any cognitive symptoms. His speech was hypophonic and dysarthric but understandable, with moderate hypomimia. His movements were moderately bradykinetic and rigid. Dyskinesias were present more than 50% of the time. He walks with assistance and using a cane, with mild postural instability.

The initial step I took was to open the dialog between the patient, his daughter, and myself. Initially, the patient was ashamed, which was a big obstacle. The patient never before volunteered these hallucinations and only talked about the sexual aspects of his life when he was asked. His daughter was surprised, but after the explanation about these symptoms in relation to PD and medications, she began to understand the actions of her father. The first pharmacological approach I did was to decrease the dosage of amantadine and pramipexole and to begin quetiapine at 12.5 mg. After 1 month on 25 mg of quetiapine, the hallucinations persisted, with increase in anxiety and fear of the recurrence of symptoms. Clonazepam at 1 mg was added, which provided a big relief for the anxiety. However, his hallucinations and REM sleep behavior disorder symptoms persisted. Finally, a trial with clozapine (25 mg) and clonazepam (1 mg) was given, providing significant but not complete relief of his hallucinations and REM sleep behavior disorder.

THE LESSON

The overlap of vivid dreams, nightmares, REM sleep behavior disorder, and psychotic manifestations such as complex hallucinations and even delusions have been explored but are still not well understood. Psychosis is a nonmotor manifestation experienced at least once by 50%–60% of the patients with advanced PD. PD psychosis tends to be persistent, becoming a risk factor for death, nursing home placement, and other complications (1,2). Although the REM sleep disorders are not included in the criteria for psychosis (3) and a previous publication contests the association of vivid dreams and PD psychosis (4), another publication showed the clear association and overlap between vivid dreams and PD psychosis (5). Another study showed a strong correlation between sleep fragmentation, sleep phenomena, and hallucinations in around 14% of the patients (6). In the same study, they found that 82% of the patients with hallucinations had some kind of sleep disorder; these data are conclusive as revealed in a previous study (7). Arnulf et al. (8) elaborated in a study where they concluded that REM periods during wakefulness were present in patients with PD and psychosis. Some studies suggest that vivid dreams precede hallucination. However, in this case, the vivid dreams, symptoms of REM sleep behavior disorder, and daytime and nighttime hallucinations were so intertwined that it made me wonder how close, really, is the relationship between dreams and hallucinations.

A prospective 2-year follow-up study showed that those patients with REM behavior disorder and recently diagnosed hallucinations seem to be older, with deterioration of executive functions and with worse motor functioning, in comparison to those without hallucinations. Moreover, patients with hallucinations and REM sleep behavior disorders tended to have more cognitive impairment and a higher rate of mortality than those without REM sleep behavior disorder and hallucinations (9). Alterations in cholinergic and dopaminergic pathways, resulting in cognitive compromise and the expression of hallucinations and vivid dreams, have been implicated in its pathogenesis (10). Serotonin has also been involved in the neuropathology of this sleep phenomenon and its correlation with hallucinations, and postmortem studies have shown high density of Lewy bodies in the subcoeruleus nucleus (8,11).

This is, perhaps, the most horrific testimonial of hallucinations and REM behavior disorder I have ever heard from a patient to date. Yet, the recognition and diagnosis (and start of treatment) were delayed because of the patient's embarrassment. Moreover, the presence of a family caregiver in all of the patient's office visits contributed to his delayed testimonial. One lesson, among many, that I learned is to try to spend a few minutes alone with each patient, regardless of how seemingly satisfied they are with the control of their symptoms.

In addition, it has been reported that visual hallucinations are far more common in PD psychosis, and while auditory and tactile hallucination do occur, they are less common and are often associated with visual hallucination (12). The case presented is therefore even more unique because of the predominance of tactile and auditory hallucinations without a visual component when he described "the rape episodes." However, he also had the combination of illusions and visual and tactile hallucinations when he described his zipper transforming into a worm, then crawling over his legs and digging under his skin.

The treatment can be as challenging as its recognition. Adjunctive medications such as amantadine, anticholinergic agents, and dopamine agonists, etc. that can contribute to PD psychosis must be tapered, if not discontinued all together. If symptoms persist, atypical antipsychotic agents may be added. In this case, clozapine provided significant relief, whereas quetiapine failed to do so. The superiority of clozapine over quetiapine in PD psychosis has been described in the literature (13). Clonazepam can also be added if REM sleep behavior and insomnia are present (14).

As has been described in the literature, PD psychosis, unfortunately, is often persistent and difficult to completely resolve, even with atypical antipsychotic agents. Unfortunately, this is one such case, among many others.

REFERENCES

1. Fernandez HH, Trieschmann ME, Okun MS. Rebound psychosis: effect of discontinuation of antipsychotics in Parkinson's disease. *Mov Disord.* 2005;20:104–105.
2. Marsh L, Williams JR, Rocco M, et al. Psychiatric comorbidities in patients with Parkinson disease and psychosis. *Neurology.* 2004;63:293–300.
3. Ravina B, Marder K, Fernandez HH, et al. Diagnostic criteria for psychosis in Parkinson's disease: report of an NINDS, NIMH work group. *Mov Disord.* 2007;22(8):1061–1068.
4. Goetz CG. Scales to evaluate psychosis in Parkinson's disease. *Parkinsonism Relat Disord.* 2009;15 (Suppl 3):S38-S41.
5. Thanvi BR, Lo TCN, Harsh DP. Psychosis in Parkinson's disease. *Postgrad Med J.* 2005;81:644–646.
6. Pappert EJ, Goetz CG, Niederman FG, et al. Hallucinations, sleep fragmentation, and altered dream phenomena in Parkinson's disease. *Mov Disord.* 1999;14:117–121.
7. Nausieda PA, Glantz R, Weber S, et al. Psychiatric complications of levodopa therapy of Parkinson's disease. *Adv Neurol.* 1984;40:271–277.
8. Arnulf I, Bonnet AM, Damier P, et al. Hallucinations, REM sleep, and Parkinson's disease: a medical hypothesis. *Neurology.* 2000;55(2):281–288.
9. Sinforiani E, Pachietti C, Zangaglia R, et al. REM behavior disorder, hallucinations and cognitive impairment in Parkinson's disease: a two year follow-up. *Mov Disord.* 2008;23(10):1441–1445.
10. D'Agostino A, De Gaspari D, Antonini A, et al. Cognitive bizarreness in the dream and waking mentation of nonpsychotic patients with Parkinson's disease. *J Neuropsychiatry Clin Neurosci.* 2010;22(4):395–400.
11. Maindreville AD, Fenelon G, Mahieux F. Hallucinations in Parkinson's disease: a follow-up study. *Mov Disord.* 2005;20(2):212–216.
12. Mack J, Rabins P, Anderson K, et al. Prevalence of psychotic symptoms in a community-based Parkinson disease sample. *Am J Geriatr Psychiatry.* 2012;20(2):123–132.
13. Miyasaki JM, Shannon K, Voon V, et al. Quality standards Subcommittee of the American Academy of Neurology. Practice parameter: evaluation and treatment of depression, psychosis, and dementia in Parkinson disease (an evidence-based review): report of the Quality Standards Subcommittee of the American Academy of Neurology. *Neurology.* 2006;66(7):996–1002.
14. Nomura T, Inoue Y, Mitani H, et al. Visual hallucinations as REM sleep behavior disorders in patients with Parkinson's disease. *Mov Disord.* 2003;18(7):812–817.

5

Can a Research Subject Be Too Enthusiastic? An Important Lesson on Parkinson Trials From a 65-Year-Old Banker

RICHARD M. ZWEIG

THE CASE

A 65-year-old banker with a 7- to 8-year history of Parkinson's disease (PD) was enthusiastic about participating in a 12-week double-blind study of an adenosine A_{2A} receptor antagonist for PD. To be eligible, "motor response complications" on carbidopa/levodopa therapy were required and documented with home diaries. At the time, medications included pramipexole 1 mg five times daily, carbidopa/levodopa 1,250 mg (levodopa dosage) divided in nine daily doses, entacapone 200 mg taken with seven of the carbidopa/levodopa dosages, and amantadine 100 mg every morning. He appeared to be meticulous about taking his medications on time and kept very neat, banker-like records. Yet he had frequent, typically not troublesome, levodopa-induced dyskinesia and 3 to 5 hours of "off time" daily, with increased bradykinesia and aching in his lower extremities. He gave informed consent and was started on study drug, with a 75% chance of being on one of the three dosages of the study medication (versus placebo), and he was delighted with the response. At the 2-week visit, he reported less aching and overall "milder offs," although on the diaries he documented similar 4 and 5 (4/5) hours of "off" on consecutive days as on the baseline diaries (3.5/5 hours). For the remainder of the study, the diaries also showed great improvement: 1/1.5 hours "off" at 4 weeks, 1/2 hours at 8 weeks, and 2/2.5 hours at the final 12-week visit. He noted less aching at each visit and mildly increased dyskinesia at some, but not all, of the visits. Throughout the study, the levodopa dosage was constant. At the final visit, he was looking forward to continuing on the study medication—now open label.

Two weeks after switching to the open label study (on the highest A_{2A} receptor antagonist dosage used in the double-blind study, as allowed per study protocol), he had decreased his carbidopa/levodopa dosage to 900 mg (levodopa), taken only six times daily, along with entacapone 200 mg with each dosage. Yet he clearly had increased dyskinesia and was "off" no more than 1 to 2 hours daily. He was able to continue on the adenosine A_{2A} antagonist for the next 3 years. By the end of the open label study, the levodopa dosage (in combination with carbidopa and entacapone) had been decreased to 100 mg six times daily plus an additional 50 mg levodopa (combined with carbidopa) typically once or twice daily as needed. For dyskinesia, the amantadine dosage had been increased to 100 mg twice daily.

Once the study was over and the adenosine A_{2A} receptor antagonist was discontinued, he almost immediately needed to increase his levodopa dosage again. When the "blind" was opened, we were not too surprised to learn that he had originally been randomized to placebo.

THE APPROACH

When recruiting for a clinical trial, the ideal subject should clearly meet all inclusion and exclusion criteria, should understand the goals and demands of the trial, and it helps if the subject is also enthusiastic about participating in the trial. This patient should have been, and by all obvious measures was, an ideal participant. But can a research subject be too enthusiastic? The 2-hour reduction in "off time" from the baseline to 12-week visit was much greater than the mean "placebo effect" in similar phase 3 studies of this agent, ranging from 0.6- to 0.9-hour reduction in four published studies (1–4). Moreover, while clearly within the inclusion range, the 4.25 mean baseline amount of "off time" in this patient was less than the mean of these studies of over 6 hours. Thus, the percent improvement was particularly large. Could it be that in his enthusiasm, this meticulous banker became even more meticulous in taking his levodopa-containing medications on time, reducing "off time" despite being on placebo?

Meanwhile, the study doctor and staff, also blinded to treatment allocation, should try to be as objective as possible, and not bias to the patient in a way that might influence outcome measures, such as diary reports. Whether or not there was a subtle (or not so subtle) bias introduced by the study staff in this instance is unclear.

In addition, the study should use outcome measures and be powered to maximize the likelihood of achieving the intended goal(s) and minimizing "type 2" error. This patient clearly responded to the adenosine A_{2A} receptor antagonist, and once it was actually started, he was able to—or better stated, he had to—reduce his levodopa dosage by about 50% while on open label study drug. While diary endpoints are valid (5) and have been used extensively in Parkinson's clinical trials, if reduction in levodopa (or "levodopa-equivalent") dosage had been a prospective endpoint, this patient's response would have been informative, despite the pronounced placebo effect. Of note, the four published studies of this agent did demonstrate modest but statistically significant reductions in "off time," corrected for placebo, of 0.64 to 1.2 hours, depending upon the dosage used (1–4).

THE LESSON

Enthusiasm is great, but in a double-blind clinical trial, enthusiasm must be tempered by objectivity by both the research subject and the study staff. Even when a response seems obvious, you do not know for sure what you do not know. The placebo response can be quite profound. Moreover, a good study design should include additional primary or secondary measures that might salvage useful information concerning efficacy of study drug, even in the setting of a pronounced placebo response based upon the primary outcome measures. Finally, at least in this one subject with PD, there is no question but that adenosine A_{2A} receptor antagonism was quite efficacious.

REFERENCES

1. LeWitt PA, Guttman M, Tetrad JW, et al. Adenosine A_{2A} receptor antagonist Istradefylline (KW-6002) reduces "off" time in Parkinson's disease: a double-blind, randomized, multicenter clinical trial (6002-US-005). *Ann Neurol.* 2008;63:295–302.
2. Stacy M, Silver D, Mendis T, et al. A 12-week, placebo-controlled study (6002-US-006) of Istradefylline in Parkinson disease. *Neurology.* 2008;70:2233–2240.
3. Hauser RA, Shulman LM, Trugman JM, et al. Study of Istradefylline in patients with Parkinson's disease on levodopa with motor fluctuations. *Mov Disord.* 2008;23:2177–2185.
4. Mizuno Y, Hasegawa K, Kondo T, et al. Clinical efficacy of Istradefylline (KW-6002) in Parkinson's disease: a randomized controlled study. *Mov Disord.* 2010;25:1437–1443.
5. Hauser RA, Friedlander J, Zesiewicz TA, et al. A home diary to assess functional status in patients with Parkinson's disease with motor fluctuations and dyskinesia. *Clin Neuropharmacol.* 2000;23:75–81.

6

Parkinson's Disease Never Presents With Freezing: Except When It Does!

NIALL QUINN

THE CASE

Having taken several transatlantic voyages on the QE2, I shall never forget when I first set eyes on Mr L, when my wife and I decided to try a cruise on a smaller ship. I do not usually make a habit of approaching unknown subjects with neurological signs, but I was very struck by Mr L's problem, which was severe start hesitation and freezing of gait—in fact, just about the most severe I had ever seen. When intending to move, he would trepidate, holding two walking sticks for what seemed like an eternity, until he suddenly broke the "spell" and shot off down the port side toward the stern, only to freeze again in a narrow gangway. He seemed to spend a lot of time going up and down in the passenger lifts but never getting off when the doors opened at the intended deck. Having witnessed this on several occasions, I decided to approach him and offer some tips to overcome his problems. Stepping over my foot, or over his inverted walking stick, and walking beside me step-for-step, right-left, right-left, with my arm around his shoulder worked brilliantly, and he was most grateful. I later recounted this to my wife, who asked if I had explained that I was a neurologist. I said "no," and she replied that Mr L must have thought it all very strange. Therefore, the next day, I approached him and told him I was a neurologist who specialized in PD, to which he replied "Oh, I have seen two neurologists and I do not have Parkinson's."

On the final night was the showtime extravaganza in the theater area. Since it was a relatively small ship, this did not incorporate "wings," relying instead on the fore-and-aft corridors on either side to hold performers waiting to enter the stage. As the finale approached, a throng of dancing girls in headdresses, ostrich feathers, and frocks were waiting to burst onto the stage for the end of the gala show. At this moment, Mr L rose to his feet and trepidated, trying to head for the toilet down the same stretch of the corridor. I feared he would be bowled over and trampled underfoot by a stampede of showgirls but, just in the nick of time, he took off at speed and made his escape.

By the time I had returned to London, I had a referral from his doctor, enclosing a letter he had received 3 months previously from one of the two neurologists he had seen. It said "… for the past 2 years, he feels that he wobbled as he walked. He has particular difficulty in initiating movement. For example, when he is standing at the edge of the road, he finds it very difficult to make the move to cross the road. When the telephone goes at home, he finds he cannot move from the spot. The result is that he tends to throw himself forward and falls. He has a little bit of tremor in his hands but is more aware of a tremor in the legs. On examination, as he walked into my room, he had to make a right turn. At this point, he froze and then struggled to make his legs move forward. There was only a little postural tremor and a rest tremor of the right leg. There was no bradykinesia. I believe he has a gait apraxia, and I suspect the most likely explanation is cerebrovascular disease (he had a past history of hypertension and coronary artery bypass grafting (CABG) 5 years previously). I do not think he will be helped by antiparkinson's medication—I have not made a further appointment to see him."

When I saw him in clinic, he told me that 15 months previously on going for a walk, his legs gave way and he fell onto his knees, and since then he had developed very troublesome freezing of gait, with a further five falls onto his knees. He had also noted a tremor in both legs at rest. A brain MRI had been normal.

On examination, his speech was a little festinant, and he had an intermittent tremor of the lower lip. In the limbs, there was minimal akinesia on the right, mild to moderate on the left, with fatiguing and decrement, and mild arm rigidity. There was an intermittent tremor present at rest, on posture, and on action in both hands, and an intermittent rest tremor of both legs. He had marked start hesitation and freezing, but once he got going, he walked normally but with reduced armswing. His pull test was abnormal because of freezing up on his toes, and propulsion and retropulsion, but underlying postural instability was probably normal.

THE APPROACH

I thought it is quite likely that he had PD and requested a dopamine transporter single-photon emission computed tomography (SPECT) scan, suggesting initially a 6-week trial of amantadine, which was unhelpful. The scan showed bilateral asymmetric impairment of putaminal tracer uptake, worse on the right. I then prescribed Sinemet plus 1/2 tablet tds, which he discontinued after 2 weeks because of an increase in tremor and nausea despite domperidone. I then started him on Madopar 62.5 plus one capsule tds, increasing gradually so that after 3 months, he was on 187.5 qds, and on this dosage, he did not freeze at all, and his tremor was improved. After 9 months on the same treatment, his parkinsonism was very mild with absolutely no freezing, and after a further 16 months, when last seen, he had very little freezing.

THE LESSON

1. PD *can* present with severe freezing but only very mild tremor and akinesia, which may be overlooked. It is important to examine such cases very carefully for evidence of true parkinsonism. Primary progressive freezing of gait is more commonly due to progressive supranuclear palsy (PSP), other degenerative diseases, or cerebrovascular disease, and it usually does not respond to levodopa. However, those rare cases of PD presenting in this way, such as Mr L, may have a dramatic and sustained beneficial response. Therefore, in my view, all such cases merit a decent trial of L-dopa.

2. Although they are "equivalent" and there are no consistent response differences between Sinemet or Madopar, some individual patients seem to tolerate one better than the other. Moreover, if the patient is reluctant to try again the preparation that they associate with side effects and/or lack of efficacy, it is useful to be able to suggest a further trial of a *"different"* medication (although this is only possible in countries in which both preparations are licensed). In addition, low doses of levodopa can initially worsen tremor, and patients should be warned about this and encouraged to persevere and to continue to gradually increase the dose until they reach an effective level, rather than stopping it.

3. It is *sometimes* okay to approach an unknown individual outside a clinical context, as with Mr L. More commonly, if someone who is obviously parkinsonian is introduced to me but perhaps may not have been diagnosed, I might introduce myself as a neurologist who specializes in Parkinson's, so that they can choose to respond in whatever way they wish.

7

From Hero to Villain: Walking the Tightrope in Impulse Control Disorders

JUNAID H. SIDDIQUI, MAYUR PANDYA, ANWAR AHMED, AND HUBERT H. FERNANDEZ

THE CASE

"It's a small town, where we live," his wife told us, "and we can't take the risk of our town pharmacists telling anyone about my husband's condition."

This 53-year-old right-handed urologist, practicing in a small Midwestern town, has been traveling to our Movement Disorders Center to avoid rumors. His story started about 4 to 5 years ago when he complained of right arm slowness and burning and numbness in his feet. An MRI of his cervical spine showed cervical stenosis, leading to a neurosurgical decompression that helped his feet paresthesias but not his arm slowing. A year later, he was seen at Movement Disorders Center, where he was also noted to have hypomimia, micrographia, and shuffling gait and was finally diagnosed with Parkinson's disease (PD).

He was started on a 0.125 mg of pramipexole three times per day, which was gradually increased to 0.5 mg three times daily. He subsequently reported feeling "back to normal." After a temporary decline in the number of surgeries he was performing, his surgical volume slowly returned to his pre-Parkinson level. He had been taking 1.5 mg of pramipexole three times per day, along with 1 mg of rasagiline daily, when his brush with fame and infamy started to unfold.

To his wife's delight, he took on a number of home projects and repairs. He first remodeled their basement—a smashing success. He then compulsively took up more and more remodeling projects at home but did them one at a time and with great detail. He added a sauna, remodeled the master bathroom, built a new outdoor deck, and added two waterfall features in the house. He even manually brought in the boulders that were used for his waterfall project. In the end, he spent almost $250,000 on remodeling projects. When his wife said that she was very pleased with all the renovations and they should hold off on further projects, he directed his energy to activities with his son.

As an avid recreational shooter, he felt that he needed more practice and made a shooting range at his backyard with the help of his son. He became obsessed with guns and "almost became a sniper" according to his wife because of his obsession with perfection. He designed a new gun and started assembling this gun with the help of his son and a friend. Still with more energy left, he started lifting weights and training for a marathon.

Professionally, things could not be better. He doubled his surgical volume from his pre-Parkinson levels. In fact, his daughter, who had recently graduated from college, decided to join her father's clinic as a manager and became overwhelmed by the increasing number of patients he would schedule on a given day. He was not only productive but also had the kindest heart and was well-loved by his patients, buying clothes and offering assistance when possible.

At this point, his wife was happy and thought that things were going in the right direction, evidenced by him spending more quality time with his son, working out, and bringing in a good income while the house was looking great.

Four months later, his symptoms peaked in several aspects. He began helping his neighbors and even people he did not know. He fixed his neighbor's extensive house wiring problem, without any prior experience with electrical repairs, simply by surfing the Internet for guidance.

On the home front, his obsession with sex grew exponentially. He would demand sex from his wife so many times that she purposely left the house every time he came home from work. Not having his wife around, he would masturbate 15 times a day. His wife became concerned when she heard that he would leave his clinic early but arrive home late. She also noticed an increasing obsession with physical fitness to the extent that he would get up at 3 a.m. and start working out after sleeping just 3 hours.

After a few weeks, he planned a vacation getaway for himself. When he returned home 4 days later, the family was shocked to see his behavior. It looked like he had neither slept nor changed his clothes. He had not shaved and was "blabbering like a maniac." His children thought that he was on drugs and he might even have a gun in his pocket. He told his family, "I have done everything for you and our family is most fortunate for having everything. 'She' does not have anything and I am going to help her, and not just her; I will help anyone who needs to be helped." Who was "*she*"?

His wife became alarmed and scoured his phone records. She found out that he had made 245 calls to a woman in the last 2 weeks. He had also sent her numerous e-mails with pornographic content. The woman was a surgery technician at his hospital and was the same woman that he spent the 4 days with on vacation. He additionally leased a car for her under his name. This was his first extramarital activity in their 31 years of marriage. After realizing the impairment in judgment, his wife immediately transferred all the money into her name and threatened to kick him out of the house. His children were appalled and did not want to speak to him. When his wife confronted the other woman about the whole matter, she threatened to tell everyone about the affair and to sue them for "unfulfilled promises" that he had made to her. Unfortunately, the news had spread about his indiscretion.

Upon hearing the details, we reduced the dose of his pramipexole to 0.75 mg three times per day. Within 1 to 2 days, he felt that his impulsivity diminished and was able to appreciate the gravity of the situation. He cried, felt remorseful, and apologized to his wife. He also said repeatedly that when on medications, he felt "in control" and his actions were "justified." Attempts to increase the dose of pramipexole resulted in a rise in libido again. He therefore reduced the dose back to 0.75 mg three times a day, resulting in reduction of his hypersexuality and impulsivity, fortunately, without much deterioration in his motor functioning. This convinced his wife that it was really the medication that was causing her husband's erratic behavior, so she reluctantly took him back. However, the news of his infidelity had spread around town, prompting him to shut down his practice to begin teaching at a local college. His children would still not speak to him.

THE APPROACH

Our patient demonstrated a mixture of impulsive and compulsive behavior, along with hypomania. His hypomania was manifested by his reduced need for sleep, hypervigilance, grandiose thinking, flight of ideas, pressured speech, and involvement with pleasurable activities with possible negative effects. His impulsive behavior was primarily hypersexuality—constantly asking for sex with his wife, masturbating 15 times per day, and then ultimately ending in an extramarital affair. His compulsive behavior, interestingly, did not reach the level of "punding" as they were all generally constructive and productive (remodeling different parts of the house, shooting at the range all day, working out, fixing electrical systems, designing and assembling a gun, etc.). These behaviors more closely resemble an extreme form of hobbyism. Punding has been defined as a fascination for manipulation of mechanical objects, etc., in a nonpurposeful manner (1), which was not exactly the case with our patient.

Conventionally, impulsive behaviors, such as hypersexuality, pathological gambling, binge eating, and compulsive shopping, have been attributed to the use of dopamine agonists (2), along with other risk factors such as young age, single, family history of impulse control disorders, etc. (3). On the other hand, compulsive behaviors, such as punding, hobbyism, and dopamine dysregulation syndrome, have been attributed to levodopa use, or at the very least, high levodopa equivalent daily dose, and not necessarily due to pramipexole or other dopamine agonists.

There are still no double-blind randomized controlled trials for impulse control disorders in PD. While the "knee jerk" treatment has been to discontinue or decrease the offending agent (typically, the dopamine agonist), this is usually easier said than done and runs the risk of "dopamine agonist withdrawal syndrome" (4). Atypical antipsychotics and amantadine have been both described to alleviate (5,6), as well as worsen (7,8), impulse control behaviors. We have recently described valproic acid, a drug often used for bipolar disorder and behavioral dyscontrol, as an agent that was able to reduce these behaviors in three PD patients without the need for adjusting PD medications (9). Therefore, for our patient, because of the prominence of hypomanic features, we decided to try valproic acid, in addition to lowering his dopamine agonist dose.

THE LESSON

One of the main lessons we learned from this memorable case is the rather unfortunate but common observation that impulsive and compulsive behaviors often run together. Our patient's impulsivity was manifested through hypersexuality, while his compulsivity was manifested through extreme hobbyism.

This case also reinforced our impression that impulsive and compulsive behaviors are often not clear cut pathological behaviors but rather are manifested in a "spectrum," ranging from productive to destructive. His hypersexuality and mild hypomania was initially under control and even productive with increased surgical volumes, going "above and beyond" the care for his patients, etc., until he engaged in an extramarital affair. Similarly, his hobbyism was initially productive, that is, remodeling his house, engaging in exercise routines, helping out his neighbors, until he became obsessed, no longer needed to sleep, and started chipping away at their life savings to sustain his "hobbies." Unfortunately, insight is often lost, at least while performing impulsive and compulsive behaviors, and the longer these behaviors go on, the more difficult it becomes to "walk on the tightrope." More often, as in our case, the patient falls off the tightrope and suffers devastating consequences.

Fortunately, in our case, we did not observe some of the other common scenarios we often experience with PD patients and impulse control disorders such as the following: continued denial and persistent lack of insight; resistance to lowering dopamine agonists; experiencing severe parkinsonism when Parkinson medications are lowered; or developing dopamine (agonist) withdrawal symptoms.

Finally, our case begs for more controlled trials for the treatment of this often devastating nonmotor complication in PD.

REFERENCES

1. Nguyen FN, Chang YL, Okun MS, et al. Prevalence and characteristics of punding and repetitive behaviors among Parkinson patients in North-Central Florida. *Int J Geriatr Psychiatry*. 2010;25:540–541.
2. Shapiro MA, Chang YL, Munson SK, et al. Hypersexuality and paraphilia induced by Selegeline in Parkinson's disease; Report of 2 cases. *Parkinsonism Relat Disord*. 2006;12:392–395.
3. Weintraub D, Koester J, Potenza MN, et al. Impulse control disorders in Parkinson disease *Arch Neurol*. 2010;67(5):589–595.
4. Rabinak CA, Nirenberg MJ. Dopamine agonist withdrawal syndrome in Parkinson disease. *Arch Neurol*. 2010;67(1):58–63.

5. Thomas A, Bonanni L, Gambi F, et al. Pathological gambling in Parkinson disease is reduced by Amantadine. *Ann Neurol.* 2010;68(3):400–404.
6. Fernandez HH, Friedman JH. Punding on L-dopa. *Mov Disord.* 1999;14(5):836–838.
7. Weintraub D, Sohr M, Poenza MN, et al. Amantadine use associated with impulse control disorders in Parkinson disease in cross-sectional study. *Ann Neurol.* 2010;68:963–968
8. Miwa H, Morita S, Nakanisha I, Kondo T. Stereotyped behaviors or punding after quetiapine administration in Parkinson's disease. *Parkinsonism Relat Disord.* 2004;10:177–180.
9. Hicks CW, Pandya MM, Itin I, Fernandez HH. Valproate for the treatment of medication-induced impulse control disorders in three patients with Parkinson's disease. *Parkinsonism Relat Disord.* 2011;17: 379–381.

8

Our Unforgettable Case of Malignant Motor
Fluctuations in a Parkinson Patient

LAURA SILVEIRA-MORIYAMA AND ANDREW J. LEES

THE CASE

This patient developed slowly progressive left arm rest tremor at the age of 37. He had no family history of neurological disorder or consanguinity. At age 38, cabergoline was initiated with good response. Shortly after the benefits of cabergoline waned, amantadine and levodopa were added. Subsequently, his levodopa requirements rapidly escalated to 1,500 mg/day regardless of efforts to restrict his intake. The patient developed early motor fluctuations and severe peak dose dyskinesias. Whenever he tried to reduce the levodopa intake, he had marked worsening of tremor, dystonia, anxiety, and dysphoria, as well as very disturbing nocturnal off periods. A challenge confirmed marked responsiveness to levodopa (motor Unified Parkinson's Disease Rating Scale [UPDRS] off = 43, on = 10).

At age 42, he was started on continuous subcutaneous apomorphine infusion. This was accompanied by a significant improvement of the florid dyskinesias and longer time "on" during the day. Nevertheless, less than a year after this, he developed distressing nocturnal "off" symptoms characterized by extreme anxiety, incapacitating rest tremor of the limbs, painful dystonia, and profuse generalized sweating. The apomorphine infusion rate was increased, and he tried 24-hour continuous infusion without benefit; clonazepam and later zopiclone were added, but his insomnia and nocturnal symptoms continued to worsen, and he became dependent on help from others for activities of daily living. While on 85 mg of apomorphine per day, he evolved with intense tremor and profuse sweating, which made siting the subcutaneous needle impossible. A few hours after this was noticed by the family, he was urgently admitted to a local hospital. He was started on oral levodopa and later apomorphine was restarted. Seven days after admission, he was transferred to the National Hospital for Neurology and Neurosurgery at Queen Square, and presented with delirium, dehydration, and prerenal azotemia (serum urea = 39.9 mmol/L and creatinine = 332 μmol/L). He had extreme and abrupt motor fluctuations with severe episodes of intense rigidity, large amplitude rest tremor, perspiration, and tachycardia alternating with periods where the tremor would abate, and he often presented dyskinesias. During these "on" periods his mobility was poor and remained dependent for functions, which represented a marked deterioration from his state 2 weeks previously. Off periods were unpredictable and prolonged, lasting from 30 minutes to many hours, but he did not respond to additional oral doses of levodopa or apomorphine boluses. He had no other focal neurological signs, and the MRI imaging of the brain was normal. Motor fluctuations appeared to be unrelated to medication use and off periods were accompanied by severe anxiety and depression, and sometimes delirium. During the next 2 weeks the severe, unrelenting, and unpredictable off periods became worse despite continuous apomorphine infusion 108 mg/day, levodopa 300 to 600 mg/day, clonazepam 1 mg/day, temazepan 10 mg/day, zopiclone 7.5 mg/day, amantadine 400 mg/day, and two courses of antibiotic therapy for a possible undiagnosed infection.

He remained on an intravenous crystalloid infusion to ensure adequate hydration; however, he had persistently impaired renal function and his serum creatine kinase (CK) levels fluctuated from 240 to 63,765 IU/L with no clear correlation to clinical status or treatment. He presented dysautonomia with fluctuations in blood pressure (from 90/60 to 140/82 mmHg), heart rate (from 60 to 161 bpm), and periods of dramatic sweating. He had at least three recorded episodes of hyperpyrexia of up to 40°C without evidence of an underlying sepsis. Despite management in the intensive care unit, he died of multiple organ failure 6 weeks after presentation and 5 years after Parkinson's symptom onset.

THE APPROACH

The occurrence of a clinical syndrome resembling neuroleptic malignant syndrome in a Parkinson's disease (PD) patient following withdrawal of antiparkinsonian drugs was first described by Toru et al. (1) in 1981. Since then many cases have been reported and two series estimated an incidence between 3% and 4% in PD patients (2,3). The condition has been called "neuroleptic malignant-like syndrome" or "malignant syndrome in Parkinson's disease" because it has a series of features in common with neuroleptic malignant syndrome (NMS), which include severe muscle rigidity, hyperthermia (up to 40°C), increased CK, autonomic instability, leukocytosis, and altered consciousness varying from drowsiness to coma (4). Some authors have called similar manifestations "acute akinesia" or "akinetic crisis" (5,6), due to the impressive speed at which the lasting akinesia develops. More recently the term "parkinsonism-hyperpyrexia syndrome" (7,8) has been used, to emphasize the hyperthermia that often accompanies the features, and the fact that it can also occur in other parkinsonian syndromes.

The pathophysiology of these conditions is largely unknown, but it is likely that dopaminergic dysfunction is the common pathway. In typical NMS, dopaminergic blockade caused by neuroleptics may play a central role in the pathogenesis of the disorder. In the malignant worsening of parkinsonism, it is hypothesized that central dopaminergic hypofunction might underlie the cardinal features (9), and most cases are triggered by abrupt withdrawal of dopaminergic therapy or poor levodopa absorption (10), although intercurrent infections (11) and dehydration (12) have also been reported as provoking factors.

Our case is unusual because the patient did not present with a sustained akinesia or a malignant state with intense parkinsonian features but rather with very severe motor fluctuations. It resembles a previous case reported by Pfeiffer and Sucha (13), in which a PD patient was observed to develop severe progressive motor fluctuations with abrupt episodes of severe, generalized tremor accompanied by profuse sweating, and tachypnoea that would last for 15 minutes to 3 hours. After that, his urine would become pink-tinged; in one of these episodes, he become very stiff and incoherent and was hospitalized with dysautonomia, hyperthermia, and severe tremor and rigidity. Despite dopaminergic drugs associated with diazepam and dantrolene, the patient became anuric and died 10 hours after admission. Linazasoro (14) reported two females (age 70 and 76; disease duration 23 and 13 years) with severe motor fluctuations (UPDRS part III of 72 and 67 in off-state) who following severe dyskinesias developed hyperthermia of 40°C, delirium, marked muscle rigidity with elevated CK, leukocytosis, and dysautonomia. There was no reduction in the dose of antiparkinsonian drugs and other causes of hyperpyrexia were ruled out. Both patients recovered with supportive measures and use of benzodiazepines. Of interest, severe dyskinesias may also induce rhabdomyolysis (15), but this is unlikely to have happened in our patient.

Prompt recognition of the malignant parkinsonian features is essential for the prognosis of this condition, which can be fatal even with aggressive treatment. There is no consensus on the diagnostic features, and there are no randomized controlled trials for the treatment. Research in this area is needed. Current good clinical practice includes withdrawal of potential triggers, prompt reinitiation or escalations of antiparkinsonian medication, rehydration when appropriate, and treatment of any identified infection (9). Datrolene, which is a peripheral muscle relaxant that inhibits intracellular release of calcium from the sarcoplasmic reticulum, can be used (7). Electroconvulsive therapy, which has been used in neuroleptic malignant syndrome as a compassionate measure (16), may be a last resort (17). Intensive care and careful supportive measures with intravenous hydration are essential.

THE LESSON

Malignant parkinsonian manifestations are a medical emergency and are potentially fatal. Further research is needed to adequately classify the various presentations, clarify the pathophysiology, and improve medical management.

Acknowledgments
The authors would like to thank Dr Dominic Paviour, Dr Andrew Evans, Dr Marianna Selikhova, and Dr David R Williams who were also involved in the care of this patient and for their comments on previous versions of this manuscript.

REFERENCES

1. Toru M, Matsuda O, Makiguchi K, Sugano K. Neuroleptic malignant syndrome-like state following a withdrawal of antiparkinsonian drugs. *J Nerv Ment Dis*. 1981;169(5), 324–327.
2. Harada T, Mitsuoka K, Kumagai R, et al. Clinical features of malignant syndrome in Parkinson's disease and related neurological disorders. *Parkinsonism Relat Disord*. 2003;9(suppl 1):S15-S23.
3. Serrano-Duenas M. Neuroleptic malignant syndrome-like, or—dopaminergic malignant syndrome—due to levodopa therapy withdrawal. Clinical features in 11 patients. *Parkinsonism Relat Disord*. 2003;9(3): 175–178.
4. Gibb WR, Lees AJ. The neuroleptic malignant syndrome—a review. *Q J Med*. 1985;56(220):421–429.
5. Onofrj M, Thomas A. Acute akinesia in Parkinson disease. *Neurology*. 2005;64(7):1162–1169.
6. Thomas A, Iacono D, Luciano AL, Armellino K, Onofrj M. Acute akinesia or akinetic crisis in Parkinson's disease. *Neurol Sci*. 2003;24(3):219–220.
7. Newman EJ, Grosset DG, Kennedy PG. The parkinsonism-hyperpyrexia syndrome. *Neurocrit Care*. 2009;10(1):136–140.
8. Kipps CM, Fung VS, Grattan-Smith P, et al. Movement disorder emergencies. *Mov Disord*. 2005; 20(3):322–334.
9. Mizuno Y, Takubo H, Mizuta E, Kuno S. Malignant syndrome in Parkinson's disease: concept and review of the literature. *Parkinsonism Relat Disord*. 2003;9(suppl 1):S3-S9.
10. Gordon PH, Frucht SJ. Neuroleptic malignant syndrome in advanced Parkinson's disease. *Mov Disord*. 2001;16(5):960–962.
11. Ikebe S, Harada T, Hashimoto T, et al. Prevention and treatment of malignant syndrome in Parkinson's disease: a consensus statement of the malignant syndrome research group. *Parkinsonism Relat Disord*. 2003;9(suppl 1):S47-S49.
12. Kuno S, Mizuta E, Yamasaki S. Neuroleptic malignant syndrome in parkinsonian patients: risk factors. *Eur Neurol*. 1997;38(suppl 2):56–59.
13. Pfeiffer RF, Sucha EL. "On-off"-induced lethal hyperthermia. *Mov Disord*. 1989;4(4):338–341.
14. Linazasoro G. Malignant syndrome in Parkinson's disease. *Parkinsonism Relat Disord*. 2003;10(2):115–116.
15. Lyoo CH, Lee MS. Rhabdomyolysis induced by severe levodopa induced dyskinesia in a patient with Parkinson's disease. *J Neurol*. 2011;258(10):1893–1894. Epub 2011 Apr 16.
16. Trollor JN, Sachdev PS. Electroconvulsive treatment of neuroleptic malignant syndrome: a review and report of cases. *Aust N Z J Psychiatry*. 1999;33(5):650–659.
17. Meagher LJ, McKay D, Herkes GK, Needham M. Parkinsonism-hyperpyrexia syndrome: the role of electroconvulsive therapy. *J Clin Neurosci*. 2006;13(8):857–859.

Gaining Movement but Losing Speech: The Unexpected Side Effects of DBS Surgery

Louis C.S. Tan and John Thomas

THE CASE

This sales executive has a history of Parkinson's disease (PD) since the age of 42 when he presented with slowness of his right upper limb. Clinical evaluation revealed the presence of a mask-like facies, cogwheel rigidity, and bradykinesia of his right upper and lower limbs. MRI brain and ceruloplasmin levels were normal. A diagnosis of PD was made. He was treated on various medications that included selegiline, bromocriptine, and levodopa with good response. After 6 years of treatment, he developed predictable wearing-off effects of his medication. In his seventh year of PD, he complained that he was slower in the afternoons and his speech was becoming less fluent, resulting in a deterioration of his work performance. His job was at stake. His medications at that time were selegiline 5 mg two times a day, bromocriptine 17.5 mg three times a day, levodopa/benserazide 125 mg three times a day, and levodopa/benserazide 62.5 mg. He complained that his levodopa lasted only 5 hours at a time, and he was keen to have a deep brain stimulation (DBS) surgery performed as he still had young children and needed to work for a few more years to accumulate enough finances for his family. After a period of counseling and consideration, the patient proceeded with DBS surgery.

Bilateral subthalamic nucleus (STN)-DBS surgery was performed at the age of 49. The DBS implantation was performed with a Cosman-Roberts-Wells functional neurosurgery (CRW-FN) stereotactic frame, while the patient was under local anesthesia with mild sedation. Stereotactic planning was done after fusion of preoperative MRI scans with the perioperative stereotactic CT scan. The STN target was directly visualized and targeted on the axial T2 MRI sequence. Target confirmation was achieved with microelectrode recording and clinical examination during direct STN stimulation via both the microelectrode and the final DBS electrode. The surgery proceeded uneventfully with the left STN explored through a single tract and the right STN explored using two tracts. The DBS implantable pulse generator (IPG) was inserted under general anesthesia, after removal of the CRW frame, during the same operative session. He recovered well postoperatively and was discharged 3 days after the surgery. DBS programming was routinely done 1 month postsurgery. The patient's Unified PD Rating Scale (UPDRS) motor score improved from 19 in the off-medications, off-stimulation state to 14.5 after programming in the off-medication state, and the patient was pleased with the improvement in his motor function. Three days after programming, the patient returned complaining that his speech had worsened and that he had more problems pronouncing and articulating words. His handwriting also had deteriorated and had gotten smaller.

THE APPROACH

His DBS parameters were adjusted and reduced to determine if his speech problems were related to the stimulation of the DBS. However, his speech problems persisted despite adjustment of the stimulation parameters and turning off his DBS. An urgent CT scan of the brain was then performed to exclude an intracranial bleed such as a subdural hematoma as a cause of his problems, and this was reported to be normal. Over the next 3 months, multiple programming sessions were performed with different stimulation parameters including reduction in voltage and frequency, the use of bipolar stimulation mode, and turning off the stimulator for up to 3 days. However, these measures together with adjustment of medications did not result in a sustained benefit for his speech. He continued to have stuttering speech, with problems in articulating words. During this period, he received intensive speech therapy to improve his speech and occupational therapy to improve his handwriting. His handwriting improved with this intensive writing therapy. However, his speech did not improve with therapy. In fact, his UPDRS rating for speech, which was scored as 1 (slight loss of expression, diction, and/or volume) preoperatively, deteriorated to 2 (monotone, slurred but understandable, moderately impaired) one month after surgery, and progressed to a score of 3 (marked impairment, difficult to understand) three months after surgery, and has remained as such up to 2 years postoperatively.

Unfortunately, about 1 year after the patient's DBS surgery, after a period of prolonged medical leave, his employers terminated him from his work as they felt that he was not able to perform the functions of his job for which communication was a key aspect.

THE LESSON

The complications associated with STN-DBS surgery may be related to the implantation of electrodes and hardware (e.g., intracranial hemorrhage), hardware-related complications (e.g., infections), alterations of higher mental function, and stimulation-related complications (1). A common stimulation-related complication is dysarthria or hypophonia, which has been reported to occur in 4% to 17% of patients (1). These complications are thought to be reversible and are related to suboptimum electrode placement. A prospective study of 32 STN-DBS patients and 12 PD controls that evaluated speech intelligibility before and after surgery found that speech intelligibility significantly deteriorated by an average of 14.2% off-medication and 16.9% on-medication 1 year after STN-DBS, compared to 3.6% and 4.5%, respectively in the control group (2). The majority of speech deterioration in the surgical group occurred between 6 months and 1 year after surgery. Similar to our patient, speech deterioration in this study was not alleviated by switching the stimulation off. The effect of STN-DBS on speech is thought to be variable and multifactorial. Factors associated with an increased risk of speech deterioration include a higher preoperative on-medication UPDRS III motor score, medial placement of left STN electrodes, and higher voltage of left STN stimulation (2). A higher left STN stimulation is thought to result in a spread of current to the internal capsule or the cerebellothalamic tracts with resultant dysarthria (2). Others have postulated a more complex disruption of the cortico-striato-thalamo-cortical loops involved in prosody as a result of stimulation (3). Furthermore, as switching off the stimulation did not improve the dysarthria in affected patients, it may be possible that surgical tract through the frontal lobe, caudate nucleus, and thalamus, or the placement of the electrode in the zona incerta (4) may have an effect on dysarthria. Alternatively, this may be due to a prolonged stimulation effect that may require more than 3 days to reverse.

Patients undergoing STN-DBS should be counseled about the risk of speech disturbance postoperatively, in addition to the usual side effects and risk of such surgery. This is particularly so for patients who expect or need to verbally communicate well for purposes of work or leisure after surgery.

REFERENCES

1. Benabid AM, Chabardes S, Mitrofanis J, Pollak P. Deep brain stimulation of the subthalamic nucleus for the treatment of Parkinson's disease. *Lancet Neurol.* 2009;8:67–81.
2. Tripoloti E, Zrinzo L, Martinez-Toreres I, et al. Effects of subthalamic stimulation on speech in consecutive patients with Parkinson disease. *Neurology.* 2011;76:80–86.
3. Klostermann F, Ehlen F, Vesper J, et al. Effects of subthalamic deep brain stimulation on dysarthrophonia in Parkinson's disease. *J Neurol Neurosurg Psychiatry.* 2008;79(5):522–529.
4. Plaha P, Javed S, Agombar D, et al. Bilateral caudal zona incerta nucleus stimulation for essential tremor: outcome and quality of life. *J Neurol Neurosurg Psychiatry.* 2011;82(8):899–904. Epub 2011 Feb 1.

10

Strength (and Fun) in Numbers: Lessons From an "Extended Family" of Parkinson Patients and Their Spouses

RONALD F. PFEIFFER

THE CASE

In this vignette, I have taken considerable liberty with the word "case." I am going to describe not one individual, but a group of individuals, a very special group of patients and their spouses who forged between them a bond that has left me with an indelible impression and endless admiration of them for their determination, their bravery, their ingenuity, their pluckiness, their drive, and their ability to have fun and continue living and enjoying productive lives in the face of an illness, Parkinson's disease (PD), that they met far too early and lived with far too long.

Who were these people? Most of the individuals with PD in this group were men, but their spouses were every bit as much a part of this story as were the patients themselves. I believe most were in their late forties or early fifties when the group was formed but some were younger and a few older. Although almost all were from Nebraska (I was on the faculty of the University of Nebraska Medical Center—UNMC—at the time), they came from different parts of the state and from different walks of life. One was a lawyer, one a highway patrolman, one a staff member at the University of Nebraska-Lincoln, another, the wife of a senior administrator at the same institution. One had been the U.S. ambassador to a collection of Caribbean countries, several were accountants, and several more were businessmen. Before PD entered their worlds, they did not know each other.

I wish I could say that I brought them together, but I did not; I was only indirectly involved, although it is true that I was the neurologist treating almost all of them. I believe that the first seed leading to formation of the group was sown in the form of a dinner for young-onset PD patients and their spouses that took place during the annual UNMC Parkinson's Disease Symposium, but what ultimately grew and blossomed was the coalescence of these amazingly talented individuals, both patients and spouses, into one of the most active and impressive associations—or perhaps "extended family" is a more appropriate term for this young-onset PD support group—that I have ever witnessed.

THE APPROACH

The individuals involved came from all corners of the state. Because of the distances involved, meetings of the group were not held frequently, typically quarterly, but when they were held, they were memorable. I use the word "meetings," but that really is not the right word to describe the times the group spent together, because the primary purpose of the group was not to sit and listen to lectures about PD (there were other venues for that), but rather to provide a sense of comradeship, of shared burden, of encouragement for and with each other, for both patients and spouses. I do not know about their expectations for the group, but in my opinion and observation, they succeeded in reaching and exceeding any conceivable goals far beyond my wildest dreams. The group would meet for an evening or often for entire weekends at various locations around the state, with each meeting being hosted by a different couple. The meetings unfailingly were characterized by sharing, caring, learning, and laughing. I particularly remember one memorable meeting at the home of one of the group's members, which was situated directly along the Platte River, right where the flocks of Sandhill Cranes were pausing in their annual autumnal southward migration. In these meetings and between them, the members of the group bonded and shared both good times and bad times with each other. They were there for each other and they understood the problems each of the others was facing.

Much of the time they spent with each other was purely social, but they certainly did not stop with that. They formed a group library to further their education regarding PD. They would periodically invite a guest speaker to their meetings. Their work and accomplishments also extended far beyond the confines of their relatively small group. The individuals in this group conceived of and were instrumental—in fact, they were the driving force—in founding the first state registry for PD in the United States, the Nebraska State Parkinson's Disease Registry. This entailed an enormous amount of work and dedication as they doggedly, and ultimately successfully, lobbied and educated state legislators and, with great effort, convinced doctors and pharmacists of the value of such a registry. As a testament to the group, this registry continues today to be an important source of data for PD research. They also provided tremendous support to our Parkinson's Disease Center, both during our annual symposium and throughout the entire year.

THE LESSON

There are several lessons that I have carried away from my experience with this wonderful group of individuals. I firmly believe that it is important for individuals with PD and their family members to know that they are not alone in facing their disease. Participation in support groups is one way of achieving this, and it is so important for treating neurologists not only to encourage their patients to become active in support groups, but also to become active in the groups themselves. To know and interact with individuals facing the same problems, who truly understand what one is going through because they are in the same boat, can be a tremendous source of strength for both patients and spouses and can be just as beneficial and invigorating for the individuals providing the support as it is for those receiving it. It is vitally important, however, that this interaction not become simply a time for patients and family members to commiserate and feel sorry for each other, but that it be a time to uplift and lighten the load for each other. I think that is what this particular young-onset support group did so very well. To know that there is someone you can call to ask a question, to get advice for a problem, to request assistance, to receive empathy—and sympathy if needed—is immensely important, but it is also vitally important to have encouragement to look on the bright side and to make the best use of the abilities that still remain. Finally, the benefit of simply having pure, unadulterated fun with friends—friends who understand what one is going through and are familiar with the limitations that PD imposes—while also accomplishing important goals for the group and for others, is of inestimable value.

Suggested Reading

Bertoni JM, Sprenkle JM, Strickland D, et al. Evaluation of Parkinson's disease in entrants on the Nebraska State Parkinson's Disease Registry. *Mov Disord.* 2006;21:1623–1626.

Due-Christensen M, Zoffmann V, Hommel E, et al. Can sharing experiences in groups reduce the burden of living with diabetes, regardless of glycaemic control? *Diabet Med.* 2012;29(2):251–256.

McRae C, Fazio E, Hartsock G, et al. Predictors of loneliness in caregivers of persons with Parkinson's disease. *Parkinsonism Relat Disord.* 2009;15:554–557.

Morris R, Morris P. Participants' experiences of hospital-based peer support groups for stroke patients. *Disabil Rehabil.* 2012;34(4):347–354. Epub 2011 Oct 12.

11

Help! My Spouse Is Out of Control! Three Cases of Dopamine Dysregulation in Parkinson's Disease

MAYUR PANDYA AND ILIA ITIN

THE CASES

Our "memorable case" is actually a case series of three patients with Parkinson's disease (PD) and dopamine dysregulation. As a consulting psychiatrist, I had been asked to evaluate the following patients by our movement disorders section. The patients' ages ranged from 44 to 57. The patients had been diagnosed with PD from 5 to 10 years, and their presentations were notable for a combination of hypersexuality, unrestrained gambling, obsessive behaviors, and/or affective instability consistent with behaviors known to be associated with treatment interventions for PD (1,2). The patients also demonstrated behaviors consistent with addictive disorders, including compulsive medication use. The patients appeared to find pleasure in their "dependent" state and had limited insight into the difficulties their surreptitious medication use had created. The following case descriptions delineate the degree of functional and psychological impairment in each of these individuals. But what made these three cases memorable to us was the treatment we used to eventually relieve their dopamine dysregulation syndromes.

Case 1

A 57-year-old man presented 5 years after diagnosis of PD with hypersexuality and episodes of "extreme excitement." His wife also expressed concern that he seemed interested in purchasing "small," irrelevant things and had begun to "take things apart," leaving their home in disarray. He additionally seemed sexually preoccupied, repeatedly expressing dissatisfaction with his spouse's lack of desire for intimacy.

Case 2

A 55-year-old man presented 10 years after diagnosis of PD with unrestrained gambling, obsessive behaviors, and hypersexuality. His wife reported significant compulsions to walk, once leaving for the night and walking almost 20 miles. He also exhibited delusions of jealousy manifesting as accusations of his wife's infidelity.

Case 3

A 44-year-old man presented 7 years after diagnosis of PD for the insertion of bilateral subthalamic nucleus deep brain stimulation (STN-DBS). Two years later, the patient reported increasing urges to spend money and gamble (although he later admitted that these tendencies began almost 5 years earlier). His wife discovered that he ultimately tapped into their 401(k) to compulsively purchase lottery tickets to "get the big score." He eventually depleted the retirement accounts, landing his family in serious financial debt.

THE APPROACH

We initially made note of the remarkable similarities in our patient presentations to that of some primary mood disorders, namely bipolar disorder. Irritability, impulsivity, goal-directed behaviors, and compromised judgment were parallel in presentations to both disorders. The option of simply reducing or discontinuing the patients' PD medications seemed unrealistic and overly simplistic. Additionally, to date, there are no definitive methods of treating dopamine dysregulation in PD. We subsequently explored the use of a traditional mood stabilizer to manage the affective instability while allowing the patients to continue with their anti-Parkinson medication (or at least easing their reluctance with the possibility of a medication taper). Based on the evidence that valproate may cause a potentiation of GABAergic activity and has an inhibitory effect on the high-frequency firing of neurons, we explored its use in our patients. Based on our observations, treatment with valproate ranging from 500 to 1,000 mg daily appeared useful in decreasing impulse control disorder (ICD) behaviors in patients with PD, which we reported in (3).

THE LESSON

We were amazed by the degree of psychiatric overlay in these patients who had no prior history of psychiatric illness. The apparent de novo nature of these aberrant behaviors had created such interpersonal strain and psychosocial chaos that the spouses and families appeared desperate for a solution. More importantly, the limited options for effective intervention made the approach even more challenging. It was also notable that all three cases were men. This gender propensity may be explained by internal pressure in younger male patients to self-medicate in an attempt to maintain optimal functioning in the setting of marital, parental, social, and/or occupational demands. Interestingly, another important lesson we learned from this case series is that despite the positive benefit observed, all three patients had varying compliance and expressed some level of resistance with continuing on valproate. This suggests that the reduction of pleasurable (and often destructive) impulses may not always be a welcome intervention in patients with PD and dopamine dysregulation.

REFERENCES

1. Weintraub D, Siderowf AD, Potenza MN, et al. Association of dopamine agonist use with impulse control disorders in Parkinson disease. *Arch Neurol.* 2006;63(7):969–973.
2. Voon V, Fox SH. Medication-related impulse control and repetitive behaviors in Parkinson disease. *Arch Neurol.* 2007;64(8):1089–1096.
3. Hicks CW, Pandya MM, Itin I, Fernandez HH. Valproate for the treatment of medication-induced impulse-control disorders in three patients with Parkinson's disease. *Parkinsonism Relat Disord.* 2011;17(5):379–381.

De Novo Parkinsonism Versus Depression: What to Treat First?

Sergio E. Starkstein

THE CASE

While the clinical management of individuals presenting with parkinsonism is still under debate, the dilemma increases when there are comorbid psychiatric conditions, such as major depression. This will be the focus of our case presentation.

Dr A, a prominent vascular surgeon, was referred by his clinician to our neuropsychiatric clinic. The referral letter stated that Dr A was troubled by increasing parkinsonian symptoms as well as increasing depression.

Dr A was a 52-year-old man, with an excellent track record in his specialty as well as a consummate runner. At presentation, Dr A reported feeling increasingly slower and stiffer since 8 months before, and he had to take extra care while performing surgery. He was worried that he would shortly be unable to work as a surgeon given these problems. He stated feeling very depressed about the prospect of having to quit his job, but also added that this was not his first depressive episode. He had suffered an episode of major depression 4 years before, after a traumatic divorce. This depression lasted for about 5 months and remitted spontaneously.

Dr A presented with blunted affect, poverty of gestures, and aprosodic speech. He showed a mild bilateral postural tremor in both hands, mild to moderate rigidity, bradykinesia in both upper limbs, gait slowness without shuffling, a mild stooped posture, and normal balance. On mental state examination, Dr A reported low mood, medial insomnia and early morning awakening, poor appetite with loss of weight, loss of interest in work and usual pastimes, loss of libido and poor energy, and severe symptoms of psychological and somatic anxiety. He denied suicide ideation but expressed concerns about not wanting to live if he would eventually become unfit to work. We concluded that Dr A had a major depressive episode with anxiety features in the context of clear parkinsonian signs.

THE APPROACH

The dilemma we faced was whether we should openly discuss with Dr A the possibility of incipient Parkinson's disease (PD) or a related movement disorder and make a referral to the Movement Disorders clinic or whether we should focus on treating his mixed depressive-anxiety syndrome first, delaying discussion of his potential movement disorder for a later date, hopefully after mood improvement. The decision was quite difficult given that Dr A asked specifically whether we thought he had PD. We answered that it was too early to make such a diagnosis and that he did not have a typical presentation of PD.

Given the severity of Dr A's depression and anxiety, we decided to start psychiatric treatment, leaving the management of his motor problem for a later time. We explained to Dr A that he was suffering a recurrence of major depression and that he may benefit from antidepressant treatment. He stated that he wanted a solution for his motor problems but accepted a short trial of antidepressants. Dr A was started on 25 mg/d of nortriptyline given the lack of contraindications and the syndromic profile of his depression (e.g., insomnia, anxiety, and loss of appetite), which may have a better response to a tricyclic rather than a selective serotonergic reuptake inhibitor (SSRI). There was also a chance that the tricyclic may diminish Dr A's tremor. At our clinic, we had experience in using tricyclics in PD with generally good results, and our choice of nortriptyline was based on its being one of the tricyclics with lowest anticholinergic side effects.

Dr A returned to our clinic 2 weeks later. There was a partial improvement of his parkinsonism. The tremor had decreased, although there still was some rigidity and bradykinesia. His gait was normal, his affect was livelier, and his prosody was improved. Depression was also improved, although Dr A still complained of low mood and worrying. Nortriptyline was increased to 50 and 75 mg/d in successive weeks.

A follow-up visit 4 weeks later showed a marked overall improvement. Physical examination was normal, with no parkinsonian signs. Dr A reported that he regained his usual surgical skills and performance. There also was a full remission of his major depression and he had no symptoms of anxiety.

THE LESSON

What is this case teaching us? First, neuropsychiatrists should take a cautious approach when assessing patients with "de novo" parkinsonism and psychiatric comorbidities. Our patient had a somewhat atypical presentation for PD, but PD was certainly a potential diagnosis and we believed that PD was a likely diagnosis in this case. The decision to treat his depression before a referral to a Movement Disorders clinic or before starting antiparkinsonian treatment was based on our belief that it would be better for the patient's well-being to become emotionally stable before undergoing formal studies or treatment for PD. We construed this case as "pseudo-parkinsonism of depression" and started to look for similar cases at our clinic. In a study that included 94 patients with primary depression and 20 healthy controls, we found parkinsonism in 20% of the depressed sample and in none of the elderly healthy controls. This syndrome of major depression and parkinsonism was significantly associated with older age, more severe depression, and more severe cognitive impairment. Those patients with full remission of depression had a significantly greater recovery in parkinsonian signs and cognitive functioning than patients who remained depressed.

13

How a Wife's Insomnia Led to Her Husband's Parkinson Diagnosis: The First Warning From REM Sleep Behavior Disorder

Arturo Del Carmen Garay and Daniel P. Cardinali

THE CASE

J.F. is an 80-year-old, right-handed white man who finally presented to us after 6 years of progressive excessive diurnal sleepiness (EDS). What prompted the consultation was his wife, who complained of her own poor sleep with frequent and unexpected awakenings during the night. Detailed interview of the couple did not reveal any significant medical or behavioral pathology for the wife. Her husband only complained of "vivid dreams," but his wife remarked that he had increasing episodes of dream-enacting behavior starting long before the clinical interview. These episodes were described by his wife as "disturbing moving nightmares," occurring with eyes closed, that included vivid dreams in confrontational episodes like playing in fight or flight scenarios (in these episodes, the patient sat up in bed shouting, kicking, trying to get away from wild animals or an attacker).

The patient had a history of prostatectomy, hypertension, and nocturia. He is physically active (daily walks) and practices yoga on daily basis. On examination, he is alert, oriented to time, person, and place. His immediate and short-term memory was mildly impaired. His speech was fluent. He had a mild decrease of facial expression. Cranial nerves were normal. Motor tone relatively increased with normal deep tendon reflexes. There was a mild decrease of repetitive movements and mild cogwheel rigidity at the left wrist. Testing of gait reveals a mild decreased arm swing on the left. He meets criteria for "mild" motor involvement according to the Hoehn and Yahr Staging of Parkinson's disease (PD, Stage 1 H&Y). Epworth Sleepiness Scale was 12/24 and polysomnography (PSG) showed increased EMG (electromyogram) phasic and tonic activity during abnormal REM sleep with enacting behavior during the study. Low doses of nocturnal clonazepam (0.5 mg) and melatonin (6 mg) reduced the motor manifestations of REM sleep behavior disorder (RBD) in this patient. EDS persists at the time of the last evaluation.

THE APPROACH

Neuropsychiatric symptoms, like vivid dreams, nightmares, and nocturnal hallucinations, or RBD, are commonly observed in PD (1–5). RBD in PD may occur as a prodromal feature, predating motor symptoms by several years (6). Its prevalence, which is thought to be 60%, has been identified in longitudinal studies and is suspected to be a predictor for dementia in longitudinal studies (7,8). RBD is characterized by loss of skeletal muscle atonia with prominent motor activity and dreaming (9,10).

Numerous cases of RBD have been found in clinically diagnosed PD patients (11,12). In several studies, RBD has demonstrated to be more frequent in males than females, but the reasons for this male predominance are not yet known (13). Loss of REM sleep atonia and/or increased locomotor drive have been suggested as likely mechanisms for the clinical expression of human RBD (14). There is tendency for the dream content to involve an aggressive, attacking, or chasing theme. Nightmare behaviors such as screaming, kicking, punching, and injuring the bed partner are quite common (15).

Nocturnal disturbance and sleep arousals as measured by actigraphy are specific to RBD seen in PD (16). A loss of orexin neurons and of cells secreting melanin-concentrating hormone in the hypothalamus of PD patients is said to be responsible for nocturnal insomnia, RBD, and hallucinations (17,18). However, changes in orexin are not found to necessarily underpin associated RBD sleep disturbances (19). Our case describes an elderly patient with unrecognized EDS and early premotor stage of PD.

Neurological nonmotor and psychiatric manifestations of PD often precede the traditionally recognized motor manifestations. Case-control and cohort studies suggest that depression and anxiety disorders are among the earliest manifestations of PD (20,21). Since sleep disturbances in parkinsonians are associated with cognitive decline and psychiatric symptoms (22), it has been suggested that attention be focused on the development of targeted interventions for early correction of nonmotor disorders (23).

The finding that a reduced expression of melatonin MT1 and MT2 receptors occurs in the amygdala and substantia nigra (SN) in patients with PD (24) indicates that there is a possibility that the melatonergic system is involved in the abnormal sleep mechanisms seen in PD as well as in its overall pathophysiology. Melatonin has been used for treating sleep problems, insomnia, and daytime sleepiness in PD patients (25,26). Melatonin 3 to 12 mg at bedtime has been shown to be effective in the treatment of RBD. This benefit has been reported in one case report (27), two open-label prospective case series of patients with RBD (28,29), and two retrospective case series (30,31). Taken together, these reports include a total of 38 patients. Thirty-one were noted to experience improvement with melatonin, two more experienced transient improvements, and one seemed to worsen. Follow-up as far as 25 months was reported. PSG showed statistically significant decreases in number of R epochs without atonia and in movement time in R. This contrasted with the persistence of tonic muscle tone in R sleep seen with patients treated with clonazepam. Because of these data, a recent clinical consensus recommended melatonin use in RBD at Level B, that is, "assessment supported by sparse high-grade data or a substantial amount of low-grade data and/or clinical consensus by the task force" (32).

The occurrence of increased sleep propensity during wakefulness (EDS) appeared as an undetected early premotor manifestation of PD and suggests a complex dysregulation of sleep/wake cycle and homeostatic/circadian inputs at early stages of PD. The co-occurrence of EDS and RBD has been proposed as early premotor manifestations of PD in a recent review (33).

THE LESSON

This is a case of a woman whose initial consultation for her own difficulty in sleeping ended up with the diagnosis of PD in her husband. This case underlies a series of important clinical lessons. Although it is known that EDS and RBD can be prodromes of synucleinopathies, the help of the partner is often needed to uncover RBD in Parkinson patients. Indeed, the partner's fragmentation of sleep can be considered an associated symptom in RBD. Thus, the investigation of the components of the circadian system (that mediates the onset and timing of REM sleep), including the pattern and timing of melatonin secretion, combined with clinicopathological assessment, could be useful for defining the chronobiological correlates of RBD in PD. EDS, RBD, and other premotor manifestations should be recognized in order to attempt to stop or slow down brain degeneration in PD with currently available and future therapies (34).

Acknowledgments
Daniel P. Cardinali is a Research Career Awardee from the Consejo Nacional de Investigaciones Científicas y Técnicas, Argentina and Emeritus Professor, University of Buenos Aires.

REFERENCES

1. Dhawan V, Healy DG, Pal S, et al. Sleep-related problems of Parkinson's disease. *Age and Ageing.* 2006; 35(3):220–228.
2. Chaudhuri KR, Healy DG, Schapira AH. Non-motor symptoms of Parkinson's disease: diagnosis and management. *Lancet Neurol.* 2006;5(3):235–245.
3. Chaudhuri KR, Pal S, DiMarco A, et al. The Parkinson's disease sleep scale: a new instrument for assessing sleep and nocturnal disability in Parkinson's disease. *J. Neurol. Neurosurg. Psychiatry.* 2002;73(6):629–635.
4. Grandas F, Iranzo A. Nocturnal problems occurring in Parkinson's disease. *Neurology.* 2004;63 (8 Suppl 3):S8-S11.
5. Dhawan V, Dhoat S, Williams AJ, et al. The range and nature of sleep dysfunction in untreated Parkinson's disease (PD). A comparative controlled clinical study using the Parkinson's disease sleep scale and selective polysomnography. *J Neurol Sci.* 2006;248(1–2):158–162.
6. Postuma RB, Gagnon JF, Montplaisir J. Clinical prediction of Parkinson's disease: planning for the age of neuroprotection. *J Neurol Neurosurg Psychiatry.* 2010;81(9):1008–1013.
7. Vendette M, Gagnon JF, Decary A, et al. REM sleep behavior disorder predicts cognitive impairment in Parkinson disease without dementia. *Neurology.* 2007;69(19):1843–1849.
8. Marion MH, Qurashi M, Marshall G, et al. Is REM sleep behaviour disorder (RBD) a risk factor of dementia in idiopathic Parkinson's disease? *J Neurol.* 2008;255(2):192–196.
9. Olson EJ, Boeve BF, Silber MH. Rapid eye movement sleep behaviour disorder: demographic, clinical and laboratory findings in 93 cases. *Brain.* 2000;123(Pt 2):331–339.
10. Boeve BF, Dickson DW, Olson EJ, et al. Insights into REM sleep behavior disorder pathophysiology in brainstem-predominant Lewy body disease. *Sleep Med.* 2007;8(1):60–64.
11. Schenck CH, Bundlie SR, Mahowald MW. Delayed emergence of a parkinsonian disorder in 38% of 29 older men initially diagnosed with idiopathic rapid eye movement sleep behaviour disorder. *Neurology.* 1996;46(2):388–393.
12. Boeve BF, Dickson DW, Olson EJ, et al. Insights into REM sleep behavior disorder pathophysiology in brainstem-predominant Lewy body disease. *Sleep Med.* 2007;8(1):60–64.
13. Ceravolo R, Rossi C, Kiferle L, et al. Nonmotor symptoms in Parkinson's disease: the dark side of the moon. *Fut Neurol.* 2010;5(6):851–871.
14. Boeve BF, Silber MH, Saper CB, et al. Pathophysiology of REM sleep behaviour disorder and relevance to neurodegenerative disease. *Brain.* 2007;130(Pt 11):2770–2788.
15. Jahan I, Hauser RA, Sullivan KL, et al. Sleep disorders in Parkinson's disease. *Neuropsychiatr Dis Treat.* 2009;5:535–540.
16. Naismith SL, Rogers NL, Mackenzie J, et al. The relationship between actigraphically defined sleep disturbance and REM sleep behaviour disorder in Parkinson's Disease. *Clin Neurol Neurosurg.* 2010;112(5):420–423.
17. Thannickal TC, Lai YY, Siegel JM. Hypocretin (orexin) and melanin concentrating hormone loss and the symptoms of Parkinson's disease. *Brain.* 2008;131(Pt 1):e87.
18. Thannickal TC, Lai YY, Siegel JM. Hypocretin (orexin) cell loss in Parkinson's disease. *Brain.* 2007; 130 (Pt 6):1586–1595.
19. Compta Y, Santamaria J, Ratti L, et al. Cerebrospinal hypocretin, daytime sleepiness and sleep architecture in Parkinson's disease dementia. *Brain.* 2009;132(Pt 12):3308–3317.
20. Weisskopf MG, Chen H, Schwarzschild MA, et al. Prospective study of phobic anxiety and risk of Parkinson's disease. *Mov Disord.* 2003;18(6):646–651.
21. Postuma RB, Gagnon JF, Montplaisir J. Clinical prediction of Parkinson's disease: planning for the age of neuroprotection. *J Neurol Neurosurg Psychiatry.* 2010;81(9):1008–1013.
22. Comella CL. Sleep disorders in Parkinson's disease: an overview. *Mov Disord.* 2007;22 Suppl 17, S367-S373.
23. Naismith SL, Rogers NL, Mackenzie J, et al. The relationship between actigraphically defined sleep disturbance and REM sleep behaviour disorder in Parkinson's Disease. *Clin Neurol Neurosurg.* 2010;112(5):420–423.
24. Adi N, Mash DC, Ali Y, et al. Melatonin MT_1 and MT_2 receptor expression in Parkinson's disease. *Med Sci Monit.* 2010;16(2):BR61-BR67.
25. Dowling GA, Mastick J, Colling E, et al. Melatonin for sleep disturbances in Parkinson's disease. *Sleep Med.* 2005;6(5):459–466.
26. Medeiros CA, Carvalhedo de Bruin PF, Lopes LA, et al. Effect of exogenous melatonin on sleep and motor dysfunction in Parkinson's disease: a randomized, double blind, placebo-controlled study. *J Neurol.* 2007;254(4):459–464.
27. Kunz D, Bes F. Melatonin effects in a patient with severe REM sleep behavior disorder: case report and theoretical considerations. *Neuropsychobiology.* 1997;36(4):211–214.

28. Kunz D, Bes F. Melatonin as a therapy in REM sleep behavior disorder patients: an open-labeled pilot study on the possible influence of melatonin on REM-sleep regulation. *Mov Disord.* 1999;14(3): 507–511.
29. Takeuchi N, Uchimura N, Hashizume Y, et al. Melatonin therapy for REM sleep behavior disorder. *Psychiatry Clin Neurosci.* 2001;55(3):267–269.
30. Boeve BF, Silber MH, Ferman TJ. Melatonin for treatment of REM sleep behavior disorder in neurologic disorders: results in 14 patients. *Sleep Med.* 2003;4(4):281–284.
31. Anderson KN, Shneerson JM. Drug treatment of REM sleep behavior disorder: the use of drug therapies other than clonazepam. *J Clin Sleep Med.* 2009;5(3):235–239.
32. Aurora RN, Zak RS, Maganti RK, et al. Best practice guide for the treatment of REM sleep behavior disorder (RBD). *J Clin Sleep Med.* 2010;6(1):85–95.
33. Iranzo A. Sleep-wake changes in the premotor stage of Parkinson disease. *J Neurol Sci.* 2011;310(1–2): 283–285.
34. Srinivasan V, Cardinali DP, Srinivasan US, et al. Therapeutic potential of melatonin and its analogs in Parkinson's disease: Focus on sleep and neuroprotection. *Ther Adv Neurol Dis.* 2011;4(5):297–317.

II

Other Parkinsonian Disorders

14

Severe Hypophonia and Parkinsonism With Hepatitis C and Elevated Mn: Lessons From a Drug Abuser

Anthony E. Lang

THE CASE

An excellent community neurologist called, asking me to see a 37-year-old Azerbaijani man on an urgent basis for parkinsonism and profound hypophonia. He had been neurologically perfectly well until June of 2005 when he began to complain of reduced sexual drive followed by a variety of other symptoms including excessive sleepiness, general slowing of movement, a change in personality (more apathetic), and jerky movements in his legs throughout the night. These symptoms were followed by a change in voice that rapidly progressed to a marked loss of volume and reduction in intelligibility. He also had noted occasional choking, changes in his handwriting (smaller) and manual dexterity as well as unsteadiness of gait. The referring neurologist had done the appropriate tests to exclude Wilson's disease. In December 2005, blood manganese level was 897 nmol/L (normal: 78–289 nmol/L) and urine manganese concentration, 2,804.3 nmol/24 hr. When repeated 5 months later, the blood manganese level had risen to 1,860 nmol/L. MRI scan showed bilateral symmetrical increased signal on T1-weighted images within the basal ganglia as well as the region of the substantia nigra, pontine tectum, and deep cerebellar nuclei.

The patient had left the Soviet Union in 1993 and immigrated to Canada from Israel in 1999. His past history included hepatitis C for which he was treated in Israel with interferon. A recent liver biopsy demonstrated significant fibrosis but no clear evidence of cirrhosis. He was taking ribavirin and pegylated-interferon alfa-2b. He worked as an "engineer" in an electronics plant; his job involved considerable soldering. He denied welding or any other exposures that might have accounted for the elevated manganese levels. He smoked three to four cigarettes per day and drank alcohol minimally. Family history was unremarkable. Treatment to date had included an unsuccessful trial of selegiline, and pramipexole 0.75 mg/d resulted in excessive daytime sleepiness and craving for sweets.

In June 2006 when I first saw him, examination revealed considerable masking of his face and profound hypophonia to the extent that his speech was barely audible. He was alert and cognitive function was unremarkable. His eye movements were not normal; there was some slowing and mild restriction in the range of his vertical saccades, and vertical optokinetic nystagmus was impaired. Horizontal saccades were also somewhat slowed. His tone was normal in the limbs with mild increase in axial muscles. There was moderate bilateral upper and lower limb bradykinesia. He arose from the chair without difficulty. He walked with short strides on a slightly wide base with the arms held abducted from the sides. Turning was difficult and postural reflexes were impaired with falling on the pull test. The remainder of the neurological examination was normal. His general exam showed no hepatosplenomegaly. He had one spider nevus on his chest. He had a scar on his left forearm, which his wife claimed was secondary to a previous operation.

THE APPROACH

The patient was admitted to hospital for further evaluation. Repeated occupational and personal history taking failed to reveal a potential source of excessive manganese exposure. Investigations confirmed the outpatient laboratory abnormalities. Other laboratory tests showed normal concentrations of blood albumin, alkaline phosphatase, gamma-glutamyl transferase, total bilirubin, ceruloplasmin, serum copper, and 24-hour urine copper. Prothrombin time was 51.8 sec (reference range: 33–43 sec); aspartate aminotransferase level, 67 U/L (reference range: 10–40 U/L); and alanine aminotransferase level, 114 U/L (reference range: 2–60 U/L). 6-[18F]-fluorodopa positron emission tomography (PET) scan revealed only a minor reduction in presynaptic uptake limited to the posterior putamen.

He was discharged on increasing doses of levodopa/carbidopa and was followed as an outpatient; he eventually reached a dose of 800/200 mg without benefit. Interestingly, about that same time Schaumburg et al. (1) reported a patient working in a metal alloy facility highly exposed to manganese who only became symptomatic of manganese neurotoxicity following moderate hepatic dysfunction from hepatitis C. Antiviral therapy resulted in normalization of blood manganese and neurological improvement. Extensive discussions with our patient's hepatologist indicated that his synthetic liver function should have been normal despite the evidence of active hepatitis C liver disease. Based on this, we entertained the possibility that the patient had an unusual selective disturbance of hepatic manganese clearance and began to explore methods of confirming this with the consideration that liver transplantation might be necessary if this could be proven.

As we continued to struggle to understand the basis of the patient's manganese toxicity, we got a report from a community social worker who expressed concerns about his psychosocial situation and "poor family support." Apparently, his wife had gone on vacation, leaving the patient alone. Community services were having a great deal of difficulty communicating with him (in large part due to his speech deficit). He had also declined community social work services, and there was concern that he was not going to be able to attend a rehabilitation program because his driver's license had been revoked and he had no other means of transportation.

When he was seen with his wife in September of 2006, they admitted that for the past 3 years he had been intravenously self-injecting a methcathinone solution (ephedrone) prepared from pseudoephedrine tablets and large amounts of potassium permanganate as an oxidant. In retrospect, the lesion on his left arm noted on first assessment had been an injection site.

Subsequent to admitting his drug abuse, the patient discontinued self-injecting ephedrone. Blood manganese levels normalized quickly and MRI scan 6 months later showed no T1 hyperintensity. He had trials of chelation with both ethylenediaminetetraacetic acid (EDTA) and trientine without benefit. A trial of amantadine provided minimal benefit. He required an electronic speech device for communication. Neuropsychological testing in 2009 revealed preserved cognitive abilities, mild executive functioning deficits, and effortful encoding and retrieval. There was mild apathy and depression. On his most recent neurological assessment in October 2010, he complained of increasing walking difficulties with shuffling and freezing, with the occasional tendency to walk on his toes. Examination continued to show the severe hypophonia along with some evidence of dysarthria. Myerson sign was present. Saccadic eye movements were somewhat slowed with some evidence of lateropulsion on vertical gaze. His face was more masked than originally. He was slow with arms held in a flexed, abducted position with minimal arm swing. Postural stability was worse than when he was originally seen with a greater tendency to fall on posterior displacements.

THE LESSON

This patient is typical of an unfortunate group of young intravenous drug abusers from Eastern Europe and Russia who have self-injected methcathinone (ephedrone) prepared at home using pseudoephedrine and large amounts of potassium permanganate as an oxidant. Remarkably, the methods for preparing the drug are widely available on the Internet. When we first came to the correct diagnosis because there had been no such cases reported from North America and only a handful from Eastern Europe, we reported our experience with him (2). Because he withheld the truth about his drug abuse, we had wondered whether his hepatic damage due to hepatitis

C might have somehow been causative as had been described in another patient (1), although a source of excessive Mn exposure had been evident in that case. In retrospect, his hepatitis C was an important clue to his IV drug history. In a recent series of similar patients from Latvia, 100% of the 23 cases were hepatitis C positive and 20 of them were HIV positive as well (3). His course has been typical of many such patients (3). Discontinuation of the drug abuse failed to result in any clinical improvement and in fact, over the following 4 years, he has shown evidence of further deterioration of gait and postural stability. This progression of symptoms has also been seen in other cases of manganese toxicity long after withdrawal from the causative exposure. The parkinsonian syndrome largely relates to the toxic effects of Mn on the GPi/SNr complex, and this accounts for the levodopa-resistant clinical picture that resembles progressive supranuclear palsy more closely than typical Parkinson's disease.

REFERENCES

1. Schaumburg HH, Herskovitz S, Cassano VA. Occupational manganese neurotoxicity provoked by hepatitis C. *Neurology.* 2006;67:322–323.
2. deBie RMA, Gladstone RM, Strafella AP, et al. Manganese-induced parkinsonism associated with methcathinone (Ephedrone) abuse. *Arch Neurol.* 2007;64(6):886–889.
3. Stepens A, Logina I, Liguts V, et al. A Parkinsonian syndrome in methcathinone users and the role of manganese. *N Engl J Med.* 2008;358(10):1009–1017.

15

Ironing Out the Details: Two Sisters With Progressive Parkinsonism and Ataxia

MATTHEW A. BOWER AND PAUL J. TUITE

As a movement disorders neurologist, I am occasionally called upon to evaluate younger individuals presenting with parkinsonism, dystonia, or ataxia. In such cases, it is important to consider genetic causes. One particular diagnostic challenge involved two sisters who presented to me at ages 18 and 20 years.

The older sister was able to relate her clinical history with some help from her mother. She was the product of a routine pregnancy and had normal motor and cognitive development. She was able to complete high school, and at age 18, she experienced the first of several significant depressive episodes. She attended 2 years of community college and maintained a B average despite being hospitalized several times for depression and suicidal ideation. Approximately 2 years after the onset of psychiatric symptoms, she developed gait difficulty, a tendency to fall, and softened speech. Her primary neurologist ordered a brain MRI, which revealed cerebellar atrophy, and she was referred for a second opinion.

Her examination at age 20 revealed hypophonia, appendicular and axial rigidity, stooped posture with shuffling gait accompanying dystonic posturing of her limbs, brisk reflexes, negative Babinski, and positive Romberg. Subtle intermittent arm tremor was noted at rest but not prominent dysmetria. Now 26 years old, her course has been marked by increasing rigidity, progressive hypophonia, and profound postural impairment.

Her younger sister, who was 18 years old at her initial evaluation, was reported to have normal cognitive and motor development until the age of 4 when she began to stutter. In kindergarten, she was "clumsy" and had delayed gross motor skills. Subsequently, she had "behavioral issues" through elementary school, and she was evaluated by a neurologist at the age of nine. A brain MRI scan at the time demonstrated cerebellar atrophy. Cognitive testing at age 12 demonstrated an IQ of 90. The patient's psychiatric health declined, and she received diagnoses of "social anxiety disorder," "elective mutism," and schizophrenia in her teenage years. She was treated with antipsychotics including risperidone, clozapine, and olanzapine. She developed extrapyramidal side effects with each of these medications. Her mother reported that her gait imbalance was stable through her teenage years.

At age 23, she had a flattened affect with paucity of speech, hypophonia, and masked facies. She had saccadic pursuits without nystagmus, lip smacking suggestive of tardive dyskinesia, and dystonic hand posturing. Her appendicular tone was increased with some accompanying contractures that reduced the range of motion. A fine distal hand tremor was present. Sensation was not reliably tested. Ankle reflexes were absent with negative Babinski. Her upper extremities were slow and dysmetric on targeted movements. Stance was wide-based, and she was unsteady with turning, requiring continual support while ambulating.

We obtained a four-generation family history (Figure 15.1). Both parents reported Northern European white ancestry without consanguinity, and no other family members were reported to have the same constellation of neurologic findings. A paternal great uncle supposedly had "mental illness" and a maternal first cousin had seizures but was otherwise healthy.

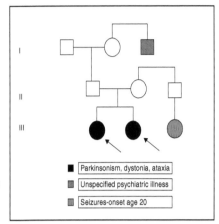

FIGURE 15.1
Abridged family history demonstrating the two affected siblings (individuals III-1 and III-2), the paternal great uncle with psychiatric findings (individual I-3) and the maternal cousin with seizures (individual III-3).

■ Parkinsonism, dystonia, ataxia

▦ Unspecified psychiatric illness

▨ Seizures-onset age 20

THE APPROACH

These sisters had a constellation of progressive cognitive deterioration along with extrapyramidal and cerebellar features, which suggested a neurodegenerative process with possible recessive transmission. The first thing to exclude was Wilson's disease (WD) as it is potentially treatable. The clinical features fit to a degree but there was an absence of dysarthria and the typical wing-beating tremor. Imaging in WD may show iron deposition in the basal ganglia (T2-weighted hypointensity), but there is often accompanying gliosis (T2-weighted hyperintensity), which was absent in this case. Also, some refer to the "face of the giant panda" sign in the midbrain and "face of the miniature panda" sign in the pons due to accompanying iron deposits in both structures, which were not seen (1). Clinical and laboratory evaluations including slit-lamp eye examination, serum ceruloplasmin, and 24-hour urine copper excluded WD.

Neuronal ceroid lipofuscinosis was another possibility as it can manifest with cerebellar atrophy. Lysosomal storage disease was also considered as was autosomal recessive parkinsonism. Extensive genetic testing excluded known causes of inherited ataxia, parkinsonism, and metabolic conditions. The facial movements in the younger sister suggested the unlikely possibility of neuroacanthocytosis, which was ruled out by the absence of acanthocytes on a peripheral smear and a normal creatine kinase level.

As we exhausted possibilities in our differential diagnoses, we considered the MRI images again. In addition to cerebellar atrophy, there was hypointensity of the globus pallidus on T2-weighted images (Figure 15.2). This hypointensity is a nonspecific finding that can be seen with a variety of disorders with increased iron deposition. This includes conditions collectively known as neurodegeneration with brain iron accumulation (NBIA) (2,3). The most common form of NBIA is NBIA1 or pantothenate kinase-associated neurodegeneration (PKAN). PKAN is caused by mutations in the *PANK2* gene (4), and it is classically associated with the "eye-of-the-tiger" sign on MRI, which was not seen with our patients (3). Individuals with PKAN may present with a variety of neurological findings including cognitive regression, spasticity, ataxia, dystonia, and optic atrophy.

Other forms of NBIA may be accompanied by cerebellar atrophy, most notably in individuals with mutations in the *PLA2G6* gene and the associated syndrome phospholipase A2

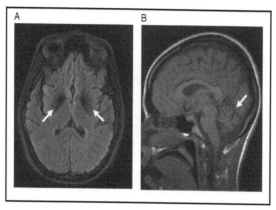

FIGURE 15.2

MRI images illustrating (A) hypointensity of the globus pallidus on T2-weighted MRI and (B) cerebellar atrophy on T1-weighted MRI.

VI-associated neurodegeneration (PLAN). Mutations in the *PLA2G6* gene were first described in individuals with infantile neuroaxonal dystrophy (INAD) in 2006 (5). INAD is characterized by onset of symptoms in the first 3 years of life. Initial symptoms include psychomotor regression and hypotonia. Clinical findings can also include optic atrophy, eye movement abnormalities, spasticity, and cognitive decline. The disease is progressive with death often occurring in the first two decades of life. Atypical forms of neuroaxonal dystrophy (NAD) have been reported with later onset (average age of onset 4.4 years) and longer survival (5–7). Atypical NAD most often presents with ataxia and gait instability. Patients often experience progressive dysphonia, dysarthria, and behavioral disturbances. While the MRI findings in my case fit well with the PLAN syndrome, the late age of presentation and slower progression did not, even with the milder atypical NAD phenotypes. A summary of the known genetic forms of NBIA is presented in Table 15.1.

At the time of the initial evaluation, sequencing of the *PANK2* gene was the only clinically available genetic test for NBIA. This testing was performed in the older sister and it was normal. Several years later, clinical testing became available for mutations in the *PLA2G6* gene. However, the late age of onset and initial mild progression in these two sisters did not fit with the classic descriptions of NAD or INAD. Nonetheless, we pursued *PLA2G6* testing thinking that these two sisters could represent an atypical, milder presentation of the PLAN spectrum of conditions. Sequence analysis of the *PLA2G6* gene in both sisters revealed a heterozygous point mutation in exon 2. This nucleotide change causes a substitution of glutamine to lysine at the second amino acid of the iPLA2-VIA protein. Unfortunately, a second mutation was not identified by this analysis. Therefore, a definitive diagnosis could not be made. This single mutation may have been an incidental finding and unrelated to this patient's diagnosis.

With time, the clinical spectrum of *PLA2G6*-related conditions broadened in the published literature. Most recently, *PLA2G6* mutations have been described in a late childhood/early adulthood onset neurodegenerative disease characterized by dystonia, parkinsonism, and psychiatric findings (8,9). This phenotype was in keeping with the clinical picture in these two

TABLE 15.1
Inherited Extrapyramidal Disorders.

GENE	INHERITANCE	CLINICAL ENTITIES	CLINICAL FINDINGS	IMAGING FINDINGS
PANK2	AR	PKAN atypical PKAN	Onset: first decade (classic form) or second to third decade (atypical form) Dystonia, rigidity, chorea, optic atrophy, retinal degeneration, and spasticity Acanthocytes on peripheral smear have been reported	"Eye-of-the-tiger" sign: T2-weighted pallidal hypointensity with central hyperintensity
		Hallervordan-Spatz, HARP	These entities are now considered part of the PKAN spectrum and these clinical terms are no longer in use	
PLA2G6	AR	PLAN	Describes the spectrum of conditions associated with *PLA2G6* mutation	
		Neuroaxonal dystrophy	Onset: 6 to 36 months Hypotonia, developmental delay, spasticity, and optic atrophy Dystrophic axons seen on nerve biopsy	Pallidal hypointensity on T2-weighted MRI Cerebellar atrophy
		Atypical neuroaxonal dystrophy	Onset: late childhood to teenage Developmental regression, spasticity, dystonia, and dysarthria	Same as above
		Dystonia parkinsonism	Onset: teenage to twenties Prominent dystonia, bradykinesia, and postural instability	Variable findings of cerebellar atrophy and pallidal hypointensity on T2-weighted MRI
		Karak syndrome	This entity is now considered a part of the PLAN spectrum, and it is no longer considered a distinct clinical entity	
CP	AR	Aceruloplasminemia	Adult onset: 25 to 60 years Dystonia, chorea, blepharospasm, and ataxia Retinal degeneration, diabetes, and anemia	Hypointensity of the striatum, thalamus, and dentate nucleus Evidence of iron accumulation in the liver

(continued)

TABLE 15.1
Inherited Extrapyramidal Disorders. (continued)

GENE	INHERITANCE	CLINICAL ENTITIES	CLINICAL FINDINGS	IMAGING FINDINGS
FTL	AD	Neuroferritinospathy	Adult onset: average age of onset in the 40s Prominent chorea, dystonia, dyarthria, and orolingual dyskinesia Less common findings include parkinsonism, brisk reflexes, and cerebellar findings Frontal/subcortical cognitive deficits	Hypointensity of the pallidum, red nucleus, caudate, putamen, and substantia nigra on T2-weighted MRI Cystic degeneration of caudate and putamen
FA2H	AR	FAHN	Onset: 1st decade of life Ataxia Spastic quadriparesis Pyramidal signs Dystonia Optic atrophy	Pallidal hypointensity on T2-weighted MRI Severe pontocerebellar atrophy Thin corpus callosum Periventricular T2-weighted hyperintensities
ATP13A2	AR	Kufor Rakeb syndrome	Onset: age 12 to 22 years Behavioral disturbances, dystonia, bradykinesia, variable cognitive deficits/ mental retardation	Diffuse cerebral atrophy Pallidal hypointensity on T2-weighted MRI

Gene: official HUGO gene symbol is provided. **Inheritance**: (AD) = autosomal dominant; (AR) = autosomal recessive. **Clinical entities**: (PKAN) = pantothenate kinase-associated neurodegeneration; (HARP) = hypoprebetalipoproteinemia, acanthocytosis, and retinitis pigmentosa; (PLAN) = phospholipase A2 VI-associated neurodegeneration; (FAHN) = fatty acid hydroxylase-associated neurodegeneration.

sisters. Interestingly, MRI evidence of iron deposition in the globus pallidus was not a consistent finding in these later-onset cases.

Given this new information, we decided to pursue additional testing that might confirm the presence of a *PLA2G6*-related condition. We were aware that a substantial proportion of mutations in the *PLA2G6* gene were actually large deletions or duplications of entire exons (10). Such deletions and duplications are not identifiable by traditional sequencing tests. A newer technology known as multiplex ligation dependent probe amplification had recently been developed and now allowed for a quantitative analysis of the *PLA2G6* gene. Deletion/duplication analysis revealed a heterozygous deletion of exon 3 in both sisters.

THE LESSON

After a long and frustrating search, we were finally able to provide this family with a definitive diagnosis. The biggest lesson that we learned from our case of these two siblings was the value of persistence and vigilance. DNA testing is a constantly evolving science. Newer technologies may help clarify prior results of uncertain significance. Ongoing review of appropriateness of diagnosis is helpful, as well as a search for new genetic tests. Access to genetic labs and genetic counselors will help in keeping oneself up to date, as well as executing unfinished diagnostic business.

From these cases, we also learned that siblings with the same autosomal recessive disorder may have striking differences in age of onset and initial clinical presentation. The initial description of phenotypes associated with gene mutations may not fully capture the broad spectrum of clinical presentations. Finally, a careful review of MRI imaging may be useful in prompting the clinician to consider NBIA and other disorders that are accompanied by iron deposition.

REFERENCES

1. Das SK, Ray K. Wilson's disease: an update. *Nat Clin Pract Neurol.* 2006;2(9):482–493.
2. Gregory A, Polster BJ, Hayflick SJ. Clinical and genetic delineation of neurodegeneration with brain iron accumulation. *J Med Genet.* 2009;46(2):73–80.
3. McNeil A, Birchall D, Hayflick SJ, Gregory A, et al. T2* and FSE MRI distinguishes four subtypes of neurodegeneration with brain iron accumulation. *Neurology.* 2008;70:1614–1619.
4. Zhou B, Westaway SK, Levinson B, et al. A novel pantothenate kinase gene (PANK2) is defective in Hallervorden-Spatz syndrome. *Nat Genet.* 2001;28(4):345–349.
5. Morgan NV, Westaway SK, Morton JEV, et al. *PLA2G6,* encoding phospholipase A₂, is mutated in neurodegenerative disorders with high brain iron. *Nat Genet.* 2006;38:752–754.
6. Gregory A, Westaway SK, Holm IE, et al. Neurodegeneration associated with genetic defects in phospholipase A2. *Neurology.* 2008;71:1042–1049.
7. Kurian MA, Morgan NV, Macpherson L, et al. Phenotypic spectrum of neurodegeneration associated with mutations in the *PLA2G6* gene (PLAN). *Neurology.* 2008;70:1623–1629.
8. Sina F, Shojaee S, Elahi E, et al. R632W mutation in PLA2G6 segregates with dystonia-parkinsonism in a consanguineous Iranian family. *Eur J Neurosci.* 2009;16(1):101–104.
9. Paisán-Ruiz C, Li A, Schneider SA, et al. Widespread Lewy body and tau accumulation in childhood and adult onset dystonia-parkinsonism cases with PLA2G6 mutations. *Neurobiol Aging.* 2012;33(4): 814–823.
10. Crompton D, Rehal PK, MacPherson L, et al. Multiplex ligation dependent probe amplification (MLPA) analysis is an effective tool for the detection of novel intragenic *PLA2G6* mutations: implications for molecular diagnosis. *Mol Genet Med.* 2010;100(2):207–212.
11. Bower MA, Bushara K, Dempsey MS, et al. Novel mutations in siblings with later-onset *PLA2G6* associated neurodegeneration (PLAN). *Mov Disord.* 2011;26(9):1768–1769.

Suggested Reading

Chinnery PF. *Neuroferritinopathy.* In: Pagon RA, Bird TC, Dolan CR, Stephens K, eds. GeneReviews [Internet]. Seattle (WA): University of Washington, Seattle; 1993–2005 Apr 25 [updated 2007 Aug 8].

Gregory A, Hayflick SJ. *Pantothenate Kinase-Associated Neurodegeneration.* In: Pagon RA, Bird TC, Dolan CR, Stephens K, eds. GeneReviews [Internet]. Seattle (WA): University of Washington, Seattle; 1993–2002 Aug 13 [updated 2010 Mar 23].

Gregory A, Hayflick SJ. *Infantile Neuroaxonal Dystrophy.* In: Pagon RA, Bird TC, Dolan CR, Stephens K, eds. GeneReviews [Internet]. Seattle (WA): University of Washington, Seattle; 1993–2008 Jun 19 [updated 2009 Sep 1].

Hayflick SJ, Hartman M, Coryell J, et al. Brain MRI in neurodegeneration with brain iron accumulation with and without PANK2 mutations. *AJNR.* 2006;27(6):1230–1233.

Kruer MC, Paisán-Ruiz C, Boddaert N, et al. Defective FA2H leads to a novel form of neurodegeneration with brain iron accumulation (NBIA). *Ann Neurol.* 2010;68(5):611–618.

Matarin MM, Singleton AB, Houlden H. *PANK2* gene analysis confirms genetic heterogeneity in neurodegeneration with brain iron accumulation (NBIA) but mutations are rare in other types of adult neurodegenerative disease. *Neurosci Lett.* 2006;407(2):162–165.

McNeill A, Pandolfo M, Kuhn J, et al. The neurological presentation of ceruloplasmin gene mutations. *Eur Neurol.* 2008;60(4):200–205.

Miyajima H. *Aceruloplasminemia.* In: Pagon RA, Bird TC, Dolan CR, Stephens K, eds. GeneReviews [Internet]. Seattle (WA): University of Washington, Seattle; 1993–2003 Aug 12 [updated 2008 May 15].

Thomas M, Hayflick SJ, Jankovic J. Clinical heterogeneity of neurodegeneration with brain iron accumulation (Hallervorden-Spatz syndrome) and pantothenate kinase-associated neurodegeneration. *Mov Disord.* 2004;19(1):36–42.

Schneider SA, Paisán-Ruiz C, Quinn NP, et al. ATP13A2 mutations (PARK9) cause neurodegeneration with brain iron accumulation. *Mov Disord.* 2010;25(8):979–984.

Schneider SA, Bhatia KP. Rare causes of dystonia parkinsonism. *Curr Neurol Neurosci Rep.* 2010; 10(6):431–439.

Zecca L, Youdim MB, Riederer P, et al. Iron, brain ageing and neurodegenerative disorders. *Nat Rev Neurosci.* 2004;5(11):863–873.

16

Acute Onset of Akinetic Mutism With Rigidity in an Elderly Psychiatric Patient: A Reminder on Catatonia

JOSEPH H. FRIEDMAN

THE CASE

I was asked to see a patient on the medical service for unresponsiveness. She was a 70-year-old woman who had been admitted to the hospital for surgery on her hip, fractured while walking her dog. The chart indicated that she had completed surgery without any problems, and seemed her normal self, conversing and behaving appropriately in the recovery room, but over the next day became mute and unresponsive to verbal or visual commands. Of particular importance was her psychiatric history. She had been treated for a disorder, variably diagnosed as bipolar or schizoaffective disorder, for 50 years and was taking trifluoperazine 4 mg, lithium carbonate 600 mg, fluoxetine 20 mg, trazodone 75 mg, and carbamazepine 200 mg daily for this. She also took levothyroxine for hypothyroidism. Before I was called, she had had a brain CT scan, which was normal, and a large number of blood tests to look for electrolyte abnormalities or signs of infection, all of which were normal.

I was asked to see her on her third day of unresponsiveness. Her vital signs were normal. She had not had a fever. She was awake, with eyes open. She was akinetic, mute, and unresponsive other than for blinking to threat and withdrawing to deep pain. Her one positive finding was symmetrically increased tone. The remainder of her neurological exam, limited by her mental state, was normal.

THE APPROACH

The first question I asked myself was whether this was a medical or psychiatric problem. She had no focal signs. Although she blinked to threat and closed her eyes, she did not respond to commands, indicating either lack of comprehension or unwillingness, at some level, to interact. To explain a lack of comprehension, she must have had global cortical involvement. She had not had a lumbar puncture (LP) to look for encephalitis, but there had been no fever and no neck stiffness. The onset was acute and full blown, without progression.

Unless a patient awakens with a new neurological disorder, brain infections should evolve and delirium or aphasia are the expected abnormalities of mental state. There were no medical processes to explain a global cortical problem. She did have increased tone, and she was on a neuroleptic, suggesting the possibility of neuroleptic malignant syndrome (NMS). NMS, however, I have always considered to be a febrile disorder (1), and although it can develop in someone on an antipsychotic for many years, it usually develops in the first few months of exposure, unlike this case. The few cases I have encountered all had profound rigidity, whereas this patient was hypertonic, but not dramatically so. The mental state in NMS is generally obtunded or cloudy, whereas this patient seemed alert. Since she seemed in no danger, as may occur with high temperatures causing heat stroke or extraordinary rigidity causing muscle damage leading to renal failure, sometimes present in NMS, there was no emergent need to treat as if this was the diagnosis.

I did not think she could be in subclinical status epilepticus, in that she was alert rather than having a clouded consciousness, she made no attempt to talk or move, and acted only to *resist* actions (2). This resistance led me to the presumptive diagnosis of *catatonia*.

Based on this presumption, intravenous lorazepam 2 mg was given (2,3). Two minutes later, she became alert and animated, exhibiting pressured speech, loose associations, and racing thoughts, confirming the diagnosis.

For unclear reasons her lorazepam was not continued, and 2 days later, she returned to her akinetic mute state. An electroencephalogram (EEG) performed then showed bilateral slowing without epileptiform activity. A bolus of normal saline was given intravenously, without any response, after which 2 mg of lorazepam was given, producing the same response as seen initially.

THE LESSON

Why does this "classic" case of catatonia belong in a book on unusual movement disorders? One psychiatric expert regards catatonia as "a motor dysregulation syndrome" (2). In this case, the patient had an akinetic-rigid syndrome associated with a behavioral alteration. Parkinsonism is an akinetic rigid syndrome, and behavioral abnormalities are the norm. But parkinsonism is rarely acute in onset, and the behavioral problems typically develop after years of the motor impairments. Secondly, catatonia may cause abnormal postures, stereotypic movements, and "waxy flexibility," which quite clearly fall into the movement disorders realm. Finally, there is an asserted connection between catatonia, lethal catatonia, and NMS (2), with NMS clearly falling into the extrapyramidal symptom complex of dopamine receptor blocking drugs.

DSM IV-TR (4) uses the term catatonia as a specific disorder, as a medical syndrome, as a subtype of schizophrenia (5), and as a modifier for affective disorders. The DSM catatonia syndrome requires the presence of the following:

● Motor immobility, including akinesia and waxy flexibility
● Excessive motor activity, such as nonpurposeful movements
● Extreme negativism as manifested by mutism or opposition to passive movements
● Peculiarities of voluntary movement such as posturing, stereotypies, mannerisms, or prominent grimacing
● Echolalia or echopraxia

Although it has been widely supposed that catatonia is a disorder of the past, perhaps akin to hebephrenic schizophrenia or encephalitis lethargica (6), this is not the case. It appears to be common in psychiatric admissions, affecting 9% of 140 consecutive admissions to one in-patient unit (7) and catatonic features were present in 38% of psychiatric admissions.

Most believe that catatonics are people who sustain odd postures for long periods of time and maintain those postures until their limbs are moved. This abnormality, termed "waxy flexibility," may be seen with catatonia but is not the defining feature and is not present in the majority of patients. Another common misconception is that catatonia is seen in schizophrenia. While there is a subcategory of schizophrenia called catatonic schizophrenia, catatonia is a syndrome that is more common in affective disorders, such as bipolar disease, as was the case here. In a prospective study over 20 years, including 180 patients with catatonia (3), affective disorders were the primary psychiatric problem in 46%, schizophrenia in 20%, schizoaffective disorders in 6%, and 16% from medical and neurological disorders.

There are two major categories of catatonia, the excited form and the nonexcited. The central feature of catatonia is negativism. Patients are usually mute, unresponsive to requests, and highly noninteractive with their environment.

The most common features of catatonia are immobility, mutism, withdrawal, negativism, posturing, grimacing, and rigidity (3). Fink et al. (2) produced a table listing 12 major features that may occur in the catatonic syndrome, which includes mutism, stupor, negativism (gegenhalten-patient voluntarily resists passive movements), posturing, waxy flexibility, stereotypy, automatic obedience, ambitendency, echophenomena, and mannerisms.

There are several fascinating aspects to catatonia. One is the discrepancy between its actual frequency, documented as common by psychiatric experts in the disorder, and the general perception of it as being rare. Another aspect is that psychiatrists state that the catatonic syndrome occurs in a variety of organic brain disorders (2) and usually goes unrecognized. The frequency of "medical catatonia" on a psychiatric unit is estimated at 20% to 25%, based on three relatively small prospective prevalence studies conducted after 1985 (8). Medical causes have included multiple sclerosis and uremia.

Having recognized one case, even capturing the response on videotape, I believe that I was quite sensitive to this potential diagnosis, yet I made this diagnosis only twice in the succeeding 10 years despite performing consults in general medical/surgical hospitals on a regular basis. There was no response to lorazepam in the medical case. However, there are reports of catatonia appearing in patients with systemic lupus erythematosis responding to treatment, and cases where catatonia developed in medically stable patients especially during liver transplantation, in whom lorazepam worked well. While severe Parkinson's disease, cortical basal ganglionic degeneration, advanced stiff person syndrome, and generalized tetanus may produce syndromes that produce signs consistent with catatonia, it is unlikely that such a categorization would be meaningful.

Differential Diagnosis for Catatonia

Nonconvulsive status epilepticus

Locked in syndrome

Severe parkinsonism (from myriad causes)

Malingering

Conversion

On recovery, patients are generally able to report what transpired during their catatonic state and often report a state of fear. This should be kept in mind when dealing with a potential catatonic patient, so that all discussions at the bedside should assume that the patient is not only alert and attentive, but terrified. Since catatonia is a syndrome, it is diagnosed by clinical criteria and is always an expression of an underlying disorder, which is usually a major mental disorder such as a mood disorder or schizophrenia, but may include medical conditions. How the classification of a syndrome of negativism in the context of a medical disorder such as encephalitis alters treatment is uncertain.

Catatonia should always be considered in patients who are seemingly awake but unresponsive, especially when no other explanation can be proffered, such as an ictal or postictal state or a drug-induced condition. It is likely that such patients, when they do not display waxy flexibility or adapt bizarre postures, will be classified as having a "functional" disorder, either malingering or conversion. The importance of recognizing catatonia versus these other psychogenic disorders is that the treatment and prognosis are very different. Catatonia is treated, with a high degree of success, with intravenous or intramuscular (IM) lorazepam, a low-risk procedure, which not only improves the catatonia but also allows for a diagnosis of the underlying psychiatric problem.

REFERENCES

1. Gillman PK. Neuroleptic malignant syndrome: mechanisms, interactions and causality. *Mov Disord.* 2010;25:1780–1790.
2. Fink M, Taylor AM. The catatonia syndrome. Forgotten but not gone. *Arch Gen Psychiatry.* 2009;66: 1173–1177.

3. Rosebush PI, Mazurek MF. Catatonia and its treatment. *Schizophr Bull.* 2010;36:239–242.
4. American Psychiatric Association. Diagnostic and statistical manual IV-TR. American Psychiatric Association Press, Washington, DC, 2000.
5. Heckers S, Tandon R, Bustillo J. Catatonia in the DSM—shall we move or not? *Schiz Bull.* 2009; 36(2):205–207.
6. Mahendra B. Where have all the catatonics gone? *Psychol Med.* 1981;11:669–671.
7. Rosebush P, Hildebrand AM, Furlong BG, Mazurek MF. Catatonic syndrome in a general psychiatric inpatient population: frequency, clinical presentation and response to lorazepam. *J Clin Psychiatry.* 1990;51:357–362.
8. Daniels J. Catatonia. *J Neuropsychiatry Clin Neurosci.* 2009;21:371–380.

Suggested Reading

Bleuler E. Dementia praecox or the group of schizophrenias. Translated by Zinkin J. International Universities Press, New York, NY, 1950. A highly readable description of cases from the perspective of 1911.
Rosenfeld MJ, Friedman JH. Catatonia responsive to lorazepam: a case report. *Mov Disord.* 1999;14:161–162. NB: this report of this case contains a videotape showing the patient before and after the lorazepam.

17

Acute Onset Parkinsonism in a Middle-Aged Alcoholic: A "Great Case"

JOSEPH H. FRIEDMAN

I learned from my residency mentor-in-chief, the great and wise Lewis P. Rowland, MD, that "when a resident tells you, 'this is a great case,' it's bad news for the patient." Obviously this stuck with me and always contrasts with another phrase I can never forget. I was working as a third-year medical student with a new intern who I did not get along with. When he took the patient's history and the patient answered some of the questions in the affirmative, having tuberculosis, for example, the intern's response was, "That's good, very good," which clearly disturbed the poor patient.

I resolved to never describe a case as "great" unless it had a positive outcome. This case is one such.

THE CASE

Mr Jones was a 45-year-old man who I was asked to see because of difficulty walking. He was a high school gym teacher who had been admitted to the medical service for pneumonia and was found to require detoxification because of a severe alcohol problem. He had been drinking about a pint of hard liquor daily for many years but had never sought treatment for alcohol abuse. He reportedly functioned normally at his job in school and gave no hint of mental or motor impairment. He had been able to demonstrate exercises and the various athletic maneuvers required in a gym class.

When I met him, he had been in the hospital for 5 days. His pneumonia had been treated with appropriate antibiotics and he was afebrile. No underlying immune disorder had been found, and he was thought to have a typical, community-acquired pneumonia. He had had no history of neurological problems, liver disease, or abuse of other drugs. His brain MRI had been obtained before I saw him and was normal. His physical examination was normal, without stigmata of alcoholism or liver disease, and his bloodwork was normal as well. His mental status was normal, as were his cranial nerves, but his motor exam showed severe parkinsonism. He had a severely masked facial expression, severe generalized akinesia, marked bradykinesia, rigidity, and a unilateral rest tremor of the fingers. His sensory exam was normal. He was unable to get out of the bed on his own and needed me to pull him up to a sitting position so that, with help, we could swing his legs over the side of the bed. I pulled him to a standing position, but he needed to hold on to me to keep from falling. His posture was markedly stooped, and his knees were flexed. He needed to hold on to me in order to walk, and when he did walk, he took very small steps, with a normal base and a flat footstrike. Turning was slow and laborious, requiring several steps. In short, he had what appeared to be severe Parkinson's disease (PD), but without any sign.

THE APPROACH

I immediately assumed the obvious that the patient had been obstreperous during his detoxification and had been given haloperidol, and, being an athlete, had required a large dose.

Nevertheless, I was still impressed that he could have become so parkinsonian so quickly, regardless of the dose. Neuroleptics usually take several days to weeks to produce parkinsonism, and there is some data to suggest that this problem is less likely, rather than more, to accompany intravenous, although not intramuscular use of the drug. But when I reviewed the chart, I found no behavior problem and no haloperidol. He had received no dopamine-blocking drugs and few other drugs that produce parkinsonism as a side effect. I then checked the history. PD is, of course, insidious in its progression, but it is common for people to notice the disorder one day, perhaps after a fall, or if they begin to tremor under stress, and think that that's the day it started, but the history almost always reveals some slowness or mobility problem that had been blamed on arthritis or old age during the preceding several months. This man, however, had been in gym class and going through his drills without problem and family members remarked on the dramatic change they saw.

The differential for acute onset parkinsonism is fairly limited. First and foremost is drug induced from an antipsychotic drug. After that the drop off to reasonable alternatives is very steep. The toxin MPTP came to prominence when it was discovered that this synthetic opiate derivative, created to produce a "high" for intravenous opiate abusers, produced acute parkinsonism by killing substantia nigra neurons. Since its disastrous side effects were recognized, there have been no cases reported in the past two decades. However, perhaps some enterprising organic chemist in New England might have invented another drug with similarly catastrophic but unrecognized side effects. However, this patient had no other drug problems and no history or signs to suggest a problem with other drugs. In older patients, rapid onset parkinsonism brings to mind Creutzfeldt-Jakob disease, which frequently causes parkinsonism, but never in isolation without dementia, and usually has features that would be atypical for PD, such as apraxia, aphasia, eye movement abnormalities, pyramidal tract or cerebellar signs, and often an abnormal brain MRI. In this case, the MRI was normal and the patient was not demented. Although CJD can advance quickly, it does not produce severe parkinsonism from a normal baseline in just a few days. Encephalitis may cause parkinsonism, and rare cases of postencephalitic parkinsonism similar to those that followed von Economo's encephalitis have been reported. However, there were no findings to suggest this as fever, other than that associated with the pneumonia, mental status changes, or findings atypical for PD. There had been no carbon monoxide poisoning or abnormalities to suggest a vasculitis. His liver testing had been normal so that chronic liver failure could not be the explanation. Wilson's and Huntington's disease do not develop acutely although their neurological abnormalities might worsen acutely with a somatic illness like pneumonia.

Luckily, I had recalled an article I had read years before, "Parkinsonism in alcohol withdrawal," and the videotape that had accompanied it (1).

THE LESSON

The first lesson was that reading journals can pay off, at least when you can remember what you read. I can recall my surprise at reading that article when it came out, which was a follow-up to an article in a medical journal that I had not seen. It registered in my memory bank because I thought that I had a lot of experience and knowledge of alcohol-related neurological syndromes, having spent several months at a New York City public hospital during my training and had never heard of parkinsonism as a consequence of alcoholism or its withdrawal. So when I read about it, I was skeptical and reviewed the videotape, so the memory had stuck with me. And this is what made the case "great." Not only did I look like a genius, since no one else in the hospital, including the alcohol-detox team, had heard of this, so that I could explain the problem, if not from a pathophysiological perspective, at least from the perspective of putting it into a described syndrome, but I could also render a prognosis. The report had followed these patients for several years, and all had recovered. At the time they were initially seen (2), there was concern that the alcohol-related brain changes were unmasking idiopathic PD prematurely, the follow-up showed this not to be the case. So I was able to diagnose and then confidently predict recovery. This appears to be a rare syndrome (3). Over the following 2 weeks in the hospital, the patient improved, without PD medications, from being barely able to walk to walking independently, which is clearly parkinsonian, but only mildly so. A month later, he had a normal examination and had, he stated, stopped drinking entirely.

So, not only can bad things happen to good people, but sometimes they can even recover. I lost track of this patient but have hoped that his brush with severe impairment helped overcome his terrible addiction, which would otherwise lead to irreversible medical problems.

REFERENCES

1. Shandling M, Carlen IL, Lang AE. Parkinsonism in alcohol withdrawal: a follow up study. *Mov Disord.* 1990;5:36–39.
2. Carlen PL, Lee MA, Jacob M, Livishitz O. Parkinsonism provoked by alcoholism. *Ann Neurol.* 1981;9:84–86.
3. Brust JCM. Substance abuse and movement disorders. *Mov Disord.* 2010;25:2010–2020.

18

A 38-Year-Old Brazilian Woman Presenting With Reversible Parkinsonism Associated With Neurocysticercosis

HÉLIO A.G. TEIVE

THE CASE

Four months before consultation, a 38-year-old woman started with diffuse, occasionally throbbing, headaches associated with nausea, which was worse while waking, together with intense pain accompanied by episodes of vomiting, diplopia, drowsiness, and torpor. Since symptoms' onset, the patient reported being slower and having bilateral hand tremor.

Because the clinical picture deteriorated, the patient was assessed in the neurology service and diagnosed with intracranial hypertension after a brain MRI that showed the presence of supratentorial hydrocephalus with evidence of intraventricular cysts (at the level of the frontal horn of the right lateral ventricle, beside the foramen of Monro, and at the level of the third ventricle), as well as edema in the midbrain periaqueductal region.

The patient received a ventriculoperitoneal (VP) shunt, and the symptoms of intracranial hypertension improved. Analysis of cerebrospinal fluid (CSF) demonstrated a mild inflammatory reaction and neurocysticercosis (NCC) as detected by positive reactions to cysticercus antigens. The patient was started on high-dose (3,200 mg orally per day) albendazole, and after 4 days of treatment, she developed mutism, hypomimia, and sialorrhea, with marked muscular rigidity and bradykinesia in association with marked resting hand tremor. A new brain MRI showed mild hydrocephalus and the presence of intraventricular cysts with edema around the cerebral aqueduct and signs of ependymitis (Figures 18.1 and 18.2).

The patient was referred to the Neurology Service at the Hospital de Clínicas, Federal University of Paraná, Curitiba, Paraná, Brazil.

THE APPROACH

Neurological examination on admission showed marked bilateral akinetic-rigid syndrome in association with predominantly resting hand tremor, marked postural instability, anarthria (mutism), and vertical ophthalmoparesis on upward gaze. Parkinsonism secondary to NCC (the form with hydrocephalus, intraventricular cysts, and cysticercosis encephalitis) aggravated by high doses of albendazole was diagnosed.

Methylprednisolone pulse therapy was then started (1 g i.v./d for 5 days) followed by 50 mg of prednisone for 15 more days, together with half a tablet of levodopa/carbidopa 250/25mg four times a day, which was supplemented 7 days later with one tablet of 200 mg entacapone four times a day, with progressive improvement in the symptoms of parkinsonism.

She then underwent an endoscopic neurosurgical procedure including monroplasty, which is the removal of the cyst, a pellucidotomy, and a third ventriculostomy. Neuropathological examination confirmed the diagnosis of NCC.

With the improvement in the clinical picture, the patient was discharged from the hospital on a prescription of one tablet of levodopa/carbidopa 250/25 mg and one tablet of entacapone 200 mg four times a day. Subsequent outpatient assessment revealed that there had been a marked

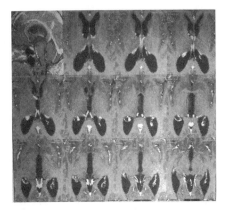

FIGURE 18.1
*Brain MRI—sagittal and axial
T1-weighted imaging showed mild
hydrocephalus and presence of
intraventricular cysts.*

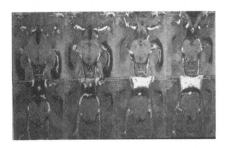

FIGURE 18.2
*Brain MRI and axial T1-weighted
imaging showed edema in the midbrain
periaqueductal area and signs of
ependymitis.*

improvement in the symptoms of parkinsonism, with no signs of intracranial hypertension. In follow-up, a new brain MRI no longer demonstrated hydrocephalus or intraventricular cysts.

Eight months later, the patient was progressively taken off entacapone and then levodopa. She remained asymptomatic and returned to normal activities of daily life.

THE LESSON

This patient presented with parkinsonism secondary to NCC with a mixed presentation (hydrocephalus with cysticercus cysts and brainstem ependymitis).

NCC is the most common helminth infection of the central nervous system, particularly in developing countries (1). Parkinsonism secondary to NCC can be related to hydrocephalus secondary to cysts of the fourth ventricle, perimesencephalic cysts, basal racemose cysts, and brainstem ependymitis due to cysticercus cysts, as well as surface cysts and ischemic lesions in the midbrain (2–4).

It was clear from the clinical description that the symptoms of parkinsonism were greatly exacerbated after albendazole treatment was started. This result has been described in the literature and occurs because cysticidal drugs can cause an intense inflammatory reaction, especially in forms of NCC involving intraventricular cysts and ependymitis/encephalitis (5).

Because it can potentially be reversed with use of steroids and levodopa, cysticercosis encephalitis should be considered in the differential diagnosis of rapidly progressive parkinsonism with atypical features (2,3).

The case described here is comparable to others already published, with the peculiarity that there was a deterioration of the symptoms of parkinsonism after the use of high doses of albendazole (2–4).

REFERENCES

1. Takayanagui OM, Jardim E. Clinical aspects of neurocysticercosis: analysis of 500 cases. *Arq Neuropsiquiatr.* 1983;41(1):50–63.
2. Sá DS, Teive HAG, Troiano AR, Werneck LC. Parkinsonism associated with neurocysticercosis. *Parkinsonism Relat Disord.* 2005;11(1):69–72.
3. Verma A, Berger JR, Bowen BC, Sanchez-Ramos J. Reversible parkinsonian syndrome complicating cysticercus midbrain encephalitis. *Mov Disord.* 1995;10(2):215–219.
4. Curran T, Lang AE. Parkinsonism syndromes associated with hydrocephalus: case report, a review of the literature, and pathophysiological hypotheses. *Mov Disord.* 1994;9(5):508–520.
5. Garcia HH, Evans CAW, Nash TE, et al. Current consensus guidelines for treatment of neurocysticercosis. *Clin Microbiol Rev.* 2002;15(4):747–756.

Suggested Reading

Troiano AR, Micheli FE, Alarcón F, Teive HAG. Movement disorders in Latin America. *Parkinsonism Relat Disord.* 2006;12(3):125–138.

19

An Apparent Case of Early Onset Parkinsonism: A Lesson on Huntington's Disease From a Bus Driver in Italy

Giovanni Abbruzzese, Monica Bandettini,
Flavio Nobili, and Paola Mandich

THE CASE

This 33-year-old bus driver was first seen in July 2006. He was directed to our Movement Disorder Clinic by his general practitioner (GP) because, a year before, he had begun to complain of low-volume speech, slowness in movement, and occasional tremors in the upper limbs. Previously, he had never suffered any symptoms and family history was apparently negative.

The neurological examination showed a slight limitation of upward gaze, his face was hypomimic, and his speech hypophonic; rigidity was widely present mostly in the upper limbs where an irregular tremor could also be observed (enhanced by emotion). Gait was moderately slow with mild bent spine, but the pull test was normal. Brisk tendon jerks were present with no Babinski sign. The UPDRS motor score was 24/108. The clinical suspicion was that of a parkinsonian syndrome with juvenile onset, and he was admitted to our hospital for further investigations.

THE APPROACH

The laboratory tests that we performed (including cerebrospinal fluid [CSF] examination and screening of copper metabolism) were normal, and the electroencephalogram (EEG) was characterized by a diffuse low-voltage fast activity. The brain MRI showed a corticosubcortical atrophy with a reduced representation of the substantia nigra (pars compacta) in the T2-weighted sequences. The neuropsychological assessment showed an initial cognitive impairment with subcortical features. SPECT with (123)I-FP-CIT (DaTSCAN) was performed and documented a widespread impairment of presynaptic nigrostriatal dopaminergic terminals with a slight asymmetry.

Because of the early onset of symptoms and the occurrence of some atypical features (e.g., the neuropsychological impairment), we decided to perform a genetic screening for "parkin" and "huntingtin" mutations.

Symptomatic treatment with dopamine-agonist drugs (pramipexole) was introduced with a moderate clinical benefit, and the patient was discharged with low-dosage (0.18 mg thrice a day) pramipexole.

A month later, the patient continued to report improvement with a reduction in rigidity and tremor. The results of genetic testing demonstrated a mutation of the "huntingtin" (*IT15*) gene with 58/17 CAG repeats. We tried to further investigate the family history and both the patient's parents agreed to undergo a testing protocol for symptomatic Huntington's disease (HD). The 62-year-old father of the patient (although fully asymptomatic) was found to be carrying a 36 CAG repeats allele (incomplete penetrance allele).

The patient continued treatment with pramipexole and amantadine (200 mg/d), and the clinical conditions remained relatively stable for 2 years. Eventually, bradykinesia and rigidity significantly worsened, the gait became wide based, and ataxic and autonomy in daily living activity was dramatically reduced.

THE LESSON

The lack of a positive family history does not exclude the diagnosis of HD since individuals with 36–39 CAG repeats may or may not exhibit symptoms but their offspring may have the disease.

HD may present with typical features of parkinsonism (akinesia, rigidity, and tremor) in the juvenile or young adult-onset parkinsonian phenotype variant (Westphal variant). Such individuals can be misdiagnosed with Parkinson's disease, catatonia, or schizophrenia.

HD (in particular, the akinetic-rigid phenotype) can be associated with decreased striatal monoaminergic terminals, suggesting the occurrence of a nigrostriatal pathology. A significant decrease of dopamine transporter in the striatum may reflect the loss of presynaptic terminals and explain a partial responsiveness to dopaminergic drugs.

Suggested Reading

Bohnen NI, Koeppe RA, Meyer P, et al. Decreased striatal monoaminergic terminals in Huntington disease. *Neurology.* 2000;54:1753–1759.

Bonelli RM, Niederwiesser G, Diez J, et al. Pramipexole ameliorates neurologic and psychiatric symptoms in a Westphal variant of Huntington's disease. *Clin Neuropharmacol.* 2002;25:58–60.

Gamez J, Lorenzo-Bosquet C, Cuberas-Borros G, et al. Does reduced [(123)I]-FP-CIT binding in Huntington disease suggest pre-synaptic dopaminergic involvement? *Clin Neurol Neurosurg.* 2010;112:870–875.

Ginovart N, Lundin A, Farde L, et al. G. PET study of the pre- and post-synaptic dopaminergic markers for the neurodegenerative process in Huntington's disease. *Brain.* 1997;120:503–514.

Ross CA, Tabrizi SJ. Huntington's disease: from molecular diagnosis to clinical treatment. *Lancet Neurol.* 2011;10:83–98.

20

A Vasculopathic Man With "Vascular Parkinsonism" Without Vasculopathy: My Humbling Case of Normal Pressure Hydrocephalus

ALBERTO J. ESPAY

THE CASE

The family doctor requested an evaluation for presumed normal pressure hydrocephalus on this 80-year-old man with progressive gait, balance, and memory impairment. About 30 months previously, he had begun to notice short-stepped gait with impairment of balance. He had accumulated multiple falls during the ensuing year, some accompanied by substantial soft tissue injury. Over the last 9 months, he became incontinent of urine. He had been twice hospitalized for sudden-onset episodes of gait freezing. He had not noted changes in speech, swallowing, visual function, or handwriting, but his daughter suggested that his short-term memory was impaired in the last few years. He had not responded to a trial with L-dopa, increased to a dose of 600 mg/d. The patient was residing at a rehabilitation facility to assist with gait and transfers. He was, however, able to bathe, dress, and feed without any assistance.

His past medical history was positive for hypertension, hypercholesterolemia, hypokalemic episodes, and "cerebral microangiopathic disease." He had stopped smoking about 40 years ago after accumulating a 60 pack/y of smoking history. His alcohol intake was restricted to social functions.

When I first saw him, he had marked lower-body-predominant parkinsonism with postural impairment and short-stride gait without stooping, clear shuffling, or festination. His base was wide and his feet were externally rotated. He had paratonia of the upper limbs but no rigidity in the legs or neck. Cognitive function based on bedside screening was mildly impaired (Folstein mini-mental state examination: 25/30; Frontal Assessment Battery: 17/18), but given the presence of frontal release signs, namely snout and palmomental reflexes, and concerns on the part of his family, a thorough neuropsychological evaluation was requested. Comparing this study with an assessment done at the onset of his symptoms, his overall cognitive functioning had dropped markedly from the average range (65th percentile) to the extremely low range (less than 1 percentile). Importantly, all executive functions (behavioral initiation, motor regulation, planning, organization, mental flexibility, problem solving, etc.) dropped from high average to less than 1 percentile. With the exception of word finding and naming skills, all other nonexecutive functions (visuospatial construction, learning, and memory) showed a similar rate of decline.

A brain MRI showed confluent punctate areas of increased T2-weighted signal affecting subcortical and periventricular white matter in a pattern consistent with chronic small vessel ischemic disease. Lateral and third ventricles were moderately dilated but not out of proportion to the degree of cortical atrophy (Figure 20.1). I was certain that his deficits were due to vascular parkinsonism (VaP) with early multi-infarct dementia. I recommended slow withdrawal from levodopa, monitor blood pressure with orthostatic measurements, tighter control of his dyslipidemia, and use of a walker for prevention of falls during ambulation.

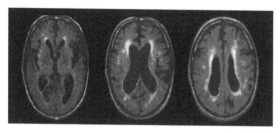

FIGURE 20.1

Axial fluid-attenuated inversion recovery brain MRI at the basal ganglia, mid-, and high-ventricular levels. My interpretation of this MRI, in part echoing the official neuroradiology report, was of increased periventricular and subcortical white matter signal suggestive of small vessel ischemic disease, and mild to moderate ventricular dilatation, felt proportionate to the apparent degree of cortical atrophy.

THE APPROACH

Despite my certainty about the diagnosis, the family of this patient fully endorsed the family physician's suggestion that his symptoms were due to normal pressure hydrocephalus (NPH). I argued that in the case of someone with a staggering progression of deficits, multiple vascular risk factors, and evidence of small-vessel ischemic disease on brain MRI, the diagnosis of VaP was almost beyond doubt. I further indicated that the increase in ventricular size was explained by the surrounding parenchymal atrophy. Succumbing to the family pressure, however, I admitted him to the hospital to appease their concerns and "confirm his ineligibility" for ventriculo-peritoneal shunt (VPS) placement by ascertaining (the lack of) gait and cognitive changes before and immediately after a 3-day external lumbar drainage (ELD).

To my surprise, his gait showed significant improvements in gait velocity and stride length (Table 20.1) and his cognitive parameters remained within abnormal range, but relatively improved over the pre-ELD measurements. Given the value of ELD in predicting ultimate response to VPS (2), this intervention was decided upon in agreement with the patient and his family. Unfortunately, he died from procedure-related complications shortly after VPS placement. The family consented to brain-only autopsy. Postmortem examination revealed a normal brain weight (1,400 g) and communicating hydrocephalus with leptomeningeal fibrosis and superficial gliosis of cerebral cortex. Unexpectedly, there were no macroinfarcts or lacunes. Lewy bodies or tau pathology were lacking. Additional neuropathology efforts, coerced by my "confidence" of the vasculopathic nature of the case, only yielded rare fibrinoid necrosis and arteriolosclerosis with focal reduction in oligodendrocytes in the basal ganglia and frontal white matter. This minimal microvascular pathology was present to an extent consistent with his advanced age. The overall neuropathological findings were most consistent with NPH and did not meet neuropathological criteria for VaP.

THE LESSON

A big dose of humility was instilled in me by this case. My reliance on a "classic" presentation of VaP was eroded by the incontrovertible weight of the evidence pointing in the direction of a shunt-responsive form of hydrocephalus. Although it has been stated that VaP and NPH may coexist and that both are part of a single pathologic spectrum, it is sobering to realize that most studies published on both disorders have not relied on clinicopathologic correlations. One of my greatest lessons was to learn of my inaccurate interpretation of the brain MRI in light

TABLE 20.1
Gait Assessments.

PARAMETERS	STRAIGHT PATH (2.6 M)			TURNING (0.7 M)		
	PRE-ELD	POST-ELD	Δ	PRE-ELD	POST-ELD	Δ
Timed gait (sec)	22	13	40.9%	15	6	60%
Cadence (steps/min)	76	92	17.4%	68	100	47.1%
Gait velocity (m/min)	7.2	12	40%	2.8	7.0	250%
Step length (cm)	9.2	12.9	28.7%	4.1	7.0	70.7%

Δ = percentage improvement; Step length × 2 ≅ stride length; ELD = external lumbar drainage.

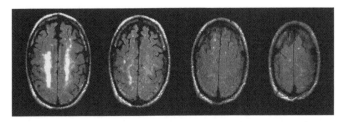

FIGURE 20.2
Axial fluid-attenuated inversion recovery brain MRI of the same patient at higher cuts shows no evidence of atrophy. The sulci are narrow and gyri are tightly packed. This information, available at the outset, had been missed.

of the known pathology. What I interpreted as microangiopathic disease must have just been transependymal exudates. Further, what I interpreted as parenchymal atrophy corresponded to a pseudoatrophic pattern that seasoned observers have attributed to a sulcal entrapment from increased subarachnoid volume. In fact, had I reviewed the apical cuts of the brain MRI appropriately, I would have concluded that there was no true atrophy (Figure 20.2). Notice how those cuts reveal tightening of the gyri rather than widening of the sulci.

This case also illustrated a shortcoming of my clinical appreciation of gait impairments as predictive of either of the disorders considered here. For all purposes, the gait pattern described (wide based, feet outwardly rotated, upright, wooden posture on walking) fits with the classic descriptions of VaP acknowledging that these descriptions were generated in the pre-MRI era and without neuropathologic confirmation (3). The VaP versus NPH dichotomy appears to have been artificially constructed to satisfy the splitters among us but, probably, bound to ultimately reward the patient lumpers in the back of the room. Ultimately, from the perspective of a treating physician, shunt responsiveness has been consistently documented even in the presence of marked periventricular and deep white matter T2-weighted hyperintensities suggestive of vascular disease, indicating that imaging-defined "small vessel ischemic disease" may be part of the broad and complex definition of "NPH" rather than a separate disorder (1,4). As such, the white matter involvement should not detract from exploring the response to fluid diversion in otherwise suitable patients, with a pseudoatrophic cortical atrophy pattern. Tighter control of already well-managed vascular risk factors, as was initially suggested for this man, may be a disappointing target of therapy for patients mischaracterized as VaP.

REFERENCES

1. Bech-Azeddine R, Hogh P, Juhler M, et al. Idiopathic normal-pressure hydrocephalus: clinical comorbidity correlated with cerebral biopsy findings and outcome of cerebrospinal fluid shunting. *J Neurol Neurosurg Psychiatry.* 2007;78:157–161.

2. Haan J, Thomeer RT. Predictive value of temporary external lumbar drainage in normal pressure hydrocephalus. *Neurosurgery.* 1988;22:388–391.

3. Thompson PD, Marsden CD. Gait disorder of subcortical arteriosclerotic encephalopathy: Binswanger's disease. *Mov Disord.* 1987;2:1–8.

4. Tullberg M, Hultin L, Ekholm S, et al. White matter changes in normal pressure hydrocephalus and Binswanger disease: specificity, predictive value and correlations to axonal degeneration and demyelination. *Acta Neurol Scand.* 2002;105:417–426.

21

Too Young for Parkinson's Disease? Levodopa-Responsive Parkinsonism in an 8-Year-Old Boy

OSCAR S. GERSHANIK

THE CASE

This patient came to our Movement Disorders Unit several years ago presenting with a slowly progressive change in his mood, followed by the insidious development of masked facies, generalized slowness of movement, gait difficulties, dysarthria, hypophonia, and drooling. He was the product of nonconsanguineous parents, his developmental milestones were within normal limits, and his past medical history was unremarkable. Family history was negative for movement disorders or other neurological conditions. The parents dated back the onset of his problems to the occurrence of two separate events in the previous year. The first was the moving out of his home of a dear uncle who had lived with them for many years, which caused significant separation anxiety. Within a few days of this event, the boy developed a febrile condition of unknown etiology that resolved spontaneously in a matter of days. From then onward, the patient's motor functioning started to deteriorate, having reached the previously described clinical picture in approximately 6 months.

THE APPROACH

Upon examination, the patient was alert and responsive, although verbal communication was markedly impaired by the presence of dysarthria and hypophonia. His face was devoid of expression, eye blinking was absent, his mouth was partly opened most of the time, and there was constant drooling of saliva. Voluntary eye movements were full, and a slight, impersistent, bilateral, jerky nystagmus was detected on lateral eye deviation. Posture was moderately flexed, involving both trunk and limbs. Gait was short stepped, with festination and propulsion, and turning was somewhat difficult. There was generalized rigidity and significant bilateral and symmetric bradykinesia with a barely detectable postural tremor in both hands. The rest of the neurological examination was within normal limits and his overall clinical examination did not reveal any abnormality.

A comprehensive imaging and laboratory work up (including urinary copper excretion and plasma ceruloplasmin) was performed, failing to reveal any structural brain changes or biochemical abnormalities.

A clinical diagnosis of "juvenile-onset parkinsonism" was made, with several possible etiologies in our minds: Dopa-responsive dystonia (DRD), autosomal recessive juvenile onset Parkinson's disease (PARK 2 or parkin parkinsonism), Kufor-Rakeb's disease (PARK 9), as our most likely candidates (1,2). We could not rule out, however, other possible secondary causes of parkinsonism, despite the failure to demonstrate structural brain changes or laboratory abnormalities. Postencephalitic parkinsonism was also considered as the patient had had a febrile condition just prior to the development of his symptoms; however, at the time of his illness, a lumbar puncture and cerebrospinal fluid (CSF) analysis had not been performed (3). We decided not to pursue this diagnosis, as no other manifestations of encephalitis were present, a significant time had elapsed since his febrile episode, and the exceptional reports of these disorders as causes of persistent parkinsonism.

We decided to put him on levodopa to determine if this case was responsive to the drug, evaluate the magnitude of the response, and observe the subsequent course of the disease. We believed, at the time, that a marked response to levodopa, and a benign course would be suggestive of either DRD or parkin parkinsonism. Genetic analysis for these conditions was not readily available then.

A few weeks after the introduction of levodopa/carbidopa (100/25 mg) up to 400 mg/d, there was dramatic improvement with an almost complete disappearance of the symptomatology. The patient regained his facial expression and was able to speak normally, drooling disappeared, his posture and movement returned to normal, and his mood improved significantly. A first step had been accomplished, having demonstrated that this was a form of levodopa-responsive parkinsonism, and due to the magnitude of the response our belief was then that the most probable diagnosis was DRD, despite the lack of family history (4). Within a few months, our enthusiasm was dampened by the development of motor fluctuations and choreatic dyskinesias, which in no way were thought to contradict our initial diagnosis as fluctuations and dyskinesias have been reported in DRD (4). Frequently these fluctuations and dyskinesias resolve with minor dose adjustments. This was not the case, however, in our patient, as the fluctuations and dyskinesias worsened despite the implementation of different pharmacological strategies (levodopa dose fractionation, addition of dopamine agonists, etc.). Moreover, choreatic dyskinesias were progressively replaced by severe dystonic-ballistic movements that presented at the beginning and end of each dose interval (diphasic dyskinesias) and caused significant disability in our patient. This pattern of response is not usually seen in DRD, and we changed our tentative diagnosis to one of the genetically determined forms of juvenile-onset Parkinson's disease. Nevertheless, we had never ruled out the possibility of a rare form of secondary parkinsonism, and the presence of minor oculomotor abnormalities in the initial examination was interpreted as a possible "red flag" alerting us to that possibility (2).

Much to our dismay, the patient progressively worsened, not only because of the severe nature of the motor fluctuations and dyskinesias, but also due to the development of ataxia, cranial dystonia, and supranuclear gaze palsy in the vertical plane. This change in the clinical picture forced us to steer away from the original diagnosis and start seriously thinking about possible causes of secondary parkinsonism associated with supranuclear gaze palsy. We believed we could readily rule out the late-onset causes of degenerative parkinsonism with supranuclear gaze palsy such as progressive supranuclear gaze palsy, corticobasal degeneration, and dementia with Lewy bodies; Gaucher's disease, among the metabolic disorders, usually develops supranuclear gaze palsy in the horizontal plane, unlike our patient who presented with significant impairment in the vertical plane (5–7). Structural lesions of the periaqueductal gray matter usually present with supranuclear gaze palsy in the vertical plane, but they are often the result of a single-hit event (e.g., vascular; although tumors in the region may result in a progressive course), do not associate levodopa-responsive parkinsonism, are not of a progressive nature, and imaging studies reveal the presence of the causative structural lesion, which was not the case in our patient (8).

We were then left with two probable etiologies that could explain our patient's condition. The least probable was brain Whipple's disease, as the patient did not exhibit any of the classical features associated with this disorder, such as oculomasticatory myorhithmia or involvement of other systems (osteoarticular, ophthalmologic, etc.), had no history of malabsorption, and to our knowledge, there has never been a case of Whipple's disease reported in the literature with levodopa-responsive parkinsonism, and moreover, at such a young age (9). The other was the so-called juvenile dystonic lipidosis, among which Niemann-Pick's type C disease is the most paradigmatic example (10,11).

We decided to perform a repeat comprehensive clinical examination, including imaging studies (brain MRI, abdominal echography) and bone marrow aspiration for microscopic analysis. Clinical examination and abdominal echography failed to reveal organomegaly, which is a common finding in Niemann-Pick type C. MRI of the brain showed mild nonspecific supra and infratentorial atrophic changes; however, microscopic examination of bone marrow aspirate showed abundant foamy macrophages and "sea-blue histiocytes," which are typical of this condition. Further to these findings, we performed a skin biopsy and confirmed the presence of cholesterol esterification block in cultured fibroblasts, thus supporting the diagnosis of Niemann-Pick type C (12).

In the following months, the patient's condition rapidly deteriorated, with marked motor impairment and cognitive deterioration, until he finally developed a severe deglutition disorder, causing aspiration pneumonia, which led to his death in a few weeks. Unfortunately, at the time we saw this patient there were no available treatment options.

THE LESSON

As the proverb goes, "all that glitters is not gold." This can easily be applied to our case since the presence of a positive and dramatic clinical response to levodopa does not necessarily mean that we are faced with a benign disorder. Keeping along the same lines, "it is never too late to learn." We have to trust our instincts and clinical experience always, and in our case, the finding of minor oculomotor abnormalities on the first examination was something that kept nagging us and made us be attentive to any significant changes in the course of the disease that could be suggestive of an alternative diagnosis. The most important lesson is that it is always "better to be safe than sorry"; therefore, we have to pay close attention to our patients and be always ready to revisit the case, think of alternative diagnoses, and perform repeat studies to keep track of potential changes that could be undetected clinically. In this case, the clue was the development of a vertical supranuclear gaze palsy in a young boy with progressive extrapyramidal features, irrespective of the presence of a dramatic response to levodopa or the absence of hepatosplenomegaly.

Crocker and Farber (1958) were perhaps the first to delineate the clinical features and boundaries of Niemann-Pick disease. Their cases showed a wide range of clinical features but were grouped together as they all had "Niemann-Pick cells" (foam-laden macrophages) and increased tissue sphingomyelin (13). Niemann-Pick disease was further divided into four types. Type A: acute neuropathic form, with onset in early infancy, rapid progression, and usually resulting in death before the age of 2 years, with both visceral involvement (hepatosplenomegaly and lung infiltration) and central nervous system (CNS) involvement (motor deterioration, progressive weakness and wasting, macular cherry-red spots, and cataracts); type B: chronic visceral form, lacking CNS involvement; type C: the chronic neuropathic form (later called juvenile dystonic lipidosis with characteristic ophthalmoplegic involvement); and type D: Nova Scotia form, which is similar to type C, but occurring in patients whose families come from Nova Scotia with Acadian ancestry, where the condition is common (14). Sphingomyelinase deficiency is usually found in types A and B, but this is not the case for types C and D (11).

Niemann-Pick type C is an autosomal recessive lysosomal neurovisceral storage disorder and is caused in 95% of the cases by a mutation in the *NPC1* gene, while the remaining 5% is due to a mutation in the *NPC2* gene. The same mutation in the *NPC1* gene is responsible for Niemann-Pick type D. The clinical manifestations of types C1 and C2 are similar because the respective genes are both involved in the handling of lipids, particularly cholesterol in lysosomes, while mutations in these genes cause a block in cholesterol esterification (15).

The presentation of Niemann-Pick disease type C (NPC) is highly heterogeneous and can manifest from the neonatal period to early adulthood. In the youngest cases, failure to thrive, jaundice, and death are common, while in infancy or early adult life, the most common presentation is a multisystem CNS disease including vertical supranuclear ophthalmoplegia, usually associated with hepatosplenomegaly. Patients with the "classic" childhood onset type C may appear normal for 1 or 2 years, until the development of the first symptoms, usually appearing between the ages of 2 to 4 years. Neurologic abnormalities gradually develop, including ataxia, grand mal seizures, and loss of previously learned speech. Spasticity, myoclonic jerks, and seizures are common. Other features include dystonia, vertical supranuclear gaze palsy, dementia, and psychiatric manifestations, while cholestatic jaundice may occur in some patients. Supranuclear gaze palsy in the vertical plain is highly suggestive of this condition. Foamy Niemann-Pick cells and "sea-blue" histiocytes with distinctive histochemical and ultrastructural appearances are found in the bone marrow. In the childhood-onset form, death usually occurs at ages 5 to 15. Adult-onset forms, with insidious onset and slower progression, have also been reported. Parkinsonism has rarely been reported, and no instance of levodopa-responsive parkinsonism with motor fluctuations and dyskinesias has been published in the literature to our knowledge (11,12).

REFERENCES

1. Paviour DC, Surtees RA, Lees AJ. Diagnostic considerations in juvenile parkinsonism. *Mov Disord.* 2004;19(2):123–135.
2. Schneider SA, Bhatia KP. Rare causes of dystonia parkinsonism. *Curr Neurol Neurosci Rep.* 2010;10(6):431–439.
3. Savant CS, Singhal BS, Jankovic J, et al. Substantia nigra lesions in viral encephalitis. *Mov Disord.* 2003;18(2):213–216.
4. Trender-Gerhard I, Sweeney MG, Schwingenschuh P, et al. Autosomal-dominant GTPCH1-deficient DRD: clinical characteristics and long-term outcome of 34 patients. *J Neurol Neurosurg Psychiatry.* 2009;80(8):839–845.
5. Ludolph AC, Kassubek J, Landwehrmeyer BG, et al,. Reisensburg Working Group for Tauopathies with parkinsonism. Tauopathies with parkinsonism: clinical spectrum, neuropathologic basis, biological markers, and treatment options. *Eur J Neurol.* 2009;16(3):297–309.
6. Nakashima H, Terada S, Ishizu H, et al. An autopsied case of dementia with Lewy bodies with supranuclear gaze palsy. *Neurol Res.* 2003;25(5):533–537.
7. Kraoua I, Stirnemann J, Ribeiro MJ, et al. Parkinsonism in Gaucher's disease type 1: ten new cases and a review of the literature. *Mov Disord.* 2009;24(10):1524–1530.
8. Karatas M. Internuclear and supranuclear disorders of eye movements: clinical features and causes. *Eur J Neurol.* 2009;16(12):1265–1277.
9. Louis ED. Whipple disease. *Curr Neurol Neurosci Rep.* 2003;3(6):470–475.
10. Martin JJ, Lowenthal A, Ceuterick C, Vanier MT. Juvenile dystonic lipidosis [variant of Niemann-Pick disease type C]. *J Neurol Sci.* 1984;66(1):33–45.
11. Coleman RJ, Robb SA, Lake BD, et al. The diverse neurological features of Niemann-Pick disease type C: a report of two cases. *Mov Disord.* 1988;3(4):295–299.
12. Héron B, Ogier H. Niemann-Pick type C disease: clinical presentations in pediatric patients. *Arch Pediatr.* 2010;17(suppl 2):S45-S49.
13. Crocker AC, Farber S. Niemann-Pick disease: a review of eighteen patients. *Medicine.* 1958;37:1–95.
14. Crocker AC. The cerebral defect in Tay-Sachs disease and Niemann-Pick disease. *J Neurochem.* 1961; 7:69430.
15. Vance, J. E. Lipid imbalance in the neurological disorder, Niemann-Pick C disease. *FEBS Lett.* 2006;580:5518–5524.

22

The Misleading Phenotypes of PD and Parkinson-Plus Syndromes: Lessons I Learned From a 59-Year-Old Woman

OSCAR S. GERSHANIK

THE CASE

It was 1998 and I was invited to a social event where a friend of mine asked me if I could pay attention to the wife of an acquaintance of his, as he had the impression that something was wrong with her. They had noticed that she was slow and her facial expression had changed significantly. As many of us in the field of movement disorders are used to observing the motor behavior of individuals outside of our offices and elaborate potential diagnosis just on the basis of observation, I agreed to his request. It was evident from the casual, undetected observation of her demeanor that everything about her was slow and that her body movements were poor and had a deliberate character; she rarely blinked and her face was lacking expression. I told my friend that, from what I could see, it was possible that she had some form of "parkinsonism," but I could not go beyond that without a formal and proper consultation and physical examination. A few weeks later, the woman in question came to my office and requested a formal medical opinion.

This 59-year-old woman told me that she had suffered an accidental fall from a stair, approximately 5 years before, without suffering any lesion according to the colleagues that had seen her at the time. From then on, she started noticing a painful weakness in that limb that became worse in the year prior to this consultation. She also perceived an occasional tremor of the right upper extremity (RUE) and a tendency to carry the arm in a flexed posture, with reduction of arm swing. She had in fact seen a neurologist before, who had not volunteered a diagnosis but had put her on levodopa, which she did not tolerate because of nausea, despite the use of domperidone. Pramipexole, up to 3 mg/d, had initially improved her considerably but at the expense of significant diurnal somnolence and nocturnal insomnia. She had been on this drug for a little over a month and felt that the improvement had been short-lived. Her past medical history was unremarkable but for the presence of mild hypertension and elevated blood cholesterol, that she controlled with low doses of enalapril and diet. She did not report experiencing reduced olfaction or REM sleep behavior disorder (RBD). Her mother had had bilateral hand tremor at an advanced age.

THE APPROACH

I proceeded to perform a detailed physical exam that showed only the presence of moderate generalized bradykinesia, hypomimia, and an asymmetric right-sided akinetic-rigid syndrome with typical ipsilateral rest tremor of her upper extremity. Other than that she appeared to be in good health, her mood was normal, and she was alert, oriented, and her discourse was fluent. She brought with her a recent MRI of the brain that was within normal limits, and a comprehensive laboratory work-up that showed no abnormalities. Applying the UK Parkinson's Disease Society Brain Bank Criteria (UK PDSBBC) led me to conclude that the most probable diagnosis in this case was Parkinson's disease (PD), and I decided to add selegiline 5 mg twice a day (1). At a follow-up visit, 3 months later, she appeared much improved; the Unified Parkinson's Disease

Rating Scale (UPDRS) part III (motor examination) had gone from 14 at the first visit to 7, which was something to be expected in a case of typical PD.

In the following 4 years, I saw her regularly at 3 to 4 month intervals, and although she remained fully independent in all of her activities (she was a very active woman, had recently been in charge of furnishing and decorating a new house, had traveled abroad several times, led a very busy social life), she had noticed a progressive worsening of the akinetic-rigid symptomatology, the tremor was more persistent, there were mild signs of involvement of the contralateral side, and she had a certain degree of postural changes with a left lateral trunk deviation. The rest of the neurologic exam did not reveal any atypical signs. I decided then that the time to introduce levodopa had come and I prescribed levodopa/carbidopa up to 400 mg in four divided doses. Once again she improved significantly, she felt her agility was almost normal, she told me her energy had come back, and her voice had recovered a normal tone and volume. She went from a UPDRS part III of 28 to 13 after the introduction of levodopa.

On her subsequent visit, things started to go wrong as she manifested increasing difficulty in finding words, which was most uncomfortable as it precluded her from carrying out a normal conversation, and her independence had been compromised because of this language limitation. Her motor functioning remained unchanged. Upon this unexpected development, I referred her to a speech therapist and a neuropsychologist for evaluation of her language and speech disorder and a full cognitive screening. To my surprise, the report came back with the conclusion that the findings were compatible with the profile usually found in primary progressive nonfluent aphasia (2). In the ensuing months, her language and speech disorder progressively worsened, her executive functions deteriorated, and she developed occasional confusional episodes. A repeat brain MRI was noncontributory. A blood perfusion single-photon emission computed tomography (SPECT) scan showed mild reduction in blood flow at the frontotemporal level.

A year later, almost 9 years into her illness, her motor functioning remained stable and her parkinsonism still had all the typical features of PD, and she had a fluctuating response to levodopa with a classic "wearing-off" phenomenon. However, she showed signs of progessive deterioration of her cognitive function, she was completely aphasic, and her behavior was quite abnormal, with disinhibition, compulsive eating (eating raw beef out of the refrigerator), confusional episodes, and hallucinations. The pattern of the dementia and her behavior were compatible with a diagnosis of a frontotemporal dementia (FTD)-like syndrome (2). I decided to gradually withdraw pramipexole and add a nocturnal dose of quetiapine 25 mg, with a resulting improvement of her behavioral disorder.

From then on, the course of the disorder went downhill. Not only was the patient unable to communicate verbally, with occasional residual palilalia, but she became profoundly demented, despite having improved her behavior with the changes introduced to her drug regime. In the following years, she developed significant gait and stability problems and required help in most of the activities of daily living. The parkinsonian symptomatology was progressively replaced by frontal release signs (paratonia, significant grasp reflexes, and imitation and utilization behaviors). In addition, she developed an asymmetric dystonic posturing of the RUE associated to myoclonic jerking and apraxia of that limb quite reminiscent of corticobasal-ganglionic degeneration (CBGD) (3).

Finally, in recent months, and almost 16 years after the onset of the first symptoms, the patient has developed extensor neck dystonia and supranuclear gaze palsy, which are compatible with a progressive supranuclear palsy (PSP) phenotype (4,5). However, despite the severity of her motor impairment, she has preserved deglutition and is still on a regular diet.

THE LESSON

Every time we see a patient with parkinsonism we are faced with the same dilemma. How can we be sure that the case in question is PD and not one of the atypical parkinsonian syndromes? In recent years, the majority of movement disorder specialists apply the UK PDSBBC, which in the hands of experienced diagnosticians gives a 98% certainty when these criteria are applied stringently (6). Among the supporting criteria, the presence of asymmetric motor signs, rest tremor, and response to levodopa appear to be the ones with the strongest predictive diagnostic value. This was the case in my patient and that is why I felt confident in providing a diagnosis of PD. As time proved me wrong, the most important lesson I learned from this case is that we must always bear in mind that the only diagnostic tool that gives a diagnosis of PD with 100% certainty is the pathologic examination of the brain. Therefore, in every instance, we have to keep a watchful eye and reexamine our patients periodically, not only to evaluate the progression of the disease but also to detect as early as possible any subtle sign or symptom that could steer us away from the original diagnosis.

The second lesson is related to the surprising phenotypic variability that the atypical parkinsonisms as a whole and the tauopathies in particular may have, which once again reinforce the concept that until we develop more reliable diagnostic tools, postmortem examination of the brain remains the only way to arrive at a definitive diagnosis in cases such as the one exemplified here.

Although it is known that tauopathies, and among them PSP, may present with different phenotypes regarded as PSP variants (PSP parkinsonism, pure akinesia, and speech apraxia, PSP with lateralized dystonic CBGD-like symptoms, and the classical Richardson syndrome), in my many years as a movement disorder specialist, this is the first time in which I have seen a case that recapitulates in its progression all the possible phenotypes that can be seen in tauopathies in general and PSP in particular. The course of the disease in this patient is somewhat similar to what Braak has postulated for PD, namely a staged progression dependent on the involvement of higher structures spreading out from a subcortical brainstem region (7). In this particular case, it is attractive to speculate that the pathology (tau accumulation) was initially restricted to the midbrain, later on affecting the left frontal cortex, progressing on to involve the frontal cortex bilaterally in the end, together with late involvement of supranuclear structures controlling vertical gaze (4).

Without pathologic confirmation, it is not possible to arrive at a definitive diagnosis in this case, but we can speculate on the basis of ruling out the possible differential diagnosis. Why am I inclined to believe this is PSP? Why not CBGD or FTD? Perhaps the most important clue is provided by the initial phenotype, namely a levodopa-responsive asymmetric parkinsonism with typical rest tremor, which according to the literature and my own clinical experience is the only tauopathy that may start with that particular clinical pattern. FTD parkinsonism is accepted to be nonresponsive to levodopa and never develops supranuclear gaze palsy. CBGD on the other hand, although it may initially show a very modest response to levodopa, has never been reported to start with a phenotype, which to the eye of an experienced movement disorder specialist can be indistinguishable from PD (3,8). Moreover, clinical diagnosis of CBGD, according to published data, has only a 23.8% positive predictive value, with the majority of cases diagnosed in life as having this disorder turned out to be something else (3).

To conclude, I would like to share with the readers the final lesson. Every case we are called upon to diagnose and manage is a challenge, and we have to accept it and deal with it to the best of our knowledge and clinical acumen and always keep an open mind and be prepared to correct our first impression.

REFERENCES

1. Hughes AJ, Daniel SE, Lees AJ. Improved accuracy of clinical diagnosis of Lewy body Parkinson's disease. *Neurology.* 2001;57(8):1497–1499.
2. Cairns NJ, Bigio EH, Mackenzie IR, et al. Consortium for frontotemporal lobar degeneration. Neuropathologic diagnostic and nosologic criteria for frontotemporal lobar degeneration: consensus of the Consortium for Frontotemporal Lobar Degeneration. *Acta Neuropathol.* 2007;114(1):5–22.
3. Ling H, O'Sullivan SS, Holton JL, et al. Does corticobasal degeneration exist? A clinicopathological re-evaluation. *Brain.* 2010;133(Pt 7):2045–2057.

4. Dickson DW, Ahmed Z, Algom AA, et al. Neuropathology of variants of progressive supranuclear palsy. *Curr Opin Neurol.* 2010;23(4):394–400.

5. Ludolph AC, Kassubek J, Landwehrmeyer BG, et al. Reisensburg Working Group for Tauopathies with Parkinsonism. Tauopathies with parkinsonism: clinical spectrum, neuropathologic basis, biological markers, and treatment options. *Eur J Neurol.* 2009;16(3):297–309.

6. Hughes AJ, Daniel SE, Ben-Shlomo Y, Lees AJ. The accuracy of diagnosis of parkinsonian syndromes in a specialist movement disorder service. *Brain.* 2002;125(Pt 4):861–870.

7. Braak H, Del Tredici K, Bratzke H, et al. Staging of the intracerebral inclusion body pathology associated with idiopathic Parkinson's disease (preclinical and clinical stages). *J Neurol.* 2002;249(suppl 3):III/1–5.

8. Constantinescu R, Richard I, Kurlan R. Levodopa responsiveness in disorders with parkinsonism: a review of the literature. *Mov Disord.* 2007;22(15):2141–2148; quiz 2295.

23

Atypical Parkinsonism With a Twist: My Memorable
Case of an Indian Woman With Levodopa-Responsive
Parkinsonism and Motor Fluctuations

KATHLEEN M. SHANNON

THE CASE

A woman from the Indian subcontinent presented at age 39 in 1986 with involuntary cramping and curling of the left foot and toes and gait difficulty. Four years prior to presentation, she noticed micrographia. Three years prior to presentation, she began to have problems with gait and balance, with spontaneous retropulsion. Two years prior to presentation, she noted soft voice, left hand tremor at rest, generalized slowing, and intermittent cramping and curling of her left foot and toes with spontaneous extension of the great toe. Curling and cramping spread to her right foot 6 months prior to presentation. She had been started on carbidopa/levodopa 10/100 three times daily with significant benefit, but had developed some end-of-dose wearing off. She complained of orthostatic dizziness without syncope. She complained of poor vision and frequent headaches. In addition to the carbidopa/levodopa, she took trihexyphenidyl 2 mg three times daily and alprazolam 0.25 mg three times daily. Family history was negative for parkinsonism, but several cousins had migraine or poor vision. Examination at that time showed reduced visual acuity (20/200 bilaterally), normal cognition, and asymmetric parkinsonism with rest tremor, rigidity, and bradykinesia. She had mildly reduced vibratory sensation in the legs. She had mild dysdiadochokinesia in the left leg and mild gait ataxia. The diagnosis of olivopontocerebellar atrophy was made at that time. Four years later, postural stability had worsened, she exhibited emotional lability, and bilateral past-pointing was noted on her cerebellar exam. Six years after her initial presentation, an ophthalmologist diagnosed retinitis pigmentosa. Eight years after her initial presentation, she complained of motor fluctuations with end-of-dose wearing off and peak-dose dyskinesias. She had developed rare visual hallucinations. Examination at that time showed moderate generalized dyskinesias, mild-to-moderate parkinsonism, very poor visual acuity, and ataxic gait with marked postural instability. Over subsequent years, she had progressive parkinsonism with motor fluctuations, gait ataxia, decreased visual acuity, and depression. She used many antiparkinsonian and other medications including carbidopa/levodopa, pergolide, bromocriptine, pramipexole, trihexyphenidyl, amantadine, and a number of psychotropic medications including fluoxetine, buspirone, and alprazolam. She saw a number of different providers over this time period. Fourteen years after onset, mild cognitive impairment was noted (MMSE 25/30). In 2005, 23 years after symptom onset, her son accompanied her to clinic for the first time and reported that the patient's brother also suffered with gait disorder and poor vision and their father was said to have neuropathy. Both affected relatives resided in India. At this time, she was wheelchair dependent with disabling ataxia and moderately severe parkinsonism with motor fluctuations and dyskinesias.

THE APPROACH

My patient presented with an atypical parkinsonism with visual deterioration and progressive ataxia but without prominent autonomic insufficiency. She saw many practitioners and carried the diagnosis of OPCA/MSA for many years. On a routine visit, her son gave the family history of progressive ataxia in a brother and neuropathy in her father. We then obtained diagnostic testing for spinocerebellar ataxia types 1, 2, 3, 6, and 7. Testing revealed an abnormality in the *SCA3/MJD* gene with 65 CAG repeats (normal < 43).

THE LESSON

Parkinson's disease (PD) and parkinsonism are diagnosed clinically. A number of diagnostic schemes have been published, and in expert hands, the accuracy of diagnosis of PD is about 90% (1). The differential diagnosis of PD includes other hereditary and sporadic neurodegenerative diseases and acquired structural and metabolic lesions (2,3). Mutations in a number of genes have convincingly been demonstrated to cause dominantly inherited PD including *alpha-synuclein, UCH-L1,* and *LRRK2* (4–9), and there are a number of other genetic associations. Several of the hereditary spinocerebellar ataxias may have a parkinsonian phenotype, including SCA2, SCA3, SCA6, SCA8, and SCA17 (10–12). In many cases, the parkinsonism is levodopa responsive, which makes differentiation from classical parkinsonism difficult.

In the present case, levodopa-responsive parkinsonism with motor fluctuations was accompanied by atypical features including early falls, retinopathy, and ataxia. Because the family history was positive only for vision loss and neuropathy, the hereditary aspect of the parkinsonism was not appreciated, and the patient carried the clinical diagnosis of olivopontocerebellar degeneration or the cerebellar subtype of multiple system atrophy for many years. Once the family history of gait disorder was unveiled, appropriate testing was performed, confirming the diagnosis of spinocerebellar ataxia type 3 (SCA3).

SCA3, also known as Machado-Joseph disease, is a dominantly inherited progressive neurodegenerative disease with protean manifestations. Three clinical subtypes are described as follows: [1] early onset with marked spasticity and dystonia, [2] pure or predominant cerebellar ataxia, and [3] late onset with peripheral neuropathy (13). Parkinsonism is a rare manifestation of SCA3 and can be levodopa responsive with motor fluctuations. Ataxia and pyramidal signs may develop later in the disease course (14). Other signs of SCA3 include abnormal oculomotor function, nystagmus, amyotrophy, spasticity, depression, cognitive impairment, sleep disorders, and autonomic dysfunction (15–21). MRI studies in SCA3 demonstrate atrophy of superior cerebellar peduncles, frontal and temporal lobes, globus pallidus, and pons (22). Survival after onset averages about 20 years (23).

REFERENCES

1. Hughes AJ, Daniel SE, Lees AJ. Improved accuracy of clinical diagnosis of Lewy body Parkinson's disease. *Neurology.* 2001;57:1497–1499.
2. Ahlskog JE. Diagnosis and differential diagnosis of Parkinson's disease and parkinsonism. *Parkinsonism Relat Disord.* 2000;7:63–70.
3. Weiner WJ. A differential diagnosis of parkinsonism. *Rev Neurol Dis.* 2005;2:124–131.
4. Clarimon J, Pagonabarraga J, Paisán-Ruiz C, et al. Tremor dominant parkinsonism: clinical description and LRRK2 mutation screening. *Mov Disord.* 2008;23:518–523.
5. Haugarvoll K, Uitti RJ, Farrer MJ, et al. LRRK2 gene and tremor-dominant parkinsonism. *Arch Neurol.* 2006;63:1346–1347.
6. Klein C, Pramstaller PP, Kis B, et al. Parkin deletions in a family with adult-onset, tremor-dominant parkinsonism: expanding the phenotype. *Ann Neurol.* 2000;48:65–71.

7. Taymans JM, Cookson MR. Mechanisms in dominant parkinsonism: the toxic triangle of LRRK2, alpha-synuclein, and tau. *Bioessays.* 2010;32:227–235.
8. Wszolek ZK, Pfeiffer RF, Tsuboi Y, et al. Autosomal dominant parkinsonism associated with variable synuclein and tau pathology. *Neurology.* 2004;62:1619–1622.
9. Zimprich A, Muller-Myhsok B, Farrer M, et al. The PARK8 locus in autosomal dominant parkinsonism: confirmation of linkage and further delineation of the disease-containing interval. *Am J Hum Genet.* 2004;74:11–19.
10. Furtado S, Payami H, Lockhart PJ, et al. Profile of families with parkinsonism-predominant spinocerebellar ataxia type 2 (SCA2). *Mov Disord.* 2004;19:622–629.
11. Khan NL, Giunti P, Sweeney MG, et al. Parkinsonism and nigrostriatal dysfunction are associated with spinocerebellar ataxia type 6 (SCA6). *Mov Disord.* 2005;20:1115–1119.
12. Tuite PJ, Rogaeva EA, St George-Hyslop PH, Lang AE. Dopa-responsive parkinsonism phenotype of Machado-Joseph disease: confirmation of 14q CAG expansion. *Ann Neurol.* 1995;38:684–687.
13. Franca MC, Jr., D'Abreu A, Nucci A, Lopes-Cendes I. Muscle excitability abnormalities in Machado-Joseph disease. *Arch Neurol.* 2008;65:525–529.
14. Buhmann C, Bussopulos A, Oechsner M. Dopaminergic response in parkinsonian phenotype of Machado-Joseph disease. *Mov Disord.* 2003;18:219–221.
15. Burk K, Abele M, Fetter M, et al. Autosomal dominant cerebellar ataxia type I clinical features and MRI in families with SCA1, SCA2 and SCA3. *Brain.* 1996;119 (Pt 5):1497–1505.
16. van de Warrenburg BP, Notermans NC, Schelhaas HJ, et al. Peripheral nerve involvement in spinocerebellar ataxias. *Arch Neurol.* 2004;61:257–261.
17. Kawai Y, Takeda A, Abe Y, et al. Cognitive impairments in Machado-Joseph disease. *Arch Neurol.* 2004;61:1757–1760.
18. Cecchin CR, Pires AP, Rieder CR, et al. Depressive symptoms in Machado-Joseph disease (SCA3) patients and their relatives. *Community Genet.* 2007;10:19–26.
19. D'Abreu A, Franca M, Jr., Conz L, et al. Sleep symptoms and their clinical correlates in Machado-Joseph disease. *Acta Neurol Scand.* 2009;119:277–280.
20. Friedman JH, Fernandez HH, Sudarsky LR. REM behavior disorder and excessive daytime somnolence in Machado-Joseph disease (SCA-3). *Mov Disord.* 2003;18:1520–1522.
21. Franca MC, Jr., D'Abreu A, Nucci A, et al. Clinical correlates of autonomic dysfunction in patients with Machado-Joseph disease. *Acta Neurol Scand.* 2010;121:422–425.
22. Murata Y, Yamaguchi S, Kawakami H, et al. Characteristic magnetic resonance imaging findings in Machado-Joseph disease. *Arch Neurol.* 1998;55:33–37.
23. Kieling C, Prestes PR, Saraiva-Pereira ML, Jardim LB. Survival estimates for patients with Machado-Joseph disease (SCA3). *Clin Genet.* 2007;72:543–545.

24

A Patient With Rapidly Progressive Dementia and Supranuclear Gaze Palsy: A Memorable Lesson on Prion Disorders

IGOR N. PETROVIC, LAURA SILVEIRA-MORIYAMA, AND ANDREW J. LEES

THE CASE

This patient was a 71-year-old woman who presented with generalized slowness and apathy over the course of 2 months. In that period of time, her family noticed that she often kept her eyes closed and was more taciturn and slower to respond to their questions. Rapidly, in the next few weeks, she developed falls, predominantly backward without loss of consciousness, and prominent forgetfulness. In the next 2 months, the imbalance and gait difficulties further progressed. She had recurrent falls backward and had sustained a fracture of the right thumb. Within 4 months of the onset, she was confined to a wheelchair. She had no hallucinations and no bladder or bowel symptoms.

The general examination was unremarkable. On neurological examination, she had an impassive face, severe apraxia of eyelid opening, slow vertical saccades with a prominent limitation of both upgaze and downgaze, a brisk jaw jerk, and a dysarthria. She had severe axial rigidity with a spinal curvature to the right, mild limb bradykinesia and rigidity, and an intermittent jerky postural tremor of the outstretched hands. She was very unsteady and unable to walk without support and had a reduced steppage gait with absent arm swing. Reflexes were brisk but her plantar responses were downgoing. On that time, a 3 weeks trial of L-dopa (400 mg/d) was negative. Unconvincing improvement was detected while on amantadine; however, she developed visual hallucinations. Quetiapine 25 mg/d was introduced with partial resolution of hallucinations. On follow-up examination, 1 year after symptom onset, she had severe limitation of vertical eye movements, apraxia of eyelid opening, and a symmetrical akinetic syndrome with marked axial rigidity. She was also anarthric. Shortly after this examination, she was admitted to a nursing home and died of pneumonia 18 months after disease onset. Myoclonus, cerebellar signs, or profound dysautonomia were never observed.

THE APPROACH

This patient in her seventies presented with gait difficulties, cognitive problems, falls backward, akinetic-rigid type of parkinsonism, and vertical supranuclear gaze palsy (VSGP), meeting the clinical diagnostic criteria for progressive supranuclear palsy (PSP, Richardson's syndrome) (1). Absence of improvement on L-dopa, as well as modest improvement on amantadine, is in accordance with this diagnosis. The aggressive deterioration raised suspicions of alternative diagnoses such as midbrain tumors; however, the MRI scan of the brain showed some modest involutional changes involving the cortex and cerebellum but was otherwise normal.

Although VSGP associated with parkinsonism and dementia is traditionally considered as the major clinical hallmark of Richardson's syndrome, this constellation of signs can be seen in a heterogeneous collection of uncommon disorders including Whipple's disease, Niemann-Pick disease type C, frontotemporal dementia associated with chromosome 17, ubiquitin-positive frontotemporal lobar degeneration, Kufor-Rakeb disease, and neurodegeneration with brain iron accumulation type 2 associated with *PLA2G6* mutation (2,3). However, none of these diagnoses that are possible to establish during the patient's life were confirmed in this case.

The final diagnosis was revealed after neuropathological examination of the brain. There was mild frontal cortical atrophy, slightly blurred appearance of globus pallidus, and mild pallor in the later half of substantia nigra. Microscopic examination demonstrated widespread, severe confluent spongiform change with patchy nerve cell loss and astrogliosis affecting all regions of the cerebral cortex and the cerebellar cortex, basal ganglia, and thalamus. The brain stem was relatively spared. Immunohistochemistry for prion protein (PRNP) showed accumulation of disease-associated PRNP that was predominantly perivacuolar with coarse deposits in the cerebral cortex. PRNP gene analysis showed that this patient was a methionine homozygote at codon 129, and protease-resistant PRNP was demonstrated on Western blotting with a type 2A isoform, confirming the MM2 subtype of sporadic Creutzfeldt-Jakob disease (sCJD). Tau, amyloid-beta, and alpha-synuclein immunohistochemical preparations did not reveal any additional pathology.

THE LESSON

Typically sCJD presents as a rapidly progressive dementia that may be accompanied by ataxia and myoclonus leading to death, usually within 12 months of disease onset (4). Searching the literature, we identified 10 cases of sCJD with PSP-like presentation similar to our case (5). Notably, the classical clinical, radiological, and laboratory findings of myoclonus, cerebellar signs, increased T2-weighted signal in the basal ganglia on MRI, periodic sharp-wave complexes on EEG, and elevated 14.3.3 protein in cerebrospinal fluid are absent in most of these cases.

In brief, those patients presented with gait impairment and/or falls, followed with VSGP and asymmetric akinetic syndrome with axial rigidity. In our case as well as in the vast majority of the cases in the literature, early and rapidly progressive cognitive decline was a distinctive feature.

PSP is a classical example of "subcortical dementia," and cognitive impairment happens in up to half of patients, but recent studies showed that in the first 2 years of the disease, cognitive impairment is present in less than a third of PSP patients, suggesting that moderate to severe dementia occurring early in the disease course should raise suspicion about an alternative diagnosis (6,7).

Ross-Russell, in 1980, described three CJD patients with apraxia of eyelid closure as well as VSGP, who, in common with our case, had extensive bilateral frontal lobe pathology and no brain stem involvement (8).

It is of interest that in our case and also in the three remaining cases in the literature, a diagnosis of the MM2 sCJD subtype was made. This finding supports the idea that different biological properties of the PrP^sc may lead to pleomorphic clinical presentations such as the Heidenhain variant of sCJD or sporadic fatal insomnia (9).

The case presented here and the literature review emphasize that sCJD can rarely mimic Richardson's syndrome with rapid progression. In patients with PSP-like presentations with aggressive course and early dementia, prion disease should always be considered, even in the absence of the other classical features of sCJD.

REFERENCES

1. Litvan I, Agid Y, Calne D, et al. Clinical research criteria for the diagnosis of progressive supranuclear palsy (Steele-Richardson-Olszewski syndrome): report of the NINDS-SPSP international workshop. *Neurology*. 1996;47:1–9.
2. Williams DR, Lees AJ. Progressive supranuclear palsy: clinicopathological concepts and diagnostic challenges. *Lancet Neurol*. 2009;8:270–279.

3. Schneider SA, Bhatia KP, Hardy J. Complicated recessive dystonia parkinsonism syndromes. *Mov Disord.* 2009;24:490–499.
4. Brown P, Gibbs CJ, Jr., Rodgers-Johnson P, et al. Human spongiform encephalopathy: the National Institutes of Health series of 300 cases of experimentally transmitted disease. *Ann Neurol.* 1994;35:513–529.
5. Petrovic IN, Martin-Bastida A, Massey L, et al. The MM2 subtype of sporadic Creutzfeldt-Jakob disease may present as progressive supranuclear palsy. Submitted.
6. Williams DR, de SR, Paviour DC, et al. Characteristics of two distinct clinical phenotypes in pathologically proven progressive supranuclear palsy: Richardson's syndrome and PSP-parkinsonism. *Brain.* 2005;128:1247–1258.
7. Josephs KA, Dickson DW. Diagnostic accuracy of progressive supranuclear palsy in the Society for Progressive Supranuclear Palsy brain bank. *Mov Disord.* 2003;18:1018–1026.
8. Russell RW. Supranuclear palsy of eyelid closure. *Brain.* 1980;103:71–82.
9. Ironside JW, Ghetti B, Head MW, et al. Prion diseases. In: Ellison DW, Louis DN, Love S, eds. *Greenfield's Neuropathology.* 8th ed. London: Hodder Arnold, 2008: 1197–1274.

25

A Lesson on Following One's Instincts: A Case of a Paraneoplastic Disorder Posing as PSP

CHRIS ADAMS AND RAJEEV KUMAR

THE CASE

We recently became more familiar with paraneoplastic disorders (PNDs) that may present as movement disorders when we saw an unusual case that resembled progressive supranuclear palsy (PSP). A 55-year-old man with a 22-pack-year history of smoking developed multiple diverse symptoms over 6 months. Initially, he noted an increased appetite and gained 22 lbs over 1 month. Next, he noticed trouble moving his eyes upward to see traffic signs when driving. As the problem worsened, his eyes would get stuck in the upgaze position, so he could not see the road. Eventually, he experienced frequent double vision. Soon thereafter, he developed sleepiness during the day, fragmented sleep at night, and symptoms of cataplexy when embarrassed or nervous. Later, he developed 30-second spells of freezing of gait (FOG) characterized by tremor and upward gaze deviation in full consciousness. These occurred up to 20 times per day. As his symptoms progressed, he became slower and clumsier, and his handwriting became illegible. On examination, the patient exhibited mild bilateral ptosis and unusual vertical supranuclear gaze palsy (SNGP) in which his eyes would become stuck when deviated upward, so that he was unable to voluntarily bring them down. Providing an object to track downward allowed him to overcome this position by using smooth pursuit mechanisms. He also had mild dysarthria, a slow lumbering gait, and mild right-hand postural and action tremor. Review of an earlier MRI scan of the patient's head was normal except for a dural-based enhancing lesion, which was suspected to be an en plaque meningioma.

THE APPROACH

We were intrigued by the subacutely progressive multifaceted presentation that did not fit neatly into any one neurological syndrome. It closely resembled several possible disorders. His slowness, clumsiness, and SNGP were suggestive of PSP. However, the tendency for his eyes to become stuck in the upgaze position, the rapid progression, and his other symptoms were inconsistent with this diagnosis. The acute nature of his symptoms and the peculiar nature of his eye movements closely resembled a PSP-like syndrome resulting from aortic arch surgeries accompanied by hypothermic cardiac arrest. The "spells" in which his eyes became stuck in the upgaze position along with tremor and FOG resembled oculogyric crises in postencephalitic parkinsonism (PEP). His appetite disturbances, sleep problems, and hormonal disturbances were suggestive of hypothalamic dysfunction, but he had an essentially unremarkable MRI scan of the head except for a possible benign meningioma.

The most common cause of progressive vertical SNGP and parkinsonism is PSP. However, the differential diagnosis includes Niemann-Pick disease type C (NPC) (1), corticobasal degeneration (CBD) (2), Whipple's disease (3), Gaucher's type I parkinsonism (4), PLA2G6 dystonia-parkinsonism (5), Kufor-Rakeb syndrome (KRD) (6), PEP (7), dementia with Lewy bodies (DLB) (8), frontotemporal dementia and parkinsonism (FTDP) (9), prion disease, progressive subcortical gliosis, primary pallidal degeneration, and dorsal midbrain syndrome. Similar to our patient's symptoms, NPC is characterized by cataplexy, dysarthria, and ptosis. In adult-onset disease, progression is slow, and patients survive into their seventies. Patients with NPC also develop cerebellar ataxia, dysphagia, hallucinations, hearing loss, epilepsy, depression, dementia, and dystonia, which our patient did not have. CBD is slowly progressive and traditionally presents with asymmetric dystonia, stimulus-sensitive myoclonus, and alien limb phenomenon, among other findings. Whipple's disease commonly presents with several symptoms not seen in our patient including abdominal pain, diarrhea, fever, discolored skin, joint pain, cognitive abnormalities, oculomasticatory myorhythmia, and weight loss. In Gaucher's type I, parkinsonism is accompanied by moderate hepatic dysfunction with hepatomegaly, low platelet count, osteopenia, osteolysis, episodic pain, diffuse yellowish skin on the face and legs, myoclonus, dementia, and arthritis, which were not seen in our patient. Mutations in *PLA2G6* and *ATP13K2* (KRD) cause young-onset autosomal recessive dystonia-parkinsonism that may also have MRI features of neurodegeneration with brain iron accumulation. Patients with *PLA2G6* mutations commonly have striking psychiatric features and cognitive decline. Patients with KRD may have oculogyric spasms similar to our patient but also commonly exhibit hyperflexia, Babinski signs, visual hallucinations, and facial-faucio-finger mini-myoclonus. PEP occurs acutely with viral infection, but delayed onset of SNGP has recently been reported to occur several years later (7). PEP may also classically cause oculogyric crises as seen in our patient. Vertical SNGP interestingly has also recently been reported in pathologically proven DLB and causes progressive cognitive decline with fluctuations in alertness and attention and hallucinations (8). FTDP may present with a PSP-like phenotype in some kindred, which is inherited in an autosomal-dominant fashion and is caused by a tau mutation. However, most patients with FTDP manifest other phenotypes usually dominated by dementia and personality change sometimes accompanied by parkinsonism, motor neuron disease, myoclonus, or epilepsy (9).

Because our patient's symptoms progressed subacutely, localized to multiple brain regions, and he lacked lesions on his MRI scan, we hypothesized that he had a PND. As a result, we checked the patient's serum and cerebrospinal fluid for multiple paraneoplastic antibodies, antineuronal nuclear autoantibody types 1, 2, and 3, antiglial/neuronal nuclear antibody type 1, Purkinje cell cytoplasmic autoantibody types 1 and 2, amphiphysin, and collapsin response-mediator protein 5 IgG. In the patient's serum, we checked for acetylcholine receptor (neuronal and muscle), N-type calcium channel, P/Q-type calcium channel, and voltage-gated potassium channel antibodies. All of these were negative; however, CSF protein and IgG index were both elevated (127 mg/dL and 15 g/d, respectively), making us concerned that he still had a PND that was antibody negative. Therefore, a fluorodeoxyglucose (18F) (FDG) positron emission tomography (PET) or computer tomography (CT) was performed, which demonstrated increased uptake in the left tonsil and a left cervical lymph node. The cervical lymph node was biopsied and was unremarkable. Therefore, we reassessed the dural-based enhancing lesion with our neuroradiologist who felt that there was a reasonable chance that the lesion represented a metastasis or other lesion rather than a meningioma. Therefore, the lesion was resected and in fact turned out to be a grade 1 meningioma. Given the multiple negative investigations, but still high suspicion for a PND, we tested serum for Ma1 and Ma2 antibodies. He was positive for both, which confirmed our clinical suspicion of a PND and encouraged us to have the left tonsil, which had high FDG uptake, resected. This revealed a poorly differentiated stage IIB squamous cell carcinoma with spread to a single lymph node. Ma-positive PNDs are characterized by cataplexy, excessive daytime sleepiness (EDS), dysarthria, and ptosis in addition to parkinsonism and vertical SNGP, which were all seen in our patient.

The standard therapy for most PNDs is first aggressive treatment of the underlying cancer. Despite radiation therapy, our patient's symptoms worsened. By 8 months after his initial presentation, he slept for much of the day, had narcolepsy, and had severe REM behavior disorder (RBD). In addition, his SNGP worsened, he became more parkinsonian, and his short-term memory was significantly worsened. There is emerging evidence of the role of immunosuppression in the treatment of PNDs, which continue to worsen despite appropriate treatment of the underlying cancer. As a result, we administered high-dose IV steroids and cyclophosphamide for

3 months, which stabilized but did not improve our patient's symptoms. We tried administering melatonin for his RBD and carbidopa-levodopa for his parkinsonism, but these were not tolerated. However, modafinil improved some symptoms of narcolepsy.

THE LESSON

We learned or reinforced three lessons during our care of this patient. Our belief in the importance of clinical neurology skills emphasizing careful examination and localization skills was reinforced. Despite many initially negative investigations, our initial clinical suspicion of a PND was found to be correct. Even though we were initially not aware that a PND could present in a fashion that resembled PSP, the subacute progression of multifocal neurologic findings led us to be highly suspicious of a PND since, in principle, PND commonly presents in this fashion.

Second, FDG PET-CT is the investigation of choice in guiding the search for underlying malignancy when the suspicion for a PND is high. Seventy percent of those with PNDs have an underlying cancer (10). A PND can develop at the very earliest stages of cancer, before symptoms referable to the cancer occur, and at this stage, the cancer may be more easily treated.

Third, PNDs present as multifocal disorders. Ma-positive PNDs usually present with EDS, impaired short-term memory, vertical SNPG, diplopia, dysarthria, unsteady gait, and parkinsonism (11). Further, Ma-positive PNDs may lack an underlying cancer and an MRI of the brain may be normal (11). In retrospect, the symptoms of our patient closely matched the symptoms of other cases with Ma-positive PNDs (12–19). However, our patient had several unusual features not previously documented in this combination, including the following: Ma1 and Ma2 antibodies, hyperphagia, both RBD and narcolepsy with cataplexy, and underlying tonsillar cancer (19). Our knowledge about rarer causes of vertical SNGP and parkinsonism has been expanded.

REFERENCES

1. Sévin M, Lesca G, Baumann N, et al. The adult form of Niemann-Pick disease type C. *Brain.* 2007;130 (Pt 1):120–133.
2. Rinne JO, Lee MS, Thompson PD, Marsden CD. Corticobasal degeneration. A clinical study of 36 cases. *Brain.* 1994;117(Pt 5):1183–1196.
3. Averbuch-Heller L, Paulson GW, Daroff RB, Leigh RJ. Whipple's disease mimicking progressive supranuclear palsy: the diagnostic value of eye movement recording. *J Neurol Neurosurg Psychiatry.* 1999;66(4):532–535.
4. Alonso-Canovas A, Katschnig P, Tucci A, et al. Atypical parkinsonism with apraxia and supranuclear gaze abnormalities in type 1 Gaucher disease. Expanding the spectrum: case report and literature review. *Mov Disord.* 2010;25(10):1506–1509.
5. Paisán-Ruiz C, Bhatia KP, Li A, et al. Characterization of PLA2G6 as a locus for dystonia-parkinsonism. *Ann Neurol.* 2009;65(1):19–23.
6. Williams DR, Hadeed A, Al-Din AS, et al. Kufor Rakeb disease: autosomal recessive, levodopa-responsive parkinsonism with pyramidal degeneration, supranuclear gaze palsy, and dementia. *Mov Disord.* 2005;20(10):1264–1271.
7. Wenning GK, Jellinger K, Litvan I. Supranuclear gaze palsy and eyelid apraxia in postencephalitic parkinsonism. *J Neural Transm.* 1997;104(8–9):845–865.
8. Louis ED, Klatka LA, Liu Y, Fahn S. Comparison of extrapyramidal features in 31 pathologically confirmed cases of diffuse Lewy body disease and 34 pathologically confirmed cases of Parkinson's disease. *Neurology.* 1997;48(2):376–380.
9. Wszolek ZK, Tsuboi Y, Ghetti B, et al. Frontotemporal dementia and parkinsonism linked to chromosome 17 (FTDP-17). *Orphanet J Rare Dis.* 2006;1:30.
10. McKeon A, Apiwattanakul M, Lachance DH, et al. Positron emission tomography-computed tomography in paraneoplastic neurologic disorders: systematic analysis and review. *Arch Neurol.* 2010;67(3):322–329.
11. Dalmau J, Graus F, Villarejo A, et al. Clinical analysis of anti-Ma2-associated encephalitis. *Brain.* 2004;127(pt 8):1831–1844.

12. Compta Y, Iranzo A, Santamaria J, et al. REM sleep behavior disorder and narcoleptic features in anti-Ma2-associated encephalitis. *Sleep.* 2007;30(6):767–769.

13. Jankovic J. Progressive supranuclear palsy: paraneoplastic effect of bronchial carcinoma. *Neurology.* 1985;35(3):446–447.

14. Matsumoto L, Yamamoto T, Higashihara M, et al. Severe hypokinesis caused by paraneoplastic anti-Ma2 encephalitis associated with bilateral intratubular germ-cell neoplasm of the testes. *Mov Disord.* 2007;22(5):728–731.

15. Castle J, Sakonju A, Dalmau J, Newman-Toker DE. Anti-Ma2-assicated encephalitis with normal FDG-PET: a case of pseudo-Whipple's disease. *Nat Clin Pract Neurol.* 2006;2(10):566–572.

16. Blumenthal DT, Salzman KL, Digr KB, et al. Early pathologic findings and long-term improvement in anti-Ma2 associated encephalitis. *Neurology.* 2006;67(1):146–149.

17. Landolfi JC, Nadkarni M. Paraneoplastic limbic encephalitis and possible narcolepsy in a patient with testicular cancer: case study. *Neuro Oncol.* 2003;5(3):214–216.

18. Tan JH, Goh BC, Tambyah PA, Wilder-Smith E. Paraneoplastic progressive supranuclear palsy syndrome in a patient with B-cell lymphoma. *Parkinsonism Relat Disord.* 2005;11(3):187–191.

19. Adams C, McKeon A, Silber MH, Kumar R. Narcolepsy, REM sleep behavior disorder, and supranuclear gaze palsy associated with Ma1 and Ma2 antibodies and tonsillar carcinoma. *Arch Neurol.* 2011;68(4):521–524.

26

A Sudden, Static, Supranuclear Syndrome After Surgical Repair of an Aortic Aneurysm in a Young Man From Thailand

Roongroj Bhidayasiri and Duang Kawahara

THE CASE

A 19-year-old man from Thailand, who previously had been healthy, underwent an aneurysmectomy and aortic valve repair for an aneurysm of the ascending aorta. The surgery seemed to have been uncomplicated and without episodes of hypotension or unexpected compromised hemodynamic function. However, the patient had one brief episode of a grand mal seizure, which was spontaneously resolved. As soon as he regained consciousness following surgery, he was found to be dysarthric and slow. Our initial examination revealed symmetrical bradykinesia and rigidity of both upper limbs associated with mild postural tremor. Axial rigidity was prominent, particularly in the neck, resulting in mild retrocollis. Moreover, an ocular examination showed supranuclear vertical gaze palsy affecting both upgaze and downgaze. Both vertical and horizontal saccades were slow. A mild "no-no" head tremor was observed, as well as action myoclonus of his left arm when it was outstretched. An additional examination revealed mild left-sided weakness and exaggerated muscle stretch reflexes. A CT scan of the brain was unremarkable (Figure 26.1) as was a spinal fluid examination. His neurological syndrome continued to progress following the initial presentation. At the 2-month follow-up examination, there was a persistent limitation of vertical gaze, bradykinesia, shuffling gait, and postural instability. Despite pronounced dysarthria, there were no sensory abnormalities, language, or cognitive deficits. Additional investigations, including a CT angiogram of aorta, carotid, and intracranial arteries, autoantibodies and the erythrocyte sedimentation rate were all within normal limits. There was no hepatosplenomegaly. The neurological syndrome stabilized 5 months after the initial presentation and has not changed significantly during the last 2 years although he has been left with considerable neurological deficits. There is no family history of Parkinson's disease or related neurodegenerative disorders.

THE APPROACH

The constellation of findings—supranuclear ophthalmoplegia, dysarthria, dystonic rigidity of the neck and upper trunk, parkinsonism, dementia, and postural instability—defines the well-known clinical description of progressive supranuclear palsy (PSP) (1). Despite substantive evidence indicating that this syndrome is most likely heterogeneous, consisting of several distinct clinical syndromes, this disorder usually occurs in the setting of chronic progressive degeneration due to the accumulation of phosphorylated tau in different brain regions. As a result, the list of clinical variants has been expanded to encompass a number of disorders that can be separated by differences in their severity, regions of pathology, and clinical features. These are linked by the accumulation of neurofibrillary tangles and a similar natural history that usually leads to death within 6 to 12 years of diagnosis (2). Moreover, cases of PSP-like syndromes have been increasingly reported in the medical literature resulting from multi-infarct disorder, drug

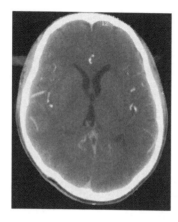

FIGURE 26.1
*Contrasted CT scan of the brain demonstrated
unremarkable findings performed 1 month after the
surgery.*

TABLE 26.1
Clinical Variants of PSP and PSP-Like Syndromes.

(1) A clinical syndrome of PSP

    (1.1) A classic PSP syndrome or Richardson's syndrome or Steele-Richardson-Olzewski's syndrome

    (1.2) PSP-parkinsonism (PSP-P)

    (1.3) PSP-pure akinesia with gait freezing (PSP-PAGF)

    (1.4) PSP-corticobasal syndrome (PSP-CBS)

    (1.5) PSP-progressive nonfluent aphasia (PSP-PNFA)

(2) PSP-like syndromes

    (2.1) Vascular PSP

    (2.2) Guadaloupean parkinsonism (5)

    (2.3) Kufor-Rakeb disease (PARK9) (16)

    (2.4) PSP-like syndrome with a novel prion protein mutation (17)

    (2.5) Intoxication

        —Occupational exposure to lead (18)

        —Amiodarone and flunarizine (19)

    (2.6) Fahr's disease [6]

    (2.7) Niemann-Pick disease type C [3]

    (2.8) Hypoxic-ischemic process [20]

    (2.9) After surgical repair of ascending aorta [13]

intoxication, Fahr's disease, and neurodegeneration (Table 26.1; 3–6). Despite increased recognition, the *acute* presentation of PSP-like syndrome in patients under 30 years of age is considered to be highly unusual. Even more perplexing was the further deterioration of his parkinsonism during the 5 months following the surgery.

    Traditional neurology emphasizes the basic neuroanatomical localization based on a detailed history and clinical signs. The combination of supranuclear vertical ophthalmoplegia, slow saccades, nuchal rigidity, and dysarthria localizes the affected region involving the pontomesencephalic tegmentum, tectum, periaqueductal gray matter, basal ganglia, and possibly superior colliculi (7,8). Based on the patient's left hemiparesis with exaggerated reflexes, he may have additional lesions in the internal capsule, corona radiata, or elsewhere along a pyramidal tract. The brief episode of the seizure also suggests transient cortical involvement. The next step would be to consider the pathophysiological process that could explain the acute presentation of these findings. Obviously, neurodegeneration, infections, and inflammation are highly unlikely to result in sudden neurological deficits. On the contrary, acute neurological presentations always favor a vascular etiology. Indeed, Winikates and Jankovic (9) describe the term vascular PSP in patients who have asymmetric and lower body parkinsonism, but all cases presented in a step-wise progressive fashion, unlike the sudden onset in our patient. Subsequent clinicopathologic studies have defined vascular PSP to be a multi-infarct disorder with demonstrated infarcts in the cerebral cortex, thalamus, basal ganglia, and cerebellum [4].

When we reviewed the literature on vascular PSP, we thought that we were close to reaching a final diagnosis on the patient. However, we were unable to explain two key findings. First, the patient had an unremarkable CT scan of the brain, which was in contrast to documented cases of vascular PSP who all had demonstrated infarcts on neuroimaging. Second, the acute presentation of the patient did not support a multi-infarct disorder as in vascular PSP. If the cause of PSP-like syndrome in our patient is due to multiple infarcts, the lesions that we presumed to be widespread involving the regions noted above should be visualized on CT images. The metallic clips of the aorta as well as the prosthetic heart valve prohibited further examination of the brain with MRI.

The seizure episode prompted us to hypothesize that the patient may have suffered a transient hypoxic event during surgery. Indeed, vulnerable brain regions following a diffuse cerebral hypoxic event can be quite selective involving bilateral basal ganglia, thalami, and/or substantia nigra that may not be evident on CT scans (10). This possibility could potentially explain the sudden onset of PSP-like features of the patient as well as a lack of demonstrated infarcts on the CT scan. In fact, a mild operative hypoxemia that is almost routine and is typically inconsequential in aortic surgeries cannot be excluded as one of several factors that could have triggered a thus-far-unexplained downstream pathophysiologic process. Another possible mechanism that has been proposed might be a perioperative microembolic event that may have occurred during aortic arch clamping (11). In addition to the location of the aortic arch, which may interfere with brain circulation, some evidence suggests that the hypothermic circulatory arrest during which the aortic surgery was performed might be responsible for causing the neurological syndromes (12).

The proposal that the patient suffered from a syndrome resembling PSP after surgical repair of the ascending aortic aneurysm is not entirely speculative. Mokri et al. (13) reported a series of seven patients who developed an unusual and fairly stereotyped biphasic neurological disorder without imaging evidence of related cerebral ischemia or infarct after uncomplicated surgery for ascending aortic aneurysm or dissection. The disease course seemed to be biphasic with a mild, nonprogressive initial phase, followed by a latent, progressive phase closely resembling a PSP phenotype. The case illustrated here does not fit completely with Mokri's report since the presentation of our patient was rather monophasic with a sudden onset, followed by a slow progression until reaching a plateau at a 5-month postoperative period. Nevertheless, the settings were very similar in a context of a distinct neurological syndrome after surgical repair of the ascending aorta. The explanation of a progressive neurological deficit after an acute event was thought to be related to a delayed tissue injury, occurring primarily in areas with selective vulnerability, which also includes midbrain dopaminergic neurons (14,15). The last, and least likely, possibility in our case is that the patient had a preexisting, mild, and unrecognized PSP or PSP-like neurodegenerative disorder that became evident only after the trauma of surgery.

THE LESSON

The combination of syndromes resembling PSP may be due to various etiologies. Despite a neurodegenerative process being the most common cause, we propose that a PSP-like syndrome may occur as a result of a diffuse cerebral hypoxia, particularly a surgical repair of an ascending aortic aneurysm. Even though this type of surgery is fairly common, this complication is quite rare. Obviously, additional predisposing factors such as individual susceptibility may be involved. While the term "progressive supranuclear palsy" infers the progressive nature of the disorder, we propose that this syndrome may not always be progressive. In this case, there was a sudden, mildly progressive presentation but a rather static course as a whole. Therefore, the term "*sudden* or *static* supranuclear palsy" may be considered in exceptional circumstances when the etiology is nonprogressive.

REFERENCES

1. Steele JC, Richardson JC, Olszewski J. Progressive supranuclear palsy. A heterogeneous degeneration involving the brain stem, basal ganglia and cerebellum with vertical gaze and pseudobulbar palsy, nuchal dystonia and dementia. *Arch Neurol.* 1964;10:333–359.
2. Williams DR, Lees AJ. Progressive supranuclear palsy: clinicopathological concepts and diagnostic challenges. *Lancet Neurol.* 2009;8:270–279.
3. Godeiro-Junior C, Inaoka RJ, Barbosa MR, et al. Mutations in npc1 in two Brazilian patients with Niemann-Pick disease type c and progressive supranuclear palsy-like presentation. *Mov Disord.* 2006;21:2270–2272.
4. Josephs KA, Ishizawa T, Tsuboi Y, et al. A clinicopathological study of vascular progressive supranuclear palsy: A multi-infarct disorder presenting as progressive supranuclear palsy. *Arch Neurol.* 2002;59:1597–1601.
5. Caparros-Lefebvre D, Sergeant N, Lees A, et al. Guadeloupean parkinsonism: A cluster of progressive supranuclear palsy-like tauopathy. *Brain.* 2002;125:801–811.
6. Kim TW, Park IS, Kim SH, et al. Striopallidodentate calcification and progressive supranuclear palsy-like phenotype in a patient with idiopathic hypoparathyroidism. *J Clin Neurol.* 2007;3:57–61.
7. Bhidayasiri R, Riley DE, Somers JT, et al. Pathophysiology of slow vertical saccades in progressive supranuclear palsy. *Neurology.* 2001;57:2070–2077.
8. Bhidayasiri R, Plant GT, Leigh RJ. A hypothetical scheme for the brainstem control of vertical gaze. *Neurology.* 2000;54:1985–1993.
9. Winikates J, Jankovic J. Vascular progressive supranuclear palsy. *J Neural Transm Suppl.* 1994;42:189–201.
10. Fujioka M, Okuchi K, Sakaki T, et al. Specific changes in human brain following reperfusion after cardiac arrest. *Stroke.* 1994;25:2091–2095.
11. Gravanis MB, Martin RP, Shah V. Thromboembolic complication of ascending aortic synthetic graft. *Heart Dis Stroke.* 1994;3:316–317.
12. Wical BS, Tomasi LG. A distinctive neurologic syndrome after induced profound hypothermia. *Pediatr Neurol.* 1990;6:202–205.
13. Mokri B, Ahlskog JE, Fulgham JR, Matsumoto JY. Syndrome resembling PSP after surgical repair of ascending aorta dissection or aneurysm. *Neurology.* 2004;62:971–973.
14. Singh V, Carman M, Roeper J, Bonci A. Brief ischemia causes long-term depression in midbrain dopamine neurons. *Eur J Neurosci.* 2007;26:1489–1499.
15. Siesjo BK, Siesjo P. Mechanisms of secondary brain injury. *Eur J Anaesthesiol.* 1996;13:247–268.
16. Rowe DB, Lewis V, Needham M, et al. Novel prion protein gene mutation presenting with subacute PSP-like syndrome. *Neurology.* 2007;68:868–870.
17. Sanz P, Nogue S, Vilchez D, et al. Progressive supranuclear palsy-like parkinsonism resulting from occupational exposure to lead sulphate batteries. *J Int Med Res.* 2007;35:159–163.
18. Mattos JP, Nicaretta DH, Rosso AL. Progressive supranuclear palsy-like syndrome induced by amiodarone and flunarizine. *Arq Neuropsiquiatr.* 2009;67:909–910.
19. Kim HT, Shields S, Bhatia KP, Quinn N. Progressive supranuclear palsy-like phenotype associated with bilateral hypoxic-ischemic striopallidal lesions. *Mov Disord.* 2005;20:755–757.

27

Asymmetric Parkinsonism With Autonomic Dysfunction and Abnormal Sphincter EMG in a 63-Year-Old English Woman: Why Not PSP?

David R. Williams

THE CASE

This patient's medical files were made available through the Queen Square Brain Bank after autopsy. Her problems started at the age of 63 when she consulted her local doctor reporting difficulty gripping objects with her right hand, a mild upper limb tremor, and deterioration of her handwriting. Her past medical history included well-controlled hypertension, type II diabetes, a vaginal hysterectomy for uterine fibroids, and a long history of smoking. At the age of 4, she had sustained a head injury following a road traffic accident, necessitating plastic surgery but no neurosurgical involvement. There was a family history of vascular disease only.

She was referred for a neurological consultation 12 months after first noticing symptoms and was reported to have had a severe, asymmetric akinetic-rigid syndrome. The initial specialist examination revealed her difficulty rising from a chair, severe hypomimia, a mild action tremor in her right upper limb, and severe bilateral cogwheel rigidity, which was worse on the right. She started Levodopa/Benserazide 300/75 mg/d, and a repeat clinical examination 4 months later revealed a marked improvement. This improvement was short-lived, and she developed impaired dexterity on the left side, postural instability, and falls forward. Her speech had also become affected; she required assistance with dressing and washing and suffered from urinary urgency and several episodes of incontinence. Sleep was disturbed by frequent nocturia.

She was reviewed 6 months later, and during her best on-period, there was severe bradykinesia on the right, marked hypomimia, moderate hypophonia, and no tremor. Postural reflexes were impaired. Her supine blood pressure was 170/80 mmHg and fell to 149/80 mmHg on standing. Eye movements were mildly limited in upgaze only and saccades were hypometric and considered to be slow. There was no ataxia, reflexes were brisk throughout, and plantars were flexor. A further increase in levodopa provided some unsustained improvement, and she eventually developed reduced blink rate and slow saccadic eye movements in all directions with preserved range of eye movements in the horizontal and down plane. Four years after developing her first symptoms, she died following a presumed pulmonary embolus after a fall that resulted in a spiral fracture to her humerus.

THE APPROACH

This patient was admitted for a number of investigations, including a levodopa challenge. A CT brain scan was performed as MRI was contraindicated because of ferromagnetic stapedal implant and was reported as normal. Autonomic function tests showed a mildly reduced postural heart rate response and a reduced rise in diastolic blood pressure on cold pressor testing. Sphincter EMG was performed at three sites and 11 motor unit potentials were analyzed. Marked polyphasia with several late components were reported. The mean duration of motor unit potentials was 15.5 ms, and 73% had a duration greater than 10 ms. This was interpreted

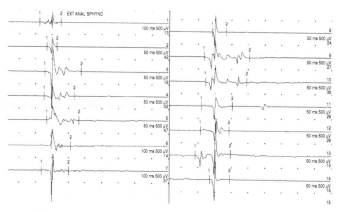

FIGURE 27.1
External anal sphincter EMG (electromyography).

as showing severe denervation changes in the external anal sphincter muscle consistent with degeneration within Onuf's nucleus with compensatory reinnervation (Figure 27.1).

The underlying diagnosis was thought to be multiple system atrophy (MSA) on the basis of the prominent autonomic features and the asymmetric partially levodopa-responsive parkinsonism. Although this patient's main problems were motor slowing and parkinsonism, a neuropsychological examination revealed poor performance in sustained attention, information processing, and executive functioning with mild impairment of verbal memory. Although the treating neurologists were uncomfortable about the clear-cut cognitive difficulties, the final designation was MSA at death. The pathological examination revealed only tau-positive glial and neuronal inclusions, with tufted astrocytes and severe atrophy of the subthalamic nucleus consistent with progressive supranuclear palsy (PSP).

THE LESSON

The diagnosis of parkinsonism when diagnostic criteria are not fully satisfied can be challenging. In our patient, asymmetric motor parkinsonism dominated the early picture, and the rapid progression and unsustained response to levodopa made idiopathic Lewy-body Parkinson's disease very unlikely (1). The most likely alternatives in this scenario were PSP and MSA, but the clinical clues that led one to a final designation were confusing in this case. On one hand, there were moderate autonomic symptoms with electrophysiological evidence of denervation of Onuf's nucleus (supporting a diagnosis of MSA), and on the other hand, there were cognitive deterioration and gaze palsy, supporting a diagnosis of PSP.

In this scenario, I find that the most helpful diagnostic approach is to (a) consider the elements of the early disease manifestations, (b) separately consider the subsequent clinical features and their progression, and (c) critically assess what information investigations are giving me.

With this approach, it is clear that the presentation was predominantly one of motor dysfunction, without prominent autonomic or cerebellar signs. Most patients with MSA will have at least moderate autonomic dysfunction by the time they have moderately severe bradykinesia (2). This patient had a systolic blood pressure drop of only 21 mmHg. Patients with PSP do not necessarily develop falls within the first 12 months, and they may even present with rest tremor and levodopa-responsive asymmetric parkinsonism. I find it useful to investigate cognitive function early in this scenario as patients with PSP-tau pathology are much more likely to perform poorly on sensitive executive function tests than patients with MSA.

In our case, the patient eventually developed frequent falls and eye-movement abnormalities. Restriction of upgaze is a nonspecific sign and can be seen in normal elderly people. Slowed saccadic eye movements are not normal and indicate dysfunction of premotor burst neurons in the rostral interstitial nucleus of the medial longitudinal fasciculus. This region is typically involved in PSP, but not MSA.

The sphincter EMG was considered diagnostic in this case, although it appears from the detailed report that it may not have been a complete study (3). Typically 10 separate motor units need to be sampled, and in this case, three pairs of duplicate units reduced the sensitivity of the study. Nevertheless, the severe degree of denervation seen on the EMG is consistent with significant loss of neurons within Onuf's nucleus. Neither diabetes nor vaginal hysterectomy many years earlier would produce such prolonged units. The reported changes are frequently seen with MSA but are not specific and can also occur in PSP. It is surprising that there was no clinical history of severe incontinence, and this may be a clue that the pathological diagnosis was not MSA.

REFERENCES

1. Köllensperger M, Geser F, Seppi K, et al. Red flags for multiple system atrophy. *Mov Disord.* 2008;23(8):1093–1099.
2. Williams DR, Lees AJ. How do patients with parkinsonism present? A clinicopathological study. *Intern Med J.* 2009;39(1):7–12.
3. Paviour DC, Williams D, Fowler CJ, et al. Is sphincter electromyography a helpful investigation in the diagnosis of multiple system atrophy? A retrospective study with pathological diagnosis. *Mov Disord.* 2005;20(11):1425–1430.

28

Tremor-Dominant Parkinsonism: Lesion or Deep Brain Stimulation?

Elisaveta Sokolov, Tipu Z. Aziz, Dipankar Nandi, and Peter G. Bain

THE CASE

A lady presented in 1993, when aged 56 years old, with right arm tremor. Her past medical history was unremarkable, except for a left hip replacement (osteoarthritis). There was a family history of parkinsonism that affected her mother and a first cousin. The tremor was resistant to propranolol, dopamine agonists, COMT inhibitors, anticholinergics, and amantadine. Consequently, treatment with co-careldopa (Sinemet-110) was instituted and gradually titrated upwards.

By 1999, in spite of treatment with Sinemet-110 q.d.s., the right-sided tremor had worsened and spread to her right leg (Table 28.1). There was mild cogwheel rigidity and bradykinesia in her right arm. She walked with reduced arm swing on the right side and had a classical parkinsonian tremor of the right hand. There were no signs in the left arm or leg. There was also mild "off-phase" dystonic clawing of her right toes. The cerebral MRI scan was normal. It was concluded that she had tremor-dominant Parkinson disease (TDPD). Consequently, in view of the poor response to medication, the issue of whether a left nucleus ventralis intermedius (Vim) thalamotomy, zona incerta (ZI) lesion, thalamic stimulation, or subthalamic nucleus (STN) stimulation should be performed was discussed.

In October 1999, a left Vim-ZI-STN lesion was performed. The procedure abolished her right-sided tremor (Table 28.1) and the clawing of her toes. The patient experienced no adverse effects, and her Sinemet-110 dose was reduced to one tablet t.d.s.

Two years later, apart from early morning rigidity, minimal tremor of her right foot (Table 28.1), and asymptomatic dystonic posturing of her right hand, her parkinsonism was well controlled on Sinemet-110 3.5 tablets/day and amantadine 100 mg o.d.

By 2009, 10 years after surgery, she had developed a left arm tremor and a mild left leg tremor. The arm tremor had gradually become more apparent, and when her medication wore off, it interfered with her activities of daily living. The left-sided tremor was suppressed by Sinemet-110 within 30 minutes but would return about 90 minutes post dose. Her daily intake of Sinemet-110 had increased to nine tablets per day, with an additional Sinemet CR® at night. She had occasional mild dyskinetic movements in the right arm and was experiencing mild generalized slowing of movement when she was "off," although her facial expression and speech remained good. During her "on" periods, her tremor was completely suppressed (Table 28.1), and she had normal facial and vocal expression, with mild bradykinesia in the left arm and a positive Froment's maneuver bilaterally. She underwent revision of her left hip replacement.

In 2010, at age 73, because of increasing left-sided tremor when her medication wore off, she underwent an assessment for further stereotactic surgery. Her neuropsychological profile was satisfactory with no specific cognitive deficits. A cerebral MRI scan showed the lesion extending from the left Vim nucleus through ZI to the dorsal STN (Figure 28.1). Her UPDRS-motor score was 41/108 in the off state when she had mild vocal impassivity, moderately severe rest and postural tremor of the left arm, mild to moderate rest tremor of the left leg, and minimal

TABLE 28.1
Tremor Severity.

DATE	UPPER LIMB TREMOR SEVERITY 0–10 RATING SCALE						LOWER LIMB TREMOR SEVERITY 0–10 RATING SCALE			
	RIGHT			LEFT			RIGHT		LEFT	
	Rest	Post	Inten	Rest	Post	Inten	Rest	Post	Rest	Post
02.03.99	6	6	2	0	0	0	4	0	4	0
11.08.99	6	6	2	0	0	0	4	0	4	0
01.10.99	Left thalamotomy performed									
01.10.99	0	0	0	0	0	0	0	0	0	0
01.02.01	0	0	0	1	2	0	0	0	0	0
03.05.02	0	0	0	0	0	0	1	0	0	0
01.05.03	0	0	0	0	0	0	1	0	0	0
11.11.08[a]	0	0	0	0	0	0	0	0	0	0
10.09.10[b]	0	0	0	4	5	0	0	0	3	1
10.09.10	Right DBS electrode inserted									
13.09.10[c]	0	0	0	0	0	0	0	0	0	0
01.10.10[d]	0	0	0	4	6	0	1	0	3	0
01.10.10[e]	0	0	0	6	8	0	1	0	3	1
01.10.10[f]	0	0	0	0	0	0	1	0	0	0

[a]In "on-medication state" thus no tremor evident.
[b]In "practically" off-medication state.
[c]Post-DBS in on-medication state with stimulation on: Contacts 1 negative, 2 positive, 1.8 V, 120 mcs, 140 Hz and impedance 1762 Ω. A microthalamotomy effect may have been present.
[d]Post-DBS in off-medication state with stimulation on (settings as above).
[e]Post-DBS off medication and off stimulation.
[f]Post-DBS off medication and stimulation on, following reprogramming to: Contacts 1 positive, 3 negative, 2.8 V, 120 mcs, 140 Hz.
Source: Adapted from Ref. 1.

intermittent tremor of the right leg (Table 28.1). There was moderate rigidity and bradykinesia in the left arm and leg but negligible on the right, with some dystonic clawing of the left foot. She could stand unaided with some difficulty. Her trunk posture was mildly flexed and gait slow with a short stride length. One hour after Madopar 250 mg dispersible, her UPDRS-motor score was 17/108. There was a mild rest and postural tremor with mild rigidity and bradykinesia in the left arm. She could stand up with her arms folded. Her truncal posture remained mildly flexed, and she walked with a good tempo and with improved stride length, with reduced arm swing on the left side and mild dystonic posturing of the right hand. Attempts to control her off-state tremor by adding entacapone and then trihexyphenidyl were limited by adverse effects, namely facial dyskinesias and diarrhea. Her left-sided off-state tremor was present for more than 50% of the waking day.

A right thalamic/ZI electrode and a deep brain stimulation (DBS) system were inserted in order to control her left-sided tremor. She experienced no adverse effects from surgery. On turning on the stimulator, total tremor suppression was obtained (Table 28.1), and the patient discharged on the following settings: channel 1 negative and 2 positive, 1.8 V, 120 mcs, 140 Hz.

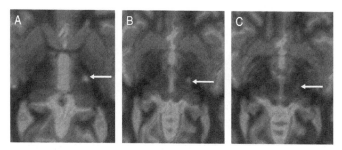

FIGURE 28.1
T2-weighted MRI images demonstrating a right-sided lesion extending from (A) Vim through (B) zona incerta to (C) the dorsal subthalamic area.

When reviewed a month later in the off-state, the tremor in her left arm and leg was similar to the pre-DBS levels in spite of stimulation (Table 28.1). Her stimulator was reprogrammed to contacts 1 negative and 3 positive, 2.8 V, 120 mcs, 140 Hz. This was well tolerated and led to complete abolition of the tremor on her left side (Table 28.1). Her Sinemet-110 dose was reduced from 11 to 8 tablets per day and trihexyphenidyl (4 mg/d) withdrawn.

THE APPROACH

In 1999, the patient's major problem was right-sided rest and postural tremor secondary to her TDPD. We debated whether the optimal surgical target would be the thalamus or STN, as the latter might reduce the possible development of rigidity and bradykinesia on the patient's right side. We felt that as the patient had TDPD, targeting the thalamus would relieve her main and virtually only symptom, namely tremor. At the time, we had begun to appreciate that ZI may be an even better target for relieving tremor than Vim, a view now widely held. Consequently, we decided to target both. Once we had made this decision, the issue became lesion versus stimulation. Although the latter is clearly safer for bilateral procedures, the evidence for that being the case for unilateral thalamic surgery was not strong, and we had some doubts about the longevity of the tremor suppression produced by thalamic stimulation at that time. The left Vim-ZI lesion in fact extended into the dorsal STN and proved to be a good decision, as even a decade later the patient's right-sided tremor was very well suppressed. Furthermore, negligible rigidity and bradykinesia and only occasional mild dyskinesia developed on the right side. The patient was delighted with these results.

THE LESSON

This fascinating case illustrates the long-term stability and effectiveness of a correctly placed Vim-ZI-STN lesion for controlling TDPD. The considerable benefit of the lesion was sustained even a decade later, without any of the maintenance requirements, pacemaker replacement surgery, or costs associated with deep brain stimulation. Furthermore, over the course of 10 years, the only other signs to appear in her right-sided limbs were asymptomatic dystonia and minimal intermittent dyskinesia of the right hand. The patient was so pleased with this effect that she would have liked a right-sided thalamotomy but was dissuaded by the risks to her speech. Nevertheless, this case demonstrates that a unilateral Vim-ZI-STN lesion may be the most successful treatment for patients with unilateral TDPD, although subsequently a contralateral DBS procedure may need to be performed because of disease progression.

Suggested Reading

Bain PG, Findley LJ. *Assessing Tremor Severity*. London, UK: Smith-Gordon; 1993.

Bain P, Aziz T, Liu X, et al. *Deep Brain Stimulation*. Oxford, UK: Oxford University Press; 2009.

Benabid AL, Pollak P, Gao D, et al. Chronic electrical stimulation of the ventralis intermedius nucleus of the thalamus as a treatment of movement disorders. *J Neurosurg.* 1996;84:203–214.

Contarino MF, Daniele A, Sibilia AH, et al. Cognitive outcomes 5 years after bilateral chronic stimulation of subthalamic nucleus in patients with Parkinson's disease. *J Neurol Neurosurg Psychiatry.* 2007;78:248–252.

Krack P, Batir A, Van Blercom N, et al. Five-year follow up of bilateral stimulation of the subthalamic nucleus in advanced Parkinson's disease. *N Eng J Med. 2003*;349:1925–1934.

Limousin P, Krack P, Pollak P, et al. Electrical stimulation of the subthalamic nucleus in advanced Parkinson's disease. *N Eng J Med.* 1998;339:1105–1111.

Merello M, Tenca E, Cerquetti D. Neuronal activity of the zona incerta in Parkinson's disease patients. *Mov Disord.* 2006;21:937–943.

Oh MY, Abosch A, Kim SH, et al. Long-term hardware-related complications of deep brain stimulation. *Neurosurgery.* 2002;50:1268–1274.

Plaha P, Ben-Shlomo Y, Patel NK, et al. Stimulation of the caudal zona incerta is superior to subthalamic nucleus stimulation in improving contralateral parkinsonism. *Brain.* 2006;129:1732–1747.

Schuurman PR, Bosch AD, Bossuyt PMM, et al. A comparison of continuous thalamic stimulation and thalamotomy for suppression of severe tremor. *N Engl J Med.* 2000;342:461–468.

The Miracle of Disappearance of Dyskinesias: The Case of an Elderly Italian Woman Who Benefited From a Stroke

GIOVANNI ABBRUZZESE, TIZIANO TAMBURINI,
LAURA AVANZINO, AND ROBERTA MARCHESE

THE CASE

Mrs V is a distinguished woman of 76 years. In the past, she had never complained of health problems (except for a trigeminal neuralgia in youth), but about 9 years ago she began to feel her right arm becoming more rigid and to complain of slowness and difficulties in fine movements of the right hand. Mrs V was directed to a neurologist who prescribed some examinations. However, the findings (including computed tomography) were normal, and the neurologist informed the patient that her problem indicated the beginning of Parkinson's disease (PD). She was prescribed with levodopa/carbidopa (200/50 mg/d), and Mrs V reported a clear clinical benefit. One year later, however, she noticed the appearance of involuntary movements affecting both upper limbs (especially the right) and the head. The dyskinesias were present for most of the day, and they were so annoying that the patient spontaneously interrupted the levodopa therapy. Discontinuation of medical treatment, however, caused a marked akinesia and rigidity, so that the patient was admitted to our department for further evaluation. The brain MRI showed white matter focal hyperintensities at the corticosubcortical level suggestive of vascular gliosis but all other investigations were negative. Levodopa therapy was reintroduced with improvement of akinesia, and the immediate reappearance of dyskinesias. She was discharged with a regimen characterized by the association of low doses of levodopa/carbidopa (150/50 mg/d) and dopamine agonists (ropinirole 6 mg/d).

In subsequent years, the patient reported a progressive increase in akinesia and rigidity with the appearance of severe fluctuations and freezing of gait, but any attempt to increase the dopaminergic therapy resulted in an intolerable enhancement of dyskinesias. Also the introduction of amantadine proved ineffective.

Involuntary movements were her major complaint and her relatives were very concerned. Indeed, dyskinesias were present throughout the day, mainly in the afternoon and evening, with such a great intensity as to interfere with activities of daily living. They were exacerbated by emotional stress and made it difficult for her to eat, to the point of causing significant weight loss. In addition, dyskinesias led to frequent emergency room admissions for respiratory failure secondary to involuntary movements.

THE APPROACH

In 2009, Mrs V was again admitted to our department in an attempt to modify the regimen and to better control the parkinsonian symptoms and dyskinesias. During the first days of hospitalization, the patient was taking only levodopa/carbidopa 150/50 mg/d, and ropinirole was switched to a prolonged release formulation with a dose of 4 mg/d. We saw a slight reduction in "off" time, but no further increase of dopamine-agonist drugs was possible because of the onset of severe orthostatic hypotension.

On the morning of the seventh day of hospitalization, we discovered her to be extremely drowsy. Brain CT scan performed in the emergency was negative for hemorrhagic lesions and other causes of sensory impairment were ruled out. There were no focal deficits and the state of consciousness showed a progressive improvement within a day or two. In the meantime, the doctors and the patient noticed the disappearance of dyskinesias, which is a "miracle," claimed the relatives. Brain MRI, performed on the third day after the acute event, showed the presence of an ischemic lesion, with minimal blood spreading, in the left thalamus (Figure 29.1). Screening of cerebrovascular risk factors was not relevant. The neurological examination was characterized only by the additional presence of a mild cervical dystonia with antecollis and lateral rotation to the right. In the following days, we gradually increased the dosage of levodopa (up to 300 mg/d) with improvement of patient mobility and persisting complete disappearance of levodopa-induced dyskinesias and motor blocks.

THE LESSON

The overall frequency of symptomatic cerebrovascular disorders in PD patients is similar to that of the control population, although the prevalence of stroke is lower in PD (3.3% vs. 6.4%) (1). However, the effects of cerebrovascular disease on parkinsonian symptoms are variable. Multiple lesions tend to impair axial functions (walking, postural stability), causing a more rapid progression (Hoehn & Yahr staging) and worsening the quality of life. Single lesions in the basal ganglia may infrequently (less than 5%) lead to a "vascular parkinsonism" (2). However, the possibility has been reported that strategically located lesions in the nuclear region may even improve PD (3).

Our case was characterized by a thalamic subacute ischemic lesion that resulted in a significant improvement of parkinsonian symptoms (bilaterally) and in the disappearance of levodopa-induced dyskinesia with a marked improvement of patient's quality of life.

It is well known that stereotactic surgery (lesions or deep brain stimulation) can result in a significant antidyskinetic effect (4). This effect, although more evident in the case of lesions affecting the globus pallidus or the subthalamic nucleus, can also occur in thalamic lesions, possibly because of functional impairment of the pallidothalamic pathway. In particular, Narabayashi et al. (5) described an improvement in drug-induced dyskinesias, when the lesion included the nucleus ventralis oralis posterior (VOP) of the thalamus.

Therefore, we believe that the miracle of disappearance of dyskinesias was due to a kind of "spontaneous vascular thalamotomy" (6), providing further confirmation of the possibility of manipulating the activity of functional circuits of the basal ganglia in patients with PD.

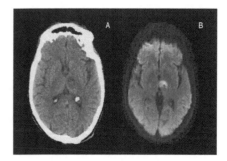

FIGURE 29.1
(A) T1-weighted and (B) DWI brain MRI shows a round inhomogeneous area in the left thalamus, probable expression of a subacute ischemic lesion (with secondary blood spreading). From Equilibri 2009;10(1):18–20.

REFERENCES

1. Nataraj A, Rajput AH. Parkinson's disease, stroke, and related epidemiology. *Mov Disord.* 2005;20:1476–1480.
2. Zijlmans JC, Daniel SE, Hughes AJ. Clinicopathological investigation of vascular parkinsonism, including clinical criteria for diagnosis. *Mov Disord.* 2004;19:630–640.
3. Krauss KJ, Grossman RG, Jankovic J. Improvement of parkinsonian signs after vascular lesion of basal ganglia circuitry. *Mov Disord.* 1997;12:124–126.
4. Guridi J, Obeso JA, Rodriguez-Oroz MC, et al. L-dopa induced dyskinesia and stereotactic surgery for Parkinson's disease. *Neurosurgery.* 2008;62:311–323.
5. Narabayashi H, Maeda T, Yokochi F. Long-term follow-up study of nucleus ventralis intermedius and ventrolateralis thalamotomy using a microelectrode technique in parkinsonism. *Appl Neurophysiol.* 1987;50:330–337.
6. Dubois B, Pillon B, De Saxce H, et al. Disappearance of parkinsonioan signs after spontaneous vascular "thalamotomy." *Arch Neurol.* 1986;43:815–817.

30

Unforgettable Lessons From a Forgetful Museum Attendant With a Supranuclear Gaze Palsy

David J. Burn

THE CASE

I was asked by a neurology fellow to see this 51-year-old right-handed male museum assistant during a weekend on call. He presented with a 5-month history of depression, followed by 6 weeks of short-term memory loss and difficulty reading due to "blurred" vision. His wife had become increasingly worried about his cognitive function, and this was corroborated by the fact that he had been sent home from work 2 weeks before because he was not coping with his job.

We determined that 18 months before, he had been investigated at a nearby hospital for persistent cough with pyrexia and was found to have syndrome of inappropriate antidiuretic hormone (SIADH; sodium 122 mmol/L, serum osmolality 258 mosmol/kg, urine osmolality 384 mosmol/kg) and mediastinal lymphadenopathy. Histological examination of a mediastinal node biopsy revealed PAS-positive material with granulomas and central necrosis. The diagnosis was uncertain at that stage, and he was managed conservatively. His other past medical history consisted of hypothyroidism (treated with thyroxine 150 mcg daily), diabetes (metformin 500 mg twice daily), gout (allopurinol 300 mg daily), and hypertension (metoprolol 50 mg twice daily). The patient was a nonsmoker and did not consume alcohol. His family history was noncontributory.

The general medical examination was unremarkable except for a fever of 38.5°C. When we tested his higher mental function, however, it revealed profound short-term memory impairment superimposed upon a background of global cognitive impairment. The Addenbrooke's Cognitive Examination score was 46/100 (mini-mental state examination [MMSE], 16/30) with marked deficits in orientation, memory, language, verbal fluency, and visuospatial orientation. Visual acuities were 6/9 on the left and 6/18 on the right. There was a significant supranuclear vertical gaze palsy, although the horizontal saccadic movements were not particularly slowed. In the limbs, there was some cog-wheeling of the right upper limb with bradykinesia, as well as a mild postural tremor.

THE APPROACH

Although superficially this man's signs resembled progressive supranuclear palsy (PSP), the rate of deterioration was highly atypical, and his pattern of cognitive dysfunction was also unusual (1). Furthermore, I could not elicit a history of falls, which are so common in PSP (2). An alternative "primary" neurodegenerative cause for his gaze palsy seemed unlikely, and we were therefore suspicious that this man had a "secondary" form of PSP, possibly inflammatory in nature, bearing in mind his recent medical history. A diagnosis of Whipple's disease, so often mentioned at grand rounds in differential diagnosis desperation, was perhaps a real possibility.

Basic laboratory investigation showed an erythrocyte sedimentation rate (ESR) of 4, C-reactive protein (CRP) less than 5, full blood count within reference range, and a hyponatremia of 122 mmol/L. Antinuclear antibody titer was 1:160. The chest X-ray on admission showed right hilar lymphadenopathy. An MRI brain scan was reported as normal (you are allowed a normal scan in Whipple's, aren't you?). An electroencephalogram (EEG) showed mild nonspecific cortical disturbance. Cerebrospinal fluid (CSF) analysis was unremarkable for cell count and glucose, although protein was elevated at 0.98 g/L and oligoclonal bands were present in the CSF, unmatched with serum. We held our breath…and then exhaled noisily when the polymerase chain reaction (PCR) for Whipple's disease came back as *negative!* A PCR for tuberculosis (TB) in the CSF as well as proteins S100 and 14-3-3 were also negative. Other negative investigations included thyroid microsomal antibodies, HIV 1 and 2 antibodies, VDRL, Lyme serology, and a vasculitic/autoimmune screen (antineutrophil cytoplasmic antibodies [ANCA], double-stranded DNA, and an extended autoantibody screen) as well as repeated venous blood cultures. Despite the CSF TB PCR result, a Heaf test was strongly positive and triple antituberculous therapy was therefore commenced. Widespread hilar lymphadenoapathy was also detected on CT.

During his admission, I noted that his parkinsonism was becoming more evident with a Unified Parkinson's Disease Rating Scale (UPDRS) III of 26 scored 2 weeks after admission. There was no symptomatic response to co-beneldopa 25/100 thrice a day, and his supranuclear ophthalmoparesis persisted. Despite receiving antimicrobial therapy, his condition acutely deteriorated with respiratory insufficiency, requiring intubation and ventilation. Given the rate of deterioration, the CT thorax findings, and the "red herring" (as it increasingly seemed) of the positive Heaf test, I became increasingly suspicious that our patient may have an underlying malignancy and that his neurological presentation was paraneoplastic in nature.

Subsequently, anti-Hu antibodies returned as strongly present in his serum and CSF. While on the intensive care unit (ICU), we requested a mediastinoscopy, and a lymph node biopsy from this procedure revealed a small-cell lung carcinoma. After discussion with the patient and his family, active treatment was withdrawn and the patient died shortly thereafter.

THE LESSON

Supranuclear gaze palsy is a rare but well-recognized presentation of paraneoplastic brain stem encephalomyelitis, but a more "overt" paraneoplastic PSP-like presentation is very uncommon. Hypokinetic presentations may be associated with anti-Ma2 encephalitis, and in young males, these should prompt a search for a testicular tumor (3). It is easy to be wise after the event, but I must confess that I had never come across either presentation previously.

Although the neurological findings in our case superficially suggested PSP as a possible diagnosis, the short history, rapid progression, presence of SIADH, mediastinal lymphadenopathy, and a spiking fever pointed us toward a possible paraneoplastic cause. Furthermore, the pattern of cognitive deficit was atypical for PSP, where a frontosubcortical pattern of involvement is typical (4). The positive Heaf test and the first biopsy findings of PAS-positive material, prompting antituberculosis treatment, were misleading, in retrospect. I do not believe, however, that this stalled our search for a unifying diagnosis, as we were never convinced that our patient had TB. Starting him on antituberculous treatment was a "safety first" measure recommended by our colleagues in "Infectious Diseases." There were no gastrointestinal or joint symptoms and, while ophthalmoparesis, obtundation, and cognitive deficits may all occur in Whipple's disease, the Whipple's PCR was negative (5). It still did not stop one hopeful trainee from mentioning this diagnosis at a grand round featuring the case, however!

A paraneoplastic cause should be considered and antibodies associated with paraneoplastic neurological disorders analyzed in cases with a rapidly progressive PSP-like syndrome, particularly when atypical features are present. You would not find many such cases during your professional career, but it may avoid you having to give a dire prognosis and make a fundamental management decision (i.e., ventilator support) within a short time, which is so hard for relatives to assimilate, as happened in our patient.

REFERENCES

1. Marras C, Lang AE, Ang LC, et al. 69-year-old man with gait disturbance and Parkinsonism. *Mov Disord.* 2001;16:548–561.

2. Litvan I, Agid Y, Jankovic J, et al. Accuracy of clinical criteria for the diagnosis of progressive supranuclear palsy (Steele-Richardson-Olszewski syndrome). *Neurology*. 1996;46(4):922–930.
3. Grant R, Graus F. Paraneoplastic movement disorders. *Mov Disord*. 2009;24:1715–1724.
4. Brown RG, Lacomblez L, Landwehrmeyer BG, et al. Cognitive impairment in patients with multiple system atrophy and progressive supranuclear palsy. *Brain*. 2010;133:2382–2393.
5. Anderson M. Neurology of Whipple's disease. *J Neurol Neurosurg Psychiatry*. 2000;68:2–5.

31

*Reversible Unilateral Parkinsonism Associated With Bipolar
Affective Disorder in a 59-Year-Old Spanish Woman*

JAIME KULISEVSKY AND ROSER RIBOSA NOGUÉ

THE CASE

Twenty years ago, we visited in the outpatient clinic a 59-year-old woman without psychiatric history who complained of a depressive state associated with general slowness initiated 15
months before consultation. The only pathological antecedent was hypercholesterolemia.

She explained that her bad mood had a subacute onset. She told us that she was doing perfectly well until a day when she suddenly collapsed in the marketplace; she rapidly regained consciousness but transiently experienced dizziness and unsteady gait. Back at home, she noticed
a slight right palpebral ptosis. Nevertheless, she did not seek medical counseling and did well
during the next 2 weeks continuing her daily routine. At that time, a marked change in her
behavior compared with her premorbid functioning was noted. She lacked motivation, became
apathetic and withdrawn, and eventually developed emotional lability, insomnia, and anorexia.
She also developed a fear of imminent death associated with fixed delusions. She believed that
her husband and the general practitioner were plotting to conceal from her a serious illness and
that her brain would drop out of her nose. A psychiatrist prescribed treatment with tricyclic
antidepressant drugs shortly followed by a combination of monoamine oxidase inhibitors and
neuroleptic drugs; however, there was no improvement for the next 14 months.

When first seen by us, she exhibited dysphoric mood, low self-esteem, hopelessness, inappropriate guilt, and insomnia but not psychotic symptoms. She had no familial or personal history
of affective disorders. On the Beck Depression Inventory, her score was 25 (severe depression).
Neuropsychological testing revealed no cognitive dysfunction. On neurological examination,
there was a mild palpebral ptosis on the right side, but ocular movements and pupillary responses
were normal. There was a moderately stooped posture. She exhibited diminished swing of the
left arm, shuffling of the left leg, and mild postural tremor, rigidity, and hypokinesia of the left
arm. Righting reflexes were moderately impaired. The remaining neurological examination was
normal.

We decided to replace tricyclic antidepressant by fluoxetine and ordered a cranial CT scan.
As the patient did not obtain a beneficial response with fluoxetine during the next month, she
voluntarily discontinued it without reassuming other medication and not returning to the outpatient clinic until 4 months after the first visit. In this visit, she claimed that her depression
was over and that the motor symptoms had spontaneously vanished. At neurological examination, she exhibited normal gait and arm swinging and had no tremor, bradykinesia, rigidity,
or postural instability. On the Beck Depression Inventory, her score was 6 (no depression). On
several follow-up examinations, depressive or parkinsonian symptoms did not reappear, and she
continued doing well until the end of the second year, when marked changes were again noted
in her behavior. She gradually became elated, hyperactive, and markedly intrusive with unfamil-
iar people. She also had logorrhea, insomnia, and moderately increased self-esteem and sexual
interest. On the Mania Scale, her score was 19 (definite mania). No parkinsonism was noted on
the neurological examination. This manic episode disappeared 4 weeks later under treatment
with lithium carbonate 1,200 mg/d. Eight months thereafter, she consulted for a new depressive

episode, similar to the previous one. When examined at this time, all the previous signs of her past left parkinsonian syndrome had reappeared. They again disappeared with improvement of the depressive episode. In the following 2 years, at least two further cycles of unilateral parkinsonism associated with depression and fading of the parkinsonism during euthymia or manic cycles were observed. She was lost for follow-up 5 years later.

THE APPROACH

In the first visit, our patient had a left parkinsonian syndrome associated with major depression. One possible diagnosis could have been a depressive episode with slowness considered an integral part of depression. However, its grossly unilateral manifestation and the clear presence of rigidity and tremor argued against this possibility. On the other hand, depression is one of the most frequent neuropsychiatric disturbances of idiopathic Parkinson's disease (PD) (1), which can precede or follow the recognition of motor symptoms. Then, idiopathic PD, with a typical unilateral presentation, could also be considered. Nevertheless, the relatively abrupt instauration of the disease, a locator sign—the unilateral ptosis—and the unusual association of de novo PD with delusional depression, all recommended the practice of a neuroimaging study to discard vascular causes. The CT scan disclosed a discrete ischemic infarction involving the right mesencephalopontine area, as well as bilateral periventricular white matter vascular changes. A magnetic resonance imaging (MRI) scan revealed changes similar to those already seen on the CT scan. A single-photon emission computed tomography (SPECT) scan with Tc-99 hexamethylpropyleneamine oxide revealed a decrease of perfusion in the centrum semiovale and basal ganglia bilaterally. Other ancillary tests such as echocardiography, ecodoppler imaging of extracranial arteries, and laboratory assessments to exclude a prothrombotic state were performed. A mild stenosis (less than 50%) in both internal carotid arteries was found. Based on these results and on the follow-up, we diagnosed our patient as having a vascular hemiparkinsonism associated with a bipolar affective disorder. Antiaggregant and hypolipemiant drugs were initiated. Mood symptoms were treated with serotonin reuptake inhibitors and lithium. No levodopa or other antiparkinsonian drugs were administered during the follow-up.

THE LESSON

From a pathophysiological standpoint, we consider this case outstanding, as it clearly demonstrates the relationship between parkinsonian symptoms and affective disorders. Depressive symptoms (major depression and dysthymia) are frequently observed in the early stages of PD, whereas rapid mood swings usually occur in advanced stages of the disease and are associated with the "on-off" phenomena (2). It has been suggested that the affective disorder is an integral part of the disease associated with neurotransmitter-related pathologic changes at the mesencephalic-forebrain region. Besides dopaminergic alterations, both serotonergic and noradrenergic changes have also been implicated (3). Both early-onset depression and the worsening of depressive symptoms during the "off" phase have been attributed to reduced levels of dopamine.

Correspondingly, a hyperdopaminergic state was postulated to explain expanded mood and occasionally mania associated with dyskinetic movements during the "on" phase (2). In our patient, the course of the affective disorder (delusional depression followed by mania) and the motor course with aggravation of parkinsonism during depression and spontaneous remission with euthymia and mania are consistent with a dysfunctional dopaminergic activity associated with the brainstem lesion. Consistently, vascular and neoplastic brainstem lesions have been reported to induce either isolated bipolar disorder (4,5) or parkinsonian symptoms without mood changes (6). Although the coexistence of these two disorders is exceptional, this patient illustrates how damage to frontal-basal ganglia-thalamocortical circuits by subcortical lesions may simultaneously provoke disorders of movement and mood regulation (7).

REFERENCES

1. Reijnders JS, Ehrt U, Weber WE, et al. A systematic review of prevalence studies of depression in Parkinson's disease. *Mov Disord.* 2008;23:183–189.
2. Kulisevsky J, Pascual-Sedano B, Barbanoj M, et al. Acute effects of immediate and controlled-release levodopa on mood in Parkinson's disease: a double-blind study. *Mov Disord.* 2007;22(1):62–67.
3. Brooks DJ, Piccini P. Imaging in Parkinson's disease: the role of monoamines in behaviour. *Biol Psychiatry.* 2006;59:908–918.
4. Turecki G, Mari Jde J, Del Porto JA. Bipolar disorder following a left basal-ganglia stroke. *Br J Psychiatry.* 1993;163:690.
5. Berthier ML. Post-stroke rapid cycling bipolar affective disorder. *Br J Psychiatry.* 1992;160:283.
6. Goldstein S, Friedman JH, Innis R, et al. Hemi-parkinsonism due to a midbrain arteriovenous malformation: dopamine transporter imaging. *Mov Disord.* 2001;16(2):350–353.
7. Berthier ML, Kulisevsky J, Gironell A, et al. Poststroke bipolar affective disorder: clinical subtypes, concurrent movement disorders, and anatomical correlates. *J Neuropsychiatry Clin Neurosci.* 1996;8(2):160–167.

32

Sudden-Onset Mutism and Parkinsonism in a Psychiatric Patient: An Unusual Case of "Central Pontine Myelinolysis"

JAIME KULISEVSKY AND ROSER RIBOSA NOGUÉ

THE CASE

This was a 41-year-old woman who had been diagnosed with paranoid schizophrenia at 20 years of age. We were called on consultation for persistent parkinsonism after what looked like a solved medical event. In her medical records, there were four admissions to the psychiatric unit due to paranoid crisis.

She lived alone and was under chronic antipsychotic therapy (haloperidol and fluphenazine decanoate injections bimonthly). In June 1996, she was taken to the emergency department because her neighbors noted that she had lost weight in a short period of time, only ingested water and liquid aliments, and two days before admission, exhibited progressive somnolence, frequent falls, and malaise. At admission, she was noted to be hypertensive (180/110 mmHg), bradipsychic, and extremely slender. No toxics were detectable in the urine test. Severe hyponatremia (104 mmol/L) and hyperosmolarity (203 mmol/L) were detected. Slow correction of the hyponatremia and intravenous fluid treatment was initiated to correct this alteration, which was fully achieved on the fourth day. However, despite an initial improvement in her general status, arterial hypertension, stupor, and fever onset were noted on the third day. A cranial CT scan and cerebrospinal fluid (CSF) analysis were done with normal results and large spectrum antibiotic treatment was started. Electroencephalogram (EEG) showed diffuse slowing. When we first saw the patient on the fifth day, she was capable of obeying simple commands but spoke no words, neurologic examination revealed no focal alterations, but her movements were extremely slow and marked axial and limb rigidity was noted. We indicated a cranial MRI. T2-weighted images showed marked hyperdense bilateral lesions in both putaminopallidal regions and slight central hyperintensity of the pons. A diagnosis of central pontine, mainly extrapontine myelinolysis (EPM), was established, and the patient was moved to our neurologic unit to complete the study and rehabilitation.

THE APPROACH

Other potential causes of hydroelectrolytic alteration, including endocrine, infectious, and autoimmune diseases, were ruled out. On the following days, she regained full consciousness, but it was evident that she was afflicted by a severe parkinsonism affecting all four limbs, which markedly limited walking. On the next week, she spontaneously regained some mobility and autonomy. At this point, she exhibited clear signs of potomania and inappropriate behavior with disinhibition. Levodopa treatment was not recommended by the consultant psychiatrist. A cerebral perfusion single-photon emission computed tomography (SPECT) detected bilateral and symmetric mild hypoperfusion in the frontal lobes and basal ganglia, which was considered the functional consequence of the basal ganglia lesions detected on MRI. Neuropsychological examination detected mild frontosubcortical alterations. A gradual spontaneous improvement of her parkinsonism was paralleled by a gradual worsening of disinhibition with repetitive language and potomanic behavior. She was discharged to a long-stay psychiatric unit and treated with clozapine. Abnormal hyperintensities slightly attenuated in a control MRI, 2 months after the beginning of parkinsonism. The patient was considered unable to live alone and remained institutionalized. At the following visits, in the outpatient clinics, both disinhibition and parkinsonism had improved. At her next visit in September 1997, potomania persisted, parkinsonism almost subsided, psychological deficits showed a discrete worsening, and a control MRI showed a noticeable vanishing of the hyperintensities. In the next months, clozapine was replaced by risperidone due to agranulocytosis. Polydipsia persisted and parkinsonism reemerged. Other antipsychotics, including typical neuroleptics such as haloperidol, were assayed by psychiatrists. When last seen as an outpatient in our Movement Disorders Clinic, a year and a half after the beginning of the disease, she exhibited a bilateral rigid-akinetic syndrome, flattening of affect, and buccolingual dyskinesias. We recommended a switch to an atypical antipsychotic and initiation of levodopa.

THE LESSON

Adams et al. (1) described central pontine myelinolysis (CPM) as a unique clinical entity in 1958 in patients who suffered from alcoholism or malnutrition. Although initially considered rare, CPM has been identified in a wide range of patients with ages ranging from 3 years old upward. Its prevalence has been highlighted by a number of large series, with one demonstrating an incidence of 3 per 1,000 in an unselected urban hospital population group (2). Two subgroups considered particularly prone to CPM appear to be alcohol abusers and liver transplantees, with some postmortem series suggesting a prevalence of up to 30% (3).

CPM is pathologically defined as a symmetric area of myelin disruption in the center of the basis pontis. Similar symmetric pathologic lesions have also been identified in extrapontine locations (EPM), such as the cerebellar and neocortical white/gray junctional areas, thalamus, subthalamus, amygdala, globus pallidus, putamen, caudate, and lateral geniculate bodies. EPM can occur in isolation, but it is found in 10% of patients with CPM (4).

Although the exact pathogenesis of this syndrome remains elusive, various mechanisms have been proposed, which may occur in isolation or in combination depending on the clinical situation such as oligodendroglial dehydration resulting in separation of the axon from its myelin sheath with subsequent myelinolysis and necrosis; oligodendroglial apoptosis owing to metabolic stress during cellular attempts to prevent osmotic dehydration especially when the predisposing illness involves nutritional deficiencies; macrophage and astroglial response to osmotic myelinolysis leading to accumulation of myelinotoxic substances augmenting demyelination. Although usually occurring in association with the rapid correction of hyponatremia, and more rarely hypernatremia and hypophosphatemia, CPM/EPM has also been reported in patients with normal sodium levels or mild derangements, as well as in hyponatremic patients with acceptable rates of sodium replacement (5).

Three presentations of myelinolysis are possible, which are as follows: isolated CPM and EPM and a combined CPM/EPM clinical picture. All three presentations occur in a similar clinical context; that is, an individual at risk for CPM/EPM (in our case, a patient with chronic hyponatremia and probable malnutrition) undergoes intravenous electrolyte management during the treatment of the underlying disease, rapidly correcting a hypoosmolar state as with hyponatremia or rapidly producing a hyperosmolar environment.

The clinical course of CPM has been classically described as biphasic, as in our patient, beginning with a generalized encephalopathy caused by the presenting hyponatremia (altered mental status, headache, myalgias, hyporeflexia, seizures), with symptoms and signs improving following serum sodium normalization. This is followed by a second phase of neurological events occurring at approximately a minimum of 2 and a maximum of 7 days (3 days in our case) after the rapid sodium correction and attributable to the onset of myelinolysis. Progressive obtundation often to coma, diplegia with pseudobulbar palsy, dysarthria, ophthalmoplegia, dysphagia, nystagmus, and ataxia can occur over several days. A "locked-in" syndrome or death can ensue (6). Clinical symptoms and signs associated with EPM are less consistent and depend on brain structures affected, but occur within a similar time frame. Akinesia and catatonia, altered mental status, emotional lability, akinetic mutism, gait disturbance, myoclonus, and extrapyramidal signs (including dystonia, choreoathetosis, rigidity, hypertonia, tremor, and a typical parkinsonian syndrome) have all been described in patients with isolated EPM (7,8).

The best treatment of CPM/EPM is prevention. Therefore, of primary importance is identifying prospectively those patients whose underlying disease places them at risk for osmotic myelinolysis. Once an osmotic derangement has been recognized, the underlying cause must be addressed. When hyponatremia is acute and above 125 mmol/L, it can be more rapidly normalized. Moreover, if the patient remains relatively asymptomatic, oral correction with an appropriate sodium diet and fluid restriction producing a slower correction rate would be the safest course.

In symptomatic acute hyponatremia, the initial rate of correction should be 1–2 mmol (mEq)/L/h for several hours; the total daily correction should not exceed 8 mmol/L/d. Treatment of other metabolic stressors should also proceed rapidly. After the onset of CPM/EPM, treatment and therefore modification of the morbidity/mortality, are best pursued by intensive support of all metabolic parameters. Assuming that myelinotoxic compounds are contributing to the myelinolytic demyelinating process in CPM/EPM, similar in this regard to patients with major immune-mediated demyelination, patients have been successfully treated with plasmapheresis, intravenous immunoglobulins, and steroid administration (9,10). Also based on the myelinotoxic mechanism, severe CPM has been successfully treated with a 6 weeks course of daily thyroid releasing hormone. Additionally in EPM, symptomatic treatment should be directed at the clinical presentation produced by the brain structure affected so that in striatal EPM with a parkinsonian picture, the usual dopaminergic compounds can relieve symptoms until lesion normalization occurs.

Fortunately, although initial reports showed very poor outcome, more recent reports suggest the contrary, mainly due to early diagnosis and improved intensive care treatment (11,12).

REFERENCES

1. Adams RD, Victor M, Mancall EL. Central pontine myelinolysis: a hitherto undescribed disease occurring in alcoholic and malnourished patients. *AMA Arch Neurol Psychiatry*. 1959;81(2):154–172.
2. Wright DG, Laureno R, Victor M. Pontine and extrapontine myelinolysis. *Brain*. 1979;102(2):361–385.
3. Singh N, Yu VL, Gayowski T. Central nervous system lesions in adult liver transplant recipients: clinical review with implications for management. *Medicine (Baltimore)*. 1994;73(2):110–118.
4. Kumar S, Fowler M, Gonzalez-Toledo E, Jaffe SL. Central pontine myelinolysis, an update. *Neurol Res*. 2006;28(3):360–366.
5. Ashrafian H, Davey P. A review of the causes of central pontine myelinosis: yet another apoptotic illness? *Eur J Neurol*. 2001;8(2):103–109.
6. Brown WD. Osmotic demyelination disorders: central pontine and extrapontine myelinolysis. *Curr Opin Neurol*. 2000;13(6):691–697.
7. Seiser A, Schwarz S, Aichinger-Steiner MM, et al. Parkinsonism and dystonia in central pontine and extrapontine myelinolysis. *J Neurol Neurosurg Psychiatry*. 1998;65(1):119–121.
8. Sajith J, Ditchfield A, Katifi HA. Extrapontine myelinolysis presenting as acute parkinsonism. *BMC Neurol*. 2006;6:33.
9. Grimaldi D, Cavalleri F, Vallone S, et al. Plasmapheresis improves the outcome of central pontine myelinolysis. *J Neurol*. 2005;252(6):734–735.
10. Deleu D, Salim K, Mesraoua B, et al. "Man-in-the-barrel" syndrome as delayed manifestation of extrapontine and central pontine myelinolysis: beneficial effect of intravenous immunoglobulin. *J Neurol Sci*. 2005;237(1–2):103–106.
11. Menger H, Jörg J. Outcome of central pontine and extrapontine myelinolysis (n = 44). *J Neurol*. 1999;246(8):700–705.
12. Kallakatta RN, Radhakrishnan A, Fayaz RK, et al. Clinical and functional outcome and factors predicting prognosis in osmotic demyelination syndrome (central pontine and/or extrapontine myelinolysis) in 25 patients. *J Neurol Neurosurg Psychiatry*. 2011;82(3):326–331.

Acute Confusion and Rapidly Progressive Dementia in Diffuse Lewy Body Disease?

EDUARDO TOLOSA AND FRANCESC VALLDEORIOLA

THE CASE

A 72-year-old man was found in the street disoriented and confused and taken to the hospital, were he was admitted. The patient's relatives had not noticed any change in the patient's mental state during the previous days or weeks, and he had been autonomous, able to manage his finances and doing his usual home duties until the day of admission. Other relevant medical or family history for neurological disorders was absent. The patient was not known to be taking antidepressants or other psychoactive drugs. On admission, examination disclosed that the patient was drowsy and had reduced attention. He was disoriented and response to questions was slow and inappropriate. He was unable to perform complex or sequential tasks. The rest of the neurological and physical examination was normal.

THE APPROACH

Routine blood analyses were normal. Toxicological screening was negative. A CT scan of the head on the day of admission and a nuclear magnetic resonance (NMR) a week later were normal except for mild generalized brain atrophy. Cerebrospinal fluid (CSF) had normal cell count, protein, and glucose values. The ensuing days, the patient became progressively more disoriented and confused, with disorganization of speech and inability to perform simple tasks on command. There were daily oscillations in attention and alertness. Delusions of persecution and visual hallucinations (spiders and people) developed. An electroencephalogram (EEG) showed 5 to 6 Hz generalized slowing but no epileptiform discharges or asymmetries. Cultures and polymerase chain reaction (PCR) testing for herpes viruses in the CSF were negative. Screening for thyroid function, antithyroid antibodies, vitamin levels, and microbiological studies with serologies for HIV, syphilis and borreliosis, autoantibodies, plasma tumoral biomarkers, onconeural antibodies, and porphyria disclosed no abnormalities. Thoracic and abdominal CT and whole-body 18F-glucose positron emission tomography (PET) scan were normal. Duodenal biopsy ruled out Whipple's disease. A second lumbar puncture was performed for 14–3-3 protein testing, which was negative. A new EEG showed diffuse slow wave activity but no periodic slow wave complexes (PSWC) were seen. A new brain MRI with T2-, diffusion-weighted imaging (DWI) and fluid-attenuated inversion recovery (FLAIR) sequences did not show high-signal abnormalities in the striatum or in the cerebral cortex. Treatment with risperidone led to an increase in confusion. Quetiapine, up to 200 mg/d, slightly improved agitation. Because of the presence of delusions and visual hallucinations, the paradoxical response to risperidone and the absence of alternative diagnosis, diffuse Lewy body disease was suspected as the cause of the confusional syndrome. A dopamine transporter single-photon emission computed tomography (DAT SPECT) could not be done because of agitation, but iodine-123-metaiodobenzylguanidine single-photon emission computed tomography (MIBG SPECT) disclosed prominent cardiac sympathetic denervation (heart-to-mediastinum ratio, 1.35). The patient's clinical condition deteriorated while in the hospital. He became progressively more disoriented and prostrated, incontinent and could hardly stand or walk even with assistance. He was not thought to have a parkinsonian syndrome. He was transferred to a nursing home 3 weeks after admission. During the next weeks, the patient became progressively disconnected from the surroundings, non-responsive to verbal stimuli and, finally, stuporous. He died as a consequence of pneumonia, 3 months after the disease onset. Permission for an autopsy was granted by the family.

Neuropathological Examination. Brain weight was 1,125 g and showed wild generalized atrophy. There was mild nigral pallor. Alpha-synuclein positive inclusions in the form of Lewy bodies and neuritis were found to be present in the olfactory bulb, pons, medulla, midbrain; nucleus *basalis* of Meynert, insula, basal ganglia, thalamus; and frontal, parietal, temporal, and occipital cortex, being specially abundant in the amygdala, transentorhinal cortex, and anterior cingulated gyrus. Alzheimer's-related pathology was found to be moderate (Stage III Braak & Braak). Staining for TDP43, negative prion protein (PrP) deposits were not identified. Alpha-synuclein gene multiplications and progranulin gene mutations were not found. The histopathological diagnosis was diffuse Lewy body disease.

THE LESSON

Clinical Summary and Neuropathological Examination

A patient is presented who developed an acute state of confusion followed by a rapidly progressive cognitive and motor decline. Most common causes of rapidly progressive neurological deterioration such as brain tumor, Creutzfeldt-Jakob disease (CJD), and paraneoplastic or infectious diseases were ruled out or could not be substantiated with laboratory or imaging tests. A Lewy body dementia was suspected by clinical grounds and imaging results.

The diagnosis of a Lewy body dementia in patients with a syndrome of rapidly developing cognitive deterioration is difficult. Symptoms are quite nonspecific and overlap with those observed in many other conditions including CJD (1,2), and no diagnostic imaging or biological tests exist to diagnose these disorders. Furthermore, the usual course of Lewy body dementias (Parkinson's disease (PD) dementia and Lewy body dementia) is slower than the one in the patient presented here, with patients usually surviving 6 to 10 years after symptom onset (3). We recently reported six cases of rapidly developing dementia leading to death within 3 to 7 months, who at autopsy were found to have diffuse Lewy body disease.

Clinical clues for the diagnosis of a Lewy body type dementia in a rapidly deteriorating patient include the presence of visual hallucinations, delusions and psychosis, a day-to-day fluctuation in mental state, hypersensitivity to neuroleptics, and prominent parkinsonism, dysautonomia, or the presence of REM behavior disorder. In some patients, transient postoperative or illness-associated confusional states have been considered to precede the full development of dementia by several months (4). Delirium at disease onset could be a marker for particularly rapid progressive cases. Three out of six cases with a rapidly developing dementia and autopsy confirmed the diagnoses of diffuse Lewy body disease presented with an acute confusional state (5).

A tentative diagnosis of a Lewy body dementia during life as the cause of the clinical syndrome of rapidly progressive cognitive and motor deterioration requires careful exclusion of other conditions that can cause the syndrome. CJD is a main cause of concern and may have an identical clinical picture to a Lewy body dementia (6–9). Cerebellar and visual signs are frequent in CJD and are not usually found in Lewy body syndromes. In addition, a recent study analyzing movement disorders in patients with suspected CJD found that the presence of hypokinesia and the absence of ataxia made the diagnosis of CJD unlikely and suggested the presence of a degenerative process (9).

Laboratory and neuroimaging tests have a prominent role in the diagnosis of a rapidly developing dementia. Cortical and basal ganglia hyperintensities in DWI and FLAIR sequences are highly specific and sensitive for CJD and have not been reported in patients with Lewy body dementias (10,11). Analysis for 14-3-3 protein in CSF is also helpful since it has a sensitivity of 94% and specificity of 84% for the clinical diagnosis of CJD (10,11). CSF studies are usually negative for 14-3-3 in patients with rapidly progressive dementia associated with Lewy bodies (12), although occasionally some patients with Lewy body syndrome with rapid disease progression could have a positive result (4). The presence of PSWC in the EEG has a sensitivity of 66% and a specificity of 74% for the diagnosis of pathologically confirmed CJD (12). PSWC, though, are not pathognomonic for CJD and have been reported in other neurodegenerative diseases, including Lewy body dementia (13,14).

DAT SPECT and myocardial scintigraphy with MIBG may prove helpful in supporting the diagnosis of a Lewy body disorder. Although abnormal DAT imaging has been reported in occasional patients with CJD (15), it consistently shows decreased striatal tracer uptake in the various Lewy body syndromes such as PD and dementia with Lewy bodies and is not found in other dementias such as Alzheimer's disease (16). Recently, abnormal myocardial scintigraphy with MIBG has been postulated as a marker for Lewy body syndromes (17), and since the pathological process of CJD presumably does not involve the cardiac plexus, MIBG SPECT could be helpful in the differential diagnosis of a rapidly developing dementia. Experience with myocardial scintigraphy in CJD and in Lewy body dementias though is still limited.

Dementia is common in the Lewy body synucleinopathies and generally evolves gradually over years. Why in some cases, as in the case reported here, the cognitive changes can have such a rapid, malignant course leading to death in a few months remains unknown.

Conclusions

1. Lewy body diseases are one cause of a rapidly developing dementia (RDD) and should be included in the differential diagnosis of confusional states. Dementia associated with Lewy bodies should be strongly considered when other known causes of persistent delirium have been ruled out.

2. Visual hallucinations and delusions, prominent cognitive fluctuations, and changes in alertness and attention like those occurring in the patient reported here are prominent features of the Lewy body dementias. Although not present in this case, spontaneous parkinsonism, prominent dysautonomia, or REM behavior disorder, common in disorders such as PD or dementia with Lewy bodies, should raise the suspicion of a Lewy body disorder.

3. CJD is the condition that most resembles a rapidly progressive Lewy body dementia. All efforts should be made to rule out this condition, which can be done reliably with the use of imaging, EEG, and biological testing. In patients with RDD, if the diagnostic workup for CJD proves negative, the presence of an altered MIBG myocardial scintigraphy, which was the case in our patient, and an abnormal DAT SPECT may support the clinical diagnosis of a Lewy body dementia.

REFERENCES

1. Kraemer C, Lang K, Weckesser M, Evers S. Creutzfeldt-Jakob disease misdiagnosed as dementia with Lewy bodies. *J Neurol.* 2005;252:861–862.
2. du Plessis DG, Larner AJ. Phenotypic similarities causing clinical misdiagnosis of pathologically-confirmed sporadic Creutzfeldt-Jakob disease as dementia with Lewy bodies. *Clin Neurol Neurosurg.* 2008;110:194–197.
3. Geser F, Wenning GK, Poewe W, McKeith I. How to diagnose dementia with Lewy bodies: state of the art. *Mov Disord.* 2005;20(suppl. 12):S11–S20.
4. Josephs KA, Ahlskog JE, Parisi JE, et al. Rapidly progressive neurodegenerative dementias. *Arch Neurol.* 2009;66:201–207.
5. Gaig C, Valldeoriola F, Gelpi E, et al. Rapidly progressive diffuse Lewy body disease. *Mov Disord.* 2011;26:1316–1323.
6. Van Everbroeck B, Dobbeleir I, De Waele M, et al. Differential diagnosis of 201 possible Creutzfeldt-Jakob disease patients. *J Neurol.* 2004;251:298–304.
7. Haik S, Brandel JP, Sazdovitch V, et al. Dementia with Lewy bodies in a neuropathologic series of suspected Creutzfeldt-Jakob disease. *Neurology.* 2000;55:1401–04.

8. Tschampa HJ, Neumann M, Zerr I, et al. Patients with Alzheimer's disease and dementia with Lewy bodies mistaken for Creutzfeldt-Jakob disease. *J Neurol Neurosurg Psychiatry.* 2001;71:33–39.
9. Edler J, Mollenhauer B, Heinemann U, et al. Movement disturbances in the differential diagnosis of Creutzfeldt-Jakob disease. *Mov Disord.* 2009;24:350–356.
10. Vrancken AF, Frijns CJ, Ramos LM. FLAIR MRI in sporadic Creutzfeldt Jakob disease. *Neurology.* 2000;55:147–148.
11. Shiga Y, Miyazawa K, Sato S, et al. Diffusion-weighted MRI abnormalities as an early diagnostic marker for Creutzfeldt-Jakob disease. *Neurology.* 2004;63:443–449.
12. Zerr I, Pocchiari M, Collins S, et al. Analysis of EEG and CSF 14–3–3 proteins as aids to the diagnosis of Creutzfeldt-Jakob disease. *Neurology.* 2000;55:811–815.
13. Byrne EJ, Lennox G, Lowe J, Godwin-Austin RB. Diffuse Lewy body disease: clinical features in 15 cases. *J Neurol Neurosurg Psychiatry.* 1989;52:709–717.
14. Yamamoto T, Imai T. A case of diffuse Lewy body and Alzheimer's diseases with periodic synchronous discharges. *J Neuropathol Exp Neurol.* 1988;47:536–548.
15. Ragno M, Scarcella MG, Cacchio G, et al. Striatal [123I] FP-CIT SPECT demonstrates dopaminergic deficit in a sporadic case of Creutzfeldt-Jakob disease. *Acta Neurol Scand.* 2009;119:131–134.
16. Walker Z, Costa DC, Walker RW, et al. Differentiation of dementia with Lewy bodies from Alzheimer's disease using a dopaminergic presynaptic ligand. *J Neurol Neurosurg Psychiatry.* 2002;73:134–140.
17. Yoshita M, Taki J, Yamada M. A clinical role for I-123 MIBG myocardial scintigraphy in the distinction between dementia of the Alzheimer's-type and dementia with Lewy bodies. *J Neurol Neurosurg Psychiatry.* 2001;71:583–588.

34

Stereotypic Movements in a Nurse Referred for the Evaluation of Parkinson's Disease

PATRICK HICKEY AND MARK STACY

THE CASE

SD is a 51-year-old woman originally from New Zealand who has spent the last 20 years in the United States as an infant care nurse. In the early 1990s, she was attacked by the mother of a patient, an incident that caused her significant emotional distress. She was eventually diagnosed with post-traumatic stress disorder and started on medication. In the initial interview, she has acknowledged always feeling somewhat depressed, even as a child, although she was never treated for depression until after this event.

Our patient has continued to struggle with depression and chronic pain over the years and has also been diagnosed with fibromyalgia. She recalls a number of medication trials for mood and pain, including methylphenidate, fluoxetine, sertraline, trazodone, escitalopram, duloxetine, citalopram, mirtazapine, aripiprazole, bupropion, quetiapine, atomoxetine, desipramine, desvenlafaxine, fluvoxamine, and lithium. Most of these medications were taken for 2 to 4 weeks before switching to an alternative agent due to lack of effect. In addition, she believes she has taken haloperidol and risperidone and other antipsychotic medications.

A few years ago, she began having "trouble moving" at work. Her walk has become slower, and she feels "stiff" when trying to perform her nursing duties. Turning around has also become "cumbersome" as she has to make a slow, complete rotation to look backward. She has the tendency to fall backward (retropulsion), although she has had no falls. A resting tremor in her right hand has emerged and intermittent, spontaneous extension of her neck (retrocollis). No increased pain is associated with these symptoms, although they do impact her work. In addition, both she and her husband have noticed the onset of two new stereotypic activities: she tends to rock to and fro when sitting and makes humming noises when concentrating.

Four months ago, she was evaluated by an outside neurologist and was diagnosed with Parkinson's disease (PD) and started on carbidopa/levodopa 25/100 mg twice daily. Since this time, she feels that her tremor has somewhat improved, although she continues to have difficulty with balance and involuntary movements. She denies worsening of her neck posture or stereotypic utterances or rocking.

Her medical history is significant for depression, hypertension, and hypercholesterolemia, which are treated with oral medications. She has had a total abdominal hysterectomy, cholecystectomy, and a left carpel tunnel release. She denies using tobacco, alcohol, or illicit drugs and exposure to toxins or head trauma. She is married without children and employed as an infant care nurse at a local hospital.

Our patient is a well-nourished female in no acute distress. She is able to provide her medical history. Her vital signs and general physical examination are unremarkable. She was able to name, repeat, follow commands, and perform calculations and extractions without difficulty. Ophthalmoscopy did not reveal a Kaiser-Fleisher ring. Her visual fields and extraocular movements were full; facial movements were symmetric, and hearing was intact to voice. Bulbar musculature examination was unremarkable. No abnormal head posture was noted. At rest, she rocks to and fro and makes occasional humming noises throughout the evaluation. She displays moderate hypomimia and mild hypophonia. No tremor is appreciated, although there is mild cogwheel rigidity at the wrists bilaterally. With finger tapping, pronation or supination, and heel tapping, she has mild bradykinesia on the left. She can arise slowly from a chair with her arms crossed, and her posture is upright. She has good stride length and height, although with an exaggerated arm swing. There is a mild degree of postural instability and body bradykinesia. Her sensory, coordination, and reflex examination is unremarkable.

THE APPROACH

PD is typified by a combination of slowed voluntary actions (bradykinesia), rigidity, resting tremor, and a loss of postural reflexes, a phenotype that is referred to clinically as parkinsonism (1). However, parkinsonism does not necessarily imply PD. In a pathologic study of 100 consecutive cases with a diagnosis of PD based on neurologic evaluation, 24 were found to have an alternate diagnosis at autopsy (2). This finding was replicated in a clinical study of 1,528 patients with parkinsonism, where more than 25% were found to have diagnoses not consistent with PD (3). Drug-induced parkinsonism (DIP) is a common cause, second only to PD, and comprises nearly 7% of all patients referred to a movement disorders center for parkinsonism (Table 34.1) (4,5).

Several groups that are more susceptible to DIP, including women (5), increasing age (6), patients with HIV (7), and those with existing extrapyramidal disorders (2), head injuries, dementia, or family history of PD (4) have been identified. Misdiagnosis in the elderly is especially common and frequently leads to additional medications being added to treat DIP symptoms as opposed to stopping the offending medication (5). This is not a trivial consequence given the potential morbidity of dopaminergic medications, especially in this population.

DIP is classically thought of as a dose-related effect of long-term exposure to traditional antipsychotic medications or antinausea medication, also termed dopamine receptor blocking drugs (DRBD). The exact mechanism of action for DRBDs is not known, although most antipsychotics work by inhibiting dopamine transmission and by binding D2 receptors in the basal ganglia with a higher affinity than dopamine or other agents (8). Because of this, it is believed that DIP results from blockade of D2 receptors, which may account for its high association with these medications (4). However, numerous drugs, including antiemetics, antidepressants, calcium channel blockers, and dopamine-depleting agents (6,7), have been implicated in producing similar effects.

Atypical antipsychotics also modify dopamine transmission, although they transiently occupy D_2 receptors and then rapidly dissociate, possibly allowing resumption of normal neurophysiology (the "fast-off D_2" theory) (9). In addition to lower affinity for dopamine receptors, strong blockade of central serotonergic and cholinergic receptors may also account for their reduced risk of extrapyramidal side effects (EPS) (8). Atypical antipsychotics convey a risk of EPS of about half that of typical agents, even in high-risk populations (10). Clozapine and quetiapine offer the lowest risk of EPS, with olanzapine and ziprasidone being better tolerated than higher dose risperidone (11). In addition, low-dose clozapine significantly improved PD-associated psychosis without worsening parkinsonism in one study (12).

Up to 60% of those exposed to DRBD will develop some degree of EPS, about one quarter of whom will experience DIP (13). In some instances, DRBD have been postulated to "unmask" underlying nigral dopaminergic dysfunction, causing symptoms in patients predisposed to parkinsonism. In these instances, patients may not improve on cessation of the offending agent (14,15). Recent genome-wide association studies have identified a number of promising candidate genes that may confer an inherent susceptibility to the development of DIP (16,17). Further genomic studies may help identify other important genetic factors.

The symptoms of DIP typically occur in a rapidly progressive fashion on exposure to a causative agent, and the majority will develop symptoms of dystonia or stereotypy within 3 weeks (18).

TABLE 34.1
Drugs Implicated in Causing Parkinsonism.

Neuroleptics	Cardiac	Chemotherapeutics
Thioridazine	Amiodarone	5-Fluorouracil
Promethazine	Methyldopa	Doxorubicin
Fluphenazine	Flunarizine	Vincristine
Mesoridazine	Cinnarizine	Tamoxifen
Trifluoperazine	Trimetazidine	Thalidomide
Chlorpromazine	Reserpine	Cyclosporine
Thiethylperazine		
Veralipride	*Other*	*Antiepileptics*
Perphenazine	Tetrabenazine	Valproic acid
Haloperidol		Pregabalin
Thiothixene	*Psychiatric*	
Molindone	SSRIs	*Antibiotics*
Loxapine	TCAs	Trimethoprim-sulfamethoxazole
Ziprasidone	MAO Inhibitors	
Aripiprazole	Bupropion	*Antifungals*
	Trazodone	Co-trimoxazole
Antiemetics	Lithium	Amphotericin B
Promethazine		
Prochlorperazine	*Hormones*	*Antivirals*
Metoclopramide	Synthroid	Vidarabine
Droperidol	Medroxyprogesterone	Acyclovir
Levosulpiride	Melatonin withdrawal	Antiretrovirals
Clebopride		
Cimetidine		

However, parkinsonism may take several months to develop in some cases (4). Motor symptoms can mimic classic PD and, at times, can be clinically indistinguishable. Rigidity, bradykinesia, tremor, and postural instability have all been described in relation to DIP; however, some features may help the clinician distinguish between the two.

Although often thought of as presenting symmetrically, between 46% and 64% patients with DIP will have noticeable asymmetry in their examination (19,20). Tremor tends to be less prevalent than rigidity, although it can be quite prominent in some. Upper extremity postural tremor is frequently as conspicuous as the classic pill-rolling and chin tremor of PD, and an action component is also common (20). Upward of 33% of patients with DIP will have postural instability, which often presents earlier than in PD (20). Concurrent orofacial and limb dyskinesias and tardive akathisia are present in 48% to 60% of those exposed to DRBD and can serve as a helpful indicator of DIP (5,18). Freezing of gait is rare, affecting less than 3% patients with DIP (18).

Many patients will not report disability as a result of drug-induced EPS (20); however, significant cognitive dysfunction, including impaired information processing capacity, has been shown to impact negatively on quality of life (21). These nonmotor symptoms can occur earlier than motor dysfunction in many.

Imaging studies are typically normal in DIP and that holds true for quantitative analysis of the dopamine transporter (DaT). ^{123}I-FP-CIT is a radioligand specific for DaT, which is located at presynaptic striatal dopaminergic terminals and serves as a marker to detect their functional loss (22). In a study of 57 patients who developed parkinsonism after exposure to a DRBA, 32 were eventually found to have DIP (23). ^{123}I-FP-CIT SPECT images were normal in more than 90% of these patients showing a high predictive value in differentiating DIP from PD unmasked by antidopaminergic medication.

THE LESSON

DIP is frequently indistinguishable from PD by clinical examination alone, especially on first encounter with a new patient. In our case, the presence of stereotypic rocking and humming provided a strong suspicion to search for previous treatment with DRBDs. Without a careful history and review of medications, this often leads to erroneous diagnoses, additional medications, and increased morbidity to the patient. Cessation of the causative agent can result in rapid improvement in symptoms and is typically the best treatment for DIP.

REFERENCES

1. Stacy M. Medical treatment of Parkinson disease. *Neurol Clin.* 2009;27:605–631.
2. Hughes AJ, Daniel SE, Kilford L, et al. Accuracy of clinical diagnosis of idiopathic Parkinson's disease: a clinico-pathological study of 100 cases. *J Neurol Neurosurg Psychiatry.* 1992;55:181–184.
3. Munhoz RP, Werneck LC, Teive HA. The differential diagnoses of parkinsonism: findings from a cohort of 1528 patients and a 10 years comparison in tertiary movement disorders clinics. *Clin Neurol Neurosurg.* 2010;112:431–435.
4. Thanvi B, Treadwell S. Drug induced parkinsonism: a common cause of parkinsonism in older people. *Postgrad Med J.* 2009;85:322–326.
5. Esper CD, Factor SA. Failure of recognition of drug-induced parkinsonism in the elderly. *Mov Disord.* 2008;23:401–404.
6. Wenning GK, Kiechl S, Seppi K, et al. Prevalence of movement disorders in men and women aged 50–89 years (Bruneck Study cohort): a population-based study. *Lancet Neurol.* 2005;4:815–820.
7. Alvarez MV, Evidente VG. Understanding drug-induced parkinsonism: separating pearls from oysters. *Neurology.* 2008;70:e32–e34.
8. Dolder CR, Jeste DV. Incidence of tardive dyskinesia with typical versus atypical antipsychotics in very high risk patients. *Biol Psychiatry.* 2003;53:1142–1145.
9. Lera G, Zirulnik J. Pilot study with clozapine in patients with HIV-associated psychosis and drug-induced parkinsonism. *Mov Disord.* 1999;14:128–131.
10. Seeman P. Atypical antipsychotics: mechanism of action. *Can J Psychiatry.* 2002;47:27–38.
11. Tarsy D, Baldessarini RJ, Tarazi FI. Effects of newer antipsychotics on extrapyramidal function. *CNS Drugs.* 2002;16:23–45.
12. Janno S, Holi M, Tuisku K, et al. Prevalence of neuroleptic-induced movement disorders in chronic schizophrenia inpatients. *Am J Psychiatry.* 2004;161:160–163.
13. Alkelai A, Greenbaum L, Rigbi A, et al. Genome-wide association study of antipsychotic-induced parkinsonism severity among schizophrenia patients. *Psychopharmacology.* 2009;206:491–499.
14. Melamed E, Achiron A, Shapira A, et al. Persistent and progressive parkinsonism after discontinuation of chronic neuroleptic therapy: an additional tardive syndrome? *Clin Neuropharmacol.* 1991;14:273–278.
15. Burn DJ, Brooks DJ. Nigral dysfunction in drug-induced parkinsonism: an 18F-dopa PET study. *Neurology.* 1993;43(3 Pt 1):552–556.
16. Greenbaum L, Smith RC, Rigbi A, et al. Further evidence for association of the *RGS2* gene with antipsychotic-induced parkinsonism: protective role of a functional polymorphism in the 3'-untranslated region. *Pharmacogenomics J.* 2009;9:103–110.
17. Hirose G. Drug induced parkinsonism: a review. *J Neurol.* 2006;253(Suppl 3):iii/22–24.
18. Hardie RJ, Lees AJ. Neuroleptic-induced Parkinson's syndrome: clinical features and results of treatment with levodopa. *J Neurol Neurosurg Psychiatry.* 1988;51:850–854.
19. Arblaster LA, Lakie M, Mutch WJ, et al. A study of the early signs of drug induced parkinsonism. *J Neurol Neurosurg Psychiatry.* 1993;56:301–303.
20. Hassin-Baer S, Sirota P, Korczyn AD. Clinical characteristics of neuroleptic-induced parkinsonism. *J Neural Transm.* 2001;108:1299–1308.
21. Kim JH, Byun HJ. Non-motor cognitive-perceptual dysfunction associated with drug-induced parkinsonism. *Hum Psychopharmacol.* 2009;24:129–133.
22. Scherfler C, Schwarz J, Antonini A. Role of DAT-SPECT in the diagnostic work up of parkinsonism. *Mov Disord.* 2007;22:1229–1238.
23. Diaz-Corrales FJ, Sanz-Viedma S, Garcia-Solis D, et al. Clinical features and 123I-FP-CIT SPECT imaging in drug-induced parkinsonism and Parkinson's disease. *Eur J Nucl Med Mol Imaging.* 2010;37:556–564.

35

Familial Albers-Schonberg's Disease (Osteopetrosis) Complicated by Dystonia and Dopa-Resistant Parkinsonism

MICHELLE FERREIRA AND NÉSTOR GÁLVEZ-JIMÉNEZ

THE CASE

Our patient is a 47-year-old school teacher initially evaluated in the mid 1990s when she came to see one of the authors (NG-J) because of a progressive 2-year history of a painful left shoulder and intermittent left hand tremors, which were initially diagnosed as "frozen shoulder." Months after her diagnosis, she endured multiple injuries to her back and head after being attacked on school grounds. Days after the injury, she developed frequent falls, stiffness of the left side of her body, and difficulty walking upstairs. Over a period of several months, her symptoms worsened, becoming slow and deliberate, with marked unsteadiness, frequent falls, left leg stiffness, and loss of left manual dexterity. Her falls were sudden and associated with the feeling of "being pulled or pushed," resulting in significant bone and soft tissue injuries. Masked facies and a dystonic (striatal) left hand later developed. The patient's medical and family history was remarkable for mild osteopetrosis in both the patient and her mother, a diagnosis initially made at the National Institute of Health 30 years before presentation. In addition, her mother recently developed a "no-no" head tremor and postural hand tremors bilaterally whose phenomenology was in keeping with that seen in patients with essential tremor.

THE APPROACH

Because of the rapid progression of symptoms, particularly the development of tremor, bradykinesia, rigidity, and imbalance, an MRI of the brain was performed to exclude anatomical or structural lesion causing secondary parkinsonism, especially with the background of multiple falls and injuries to her body. Bilateral posterior-ventral pallidal hyperintensities in the proton-weighted MR images suggestive of early calcification were found (Figure 35.1). At this point, we were intrigued by her previous diagnosis of mild osteopetrosis and the possible relationship between osteopetrosis and her new symptoms.

We performed lumbosacral and hand x-rays that demonstrated increased bone density, consistent with the diagnosis of osteopetrosis (Figures 35.2 and 35.3). Routine laboratory work, including blood cell and platelet count, hemoglobin and hematocrit, electrolytes, renal and liver functions, calcium, and phosphorus levels, was normal. Serum ceruloplasmin and copper, 24-hour urinary copper excretion along with a slit lamp and dilated eye examination, were normal. We performed Tc-99 134 single photon emission computed tomography (SPECT) and fluorodeoxyglucose (FDG) positron emission tomography (PET) scans, which demonstrated asymmetric decreased uptake in the right frontal, anterior parietal, and upper temporal areas, which are commonly seen in patients with parkinsonism. Neither her parkinsonian symptomatology nor her hand dystonia improved with trihexyphenidyl alone or in combination with carbidopa or levodopa, despite high doses.

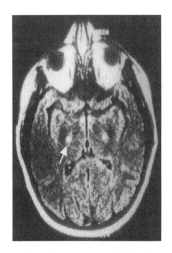

FIGURE 35.1
MRI of the brain demonstrated bilateral pallidal increased signal intensity in the proton-weighted imaging suggestive of early calcification (arrow).

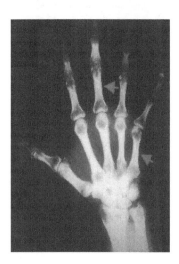

FIGURE 35.2
Lumbosacral and hand x-rays demonstrated increased bone density (arrows).

THE LESSON

We present a woman with osteopetrosis complicated by dystonia, dopa-resistant parkinsonism, and basal ganglia calcifications. Osteopetrosis is a rare familial autosomal bone disorder characterized by increase in bone density due to dysfunctional osteoclastic activity, reabsorption, and remodeling. The infantile form may be characterized by hepatosplenomegaly, anemia occasionally requiring blood transfusions, and entrapment syndromes such as optic nerve atrophy, deafness, and hydrocephalus. Radiologically, patients demonstrate increased bone density of the

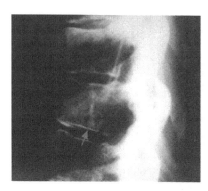

FIGURE 35.3
Lumbosacral and hand x-rays demonstrated increased bone density (arrow).

cortical laminae, which was seen in our patient's lumbosacral and hand x-rays. Our patient had the milder adult form of this disease, which usually presents with recurrent fractures because of increased bone fragility and hypersplenism resulting in anemia and thrombocytopenia. Patients with osteopetrosis and renal tubular acidosis (RTA) with carbonic anhydrase II (CAII) deficiency (autosomal recessive) have added features of hyperchloremic metabolic acidosis, normal to decreased serum potassium, increased urinary pH, and bicarbonate urinary loss. Asymptomatic calcifications of the basal ganglia have been described in adults with this syndrome. However, dystonia and parkinsonism have not been previously reported.

Basal ganglia calcifications may be found in ~0.4% to 0.6% of brain computed tomography (CT) scans of otherwise asymptomatic elderly individuals (1). According to Hume-Adams, a mild degree of calcification in and around blood vessels in the lentiform nucleus, less frequently in the hippocampus, dentate nucleus, and striate cortex, is an incidental pathologic finding, without associated symptoms, in elderly brains (2). The heaviest calcifications are found in the globus pallidus, putamen, caudate nucleus, internal capsule, thalamus, and dentate nuclei of the cerebellum. Some of these patients may have psychiatric or behavioral symptoms such as depression but others may have parkinsonism, chorea, and dystonia. Among the many causes of basal ganglia calcifications, hypoparathyroidism ranks as one of the most common causes of such radiologic findings (3,4). Patients with hypoparathyroidism may have a constellation of symptoms, including rest tremor, bradykinesia, rigidity, postural instability, chorea, dementia, and ideomotor apraxia (1) (see Table 35.1) (3–5).

Osteopetrosis has been reported as a cause of asymptomatic basal ganglia calcifications (1,6–8). Most severe cases present in the pediatric age group with symptoms related to organomegaly, anemia, and entrapment caused by bone growth and recurrent fractures. The combination of rental tubular acidosis, carbonic anhydrase deficiency, and osteopetrosis with hyperchloremic metabolic acidosis has also been reported in adults with asymptomatic basal ganglia calcifications (5,8,9). Other neurologic abnormalities reported in osteopetrosis include syringohydromyelia, optic nerve atrophy, deafness, and hydrocephalus.

Three different structural mutations have been identified in patients with carbonic anhydrase deficiency and osteopetrosis. These include a missense mutation in two families, a splice junction mutation in intron 5 in one of these families, a splice junction mutation in intron 2 for homozygous Arabic families, and a single base deletion in exon 7 in Caribbean Hispanics.

Our patient has the adult milder form of osteopetrosis with the unusual association of focal dystonia and an akinetic-rigid syndrome resistant to levodopa treatment. Her brain MRI demonstrated bilateral posterior-ventral putaminal calcifications along with FDG-PET evidence of

TABLE 35.1
Causes for Basal Ganglia Calcifications.

Idiopathic

Hypoparathyroidism

Pseudohypoparathyroidism

Infections (toxoplasmosis, rubella, CMV, cysticercosis, AIDS)

Familial striatopallidal calcification (Fahr's disease)

Birth anoxia

Small vessel ischemic vascular disease with microhemorrhages (i.e., PRES, chronic hypertension, and hypertensive encephalopathy)

Microencephaly

CO intoxication

Cockayne's syndrome

Mitochondrial cytopathies

Tuberous sclerosis

Lead poisoning

Calcification of the substantia nigra

Down syndrome

Familial encephalopathies

CMV, cytomegalovirus; PRES, posterior reversible encephalopathy syndrome; CO, carbon monoxide.

decreased uptake in the contralateral prefrontal, anterior-parietal, and a parietotemporal area akin to what is usually seen in patients with idiopathic Parkinson's disease. Lesions in the basal ganglia, thalamus, and other related structures are known to be responsible for a variety of movement disorders. Therefore, it is likely that her dystonia and parkinsonian symptoms are related to the basal ganglia calcifications. Reported cases of basal ganglia calcifications, especially in patients with hypoparathyroidism, have been reported to produce an akinetic-rigid syndrome (1,4,10).

In conclusion, osteopetrosis, a systemic carbonic anhydrase deficiency disease, with RTA and hyperchloremic metabolic acidosis, may result in symptomatic basal ganglia calcifications. This condition should be included under the causes of symptomatic parkinsonism and dystonia.

REFERENCES

1. Gálvez-Jiménez N, Hanson MR, Cabral J. Dopa-resistant parkinsonism, oculomotor disturbances, chorea, mirror movements, dyspraxia, and dementia: the expanding clinical spectrum of hypoparathyroidism. A case report. *Mov Disord.* 2000;15:1273–1276.
2. Adams JH, Corsellis AN, Duchen LW, eds. *Adams Greenfield's Neuropathology.* New York, NY: Wiley, 1984.
3. Rossi M, Morena M, Zanardi M. Calcification of the basal ganglia and Fahr disease. Report of two clinical cases and review of the literature. *Recenti Prog Med.* 1993;84:192–198.
4. Verulashvili IV, Glonti LSh, Miminoshvili DK, et al. Basal ganglia calcification: clinical manifestations and diagnostic evaluation. *Georgian Med News.* 2006:39–43.
5. Patel PJ. Some rare causes of intracranial calcification in childhood: computed tomographic findings. *Eur J Pediatr.* 1987;146:177–180.

6. Cumming WA, Ohlsson A. Intracranial calcification in children with osteopetrosis caused by carbonic anhydrase II deficiency. *Radiology.* 1985;157:325–327.
7. Harrington MG, Macpherson P, McIntosh WB, et al. The significance of the incidental finding of basal ganglia calcification on computed tomography. *J Neurol Neurosurg Psychiatry.* 1981;44:1168–1170.
8. Ohlsson A, Cumming WA, Paul A, et al. Carbonic anhydrase II deficiency syndrome: recessive osteopetrosis with renal tubular acidosis and cerebral calcification. *Pediatrics.* 1986;77:371–381.
9. Whyte MP, Murphy WA, Fallon MD, et al. Osteopetrosis, renal tubular acidosis and basal ganglia calcification in three sisters. *Am J Med.* 1980;69:64–74.
10. Vega MG, de Sousa AA, de Lucca Júnior F, et al. Extrapyramidal syndrome and hypoparathyroidism. On the identity of Fahr disease. *Arq Neuropsiquiatr.* 1994;52:419–426.

III

Tremors

36

Not "X"-actly a Simple Tremor

HAITHAM M. HUSSEIN, MATTHEW A. BOWER, AND PAUL J. TUITE

I was recently asked by a colleague to evaluate a 63-year-old man with a 16-year history of neurologic symptoms, including tremor, gait difficulty, and cognitive decline. The patient was accompanied to clinic by his wife of 28 years. When I asked him why he had come to me for an evaluation, he indicated that he was concerned about having an inherited condition. Previously, his neurologic findings had been attributed to moderate alcohol consumption and occupational exposures in his work as a chemist and as a furniture maker.

I turned our conversation to the patient's neurologic history. He first noticed a lack of stamina, which manifested as a decline in his cycling abilities, at age 46. In the same year, he developed a rhythmic hand tremor. At first, the tremor was intermittent and task specific. He reported difficulty in approaching targets such that when he brushed his teeth, he would hit his nose with his toothbrush. His handwriting became difficult to read, and he would spill beverages when holding a cup. While caffeine and anxiety aggravated his tremor, alcohol did not provide benefit. He was diagnosed with essential tremor and treated with propranolol up to 120 mg daily. After initial improvement, his symptoms recurred several months later.

Three years later, his gait became unsteady such that he began bumping into doors and walls. His imbalance was pronounced in darkness. A few years later, he started falling. Initially, falls were infrequent, but within 7 years of onset, he was falling one to two times per month. He always felt that his left leg was less coordinated than the right. He noticed that initially he could tap his right foot rhythmically while playing the clarinet but could never follow a rhythm with the left foot.

Seven years after symptom onset, he was referred to a neurologist who also thought he had essential tremor, especially after learning that his mother developed a similar tremor at the age of 55 years. His neurologic examination at that time showed a peripheral neuropathy (confirmed on nerve conduction studies) and cerebellar findings, which his neurologist attributed to alcohol intake because no clear cause could be found (he had been consuming one glass of wine with dinner three to four nights a week). Laboratory studies and brain MRI were normal. The patient tried multiple medications without lasting benefit.

Over the next 3 years, he had increasing accidents while engaged in his woodworking business. He stopped riding bicycles. His speech became slow and interrupted. Ten years after the onset of symptoms, he underwent left thalamic deep brain stimulation (DBS) implantation, which improved his right-hand shaking such that he could continue woodworking. However, his gait did not improve. He also continued to have difficulty with fine movements and dexterity. His tremor returned 5 years after DBS surgery. Because of his lack of coordination, he stopped woodworking and started a computer-based business.

Twelve years after onset, the patient began noticing difficulty with cognition. Initially, he noticed a decline in retention from reading. He lost the ability to multitask such that he was no longer able to perform activities while talking to people. He became more reliant on calendars and notes. Family and friends noticed that he would repeat himself. His ability to make calculations worsened; however, he could still balance his checkbook and pay bills. He became more irritable. He did not have any difficulty with comprehension or expression. A neuropsychological evaluation showed impairment in memory and executive functions. The patient's medical history was otherwise noncontributory.

After obtaining the patient's medical history, I examined him. He scored 22 of 26 on the Montreal Cognitive Assessment. Although his tremor prevented him from performing drawing tasks, he performed well on attention measures. He had difficulty with recall. His speech was slow and deliberate with a staccato quality. Muscle appearance, tone, and power were normal, and he had a high-frequency, high-amplitude postural hand tremor. He had great difficulty drawing the Archimedes' spiral because of tremulousness (Figure 36.1). Finger-to-nose and heel-to-shin tests demonstrated decomposition of movement and dysmetria. He also had dysdiadochokinesia and nonrhythmical finger and foot tapping. His incoordination was slightly worse on the left side. On sensory examination, he had glove and stocking hypoesthesia to pin prick and reduced vibration at the toes. Deep tendon reflexes were lost in ankles, knees, and brachioradialis. Trace biceps reflexes were elicited with facilitation. Plantars were flexor bilaterally. Romberg was positive. His gait was wide based, and he could not stand with feet together even with eyes open. He could not sit upright with arms folded in front of his chest without back support.

THE APPROACH

I thought that this man must have a multifocal disorder that involves central (extrapyramidal system causing tremor; cerebellum causing ataxia; cortical/subcortical causing cognitive impairment) and peripheral (length-dependent large fiber polyneuropathy) nervous systems. It was clear that the dual diagnosis of essential tremor- and alcohol-induced neuropathy and cerebellar syndrome was not enough to explain progression of symptoms despite cessation of alcohol for 10 years. The occupational exposures to benzene, acrylamide, chloroform, and methanol was brief and did not temporally correlate with his symptoms. The progressive course of his illness suggested a neurodegenerative process was the culprit. Friedreich's ataxia was unlikely given the late onset and absence of accompanying cardiac involvement, scoliosis, and diabetes. Spinocerebellar ataxia 19 (SCA19) was a better fit with cognitive impairment, hyporeflexia, and ataxia; however, onset is typically younger, and the neuropathy is very mild or not existent. The diagnosis of dentatorubral-pallidoluysian atrophy was considered, but usually individuals

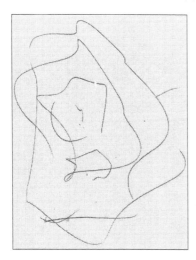

FIGURE 36.1
Archimedes' spiral attempted by patient. Instead of the typical rhythmical shakiness seen by essential tremor patients, this drawing shows gross inaccuracies, which are more in keeping with cerebellar impairments.

manifest with chorea, seizures, and myoclonus in addition to ataxia. Primary progressive multiple sclerosis seemed an unlikely cause because the patient had a normal MRI 7 years prior and the peripheral neuropathy is not a finding. Inherited metabolic conditions such as ceroid lipofuscinosis or 3-methylglutaconic aciduria seemed unlikely because of the late age of onset. Multiple system atrophy (MSA)—cerebellar subtype—was another possibility; however, the presence of a family history prompted us to consider an inherited condition that could mimic MSA.

Mutations in the fragile X mental retardation 1 (*FMR1*) gene were first described in male children with severe mental retardation (1). On the basis of the classic cytogenetic finding of a fragile site involving chromosome band Xq27, the condition was initially termed "fragile X syndrome." The underlying genetic mechanism of the fragile X syndrome is the expansion of an unstable CGG repeat in the promoter region of the *FMR1* gene. Expansions ≥200 CGG repeats lead to methylation and subsequent silencing of the *FMR1* gene, resulting in the typical fragile X syndrome phenotype (severe mental retardation, macroorchidism, and mitral valve prolapse). In the past, carriers of intermediate number of repeats in the *FMR1* gene (55–200 repeats)—termed "premutation carriers"—were believed to be asymptomatic (1). Recently, it has been recognized that premutation carriers can manifest alternative phenotypes. Female premutation carriers were first noted to have premature ovarian failure (2). Later reports identified a neurodegenerative syndrome in the maternal grandfathers of classic fragile X syndrome probands (3). The neurodegenerative phenotype is characterized by action tremor, gait ataxia, memory impairment, executive dysfunction, neuropathy, autonomic failure, and parkinsonism—fragile X tremor ataxia syndrome (FXTAS). It has since been documented that neurologic findings may be present in both male and female premutation carriers (4). This seemed to fit our patient best!

THE LESSON

Three additional pieces of information helped establish the diagnosis in our unique case:

- His previous brain MRI had been reported as normal, but no MRI had been performed in more than 7 years because of the presence of a DBS lead. With the use of a "send and receive" head coil, it was possible to demonstrate classic MRI findings (5) of FXTAS (Figure 36.2).
- A detailed review of a four-generation pedigree provided crucial information (Figure 36.3).
- Finally, genetic testing confirmed the diagnosis. Polymerase chain reaction and Southern analysis demonstrated the presence of an unmethylated premutation *FMR1* allele with 98 CGG repeats (Figure 36.4).

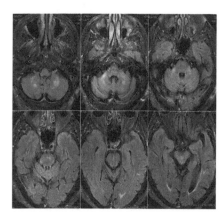

FIGURE 36.2
Brain MRI. Fluid attenuated inversion recovery (FLAIR) sequence showing white matter T2 hyperintensity signal changes in bilateral cerebellar peduncles along with cerebellar and cerebral white matter. There is also diffuse brain volume loss.

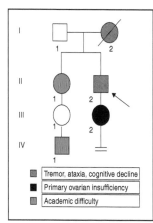

FIGURE 36.3

Family pedigree. The patient (indicated by arrow) reported that his mother (individual I-2) had dementia, gait imbalance, and a tremor at 55 years of age, which was thought to be due to normal pressure hydrocephalus or Alzheimer disease. Although a shunt briefly improved symptoms, symptoms recurred and progressed after 1 month. She eventually became bed bound and died at the age of 90 years. Per the patient's report, his mother had cerebellar atrophy by MRI. In addition, the patient's 25-year-old daughter (individual III-2) developed early menopause related to primary ovarian insufficiency, which has been reported in female carriers of FMR1 premutations (3). The patient's sister (individual II-1) had struggled in school, whereas the patient's great nephew (individual IV-1) was being evaluated for developmental delays.

■ Tremor, ataxia, cognitive decline
■ Primary ovarian insufficiency
■ Academic difficulty

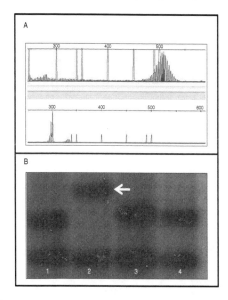

FIGURE 36.4

Molecular genetic analysis of the FMR1 gene. (A) PCR analysis of the CGG repeat of the FMR1 gene. Top panel: patient's results show a PCR product in excess of 500 base pairs, corresponding to an FMR1 allele with 98 CGG repeats. Bottom panel: normal control PCR reaction from a female with 29 and 39 CGG repeats. Note that all PCR products include 220 base pairs of non-CGG repeat DNA. (B) Southern blot analysis of the CGG repeat region of the FMR1 gene using ECOR1 restriction enzyme and the methylation-sensitive BSSHII restriction enzyme. From left to right: lanes 1,3,4 = normal males. Lane 2 = patient's FMR1 allele demonstrating larger band corresponding to the presence of an expanded and unmethylated FMR1 allele (white arrow).

I met with the patient and his wife several weeks after these evaluations were completed. After learning that he had FXTAS, they were immediately concerned about their daughter. The finding of a premutation in the *FMR1* gene meant that his daughter is an obligate carrier and that his sister and niece may also be carriers. On the other hand, this diagnosis finally liberated the patient from his guilt that alcohol use and occupational exposures caused his illness.

We learned several important lessons from our case:

❦ The combination of tremor and ataxia should raise suspicion of a neurodegenerative disease. Adding peripheral neuropathy shortened our differential diagnosis significantly.
❦ Seemingly unrelated findings in the family history (i.e., premature ovarian failure) may provide vital clues in establishing the correct diagnosis.
❦ Hereditary disorders profoundly impact patients and their families. When we make such diagnoses, we should be prepared to address how it affects families. Involvement of psychologists and genetic counselors may be appropriate before and after genetic testing.

REFERENCES

1. Fu YH, Kuhl DP, Pizzuti A, et al. Variation of the CGG repeat at the fragile X site results in genetic instability: resolution of the Sherman paradox. *Cell*. 1991;67:1047–1058.
2. Sherman SL. Premature ovarian failure in the fragile X syndrome. *Am J Med Genet*. 2000;97:189–194.
3. Hagerman RJ, Leehey M, Heinrichs W, et al. Intention tremor, parkinsonism, and generalized brain atrophy in male carriers of fragile X. *Neurology*. 2001;57:127–130.
4. Chonchaiya W, Nguyen DV, Au J, et al. Clinical involvement in daughters of men with fragile X-associated tremor ataxia syndrome. *Clin Genet*. 2010;78:38–46.
5. Cohen S, Masyn K, Adams J, et al. Molecular and imaging correlates of the fragile X-associated tremor/ataxia syndrome. *Neurology*. 2006;67:1426–1431.

Suggested Reading

Berry-Kravis E, Abrams L, Coffey SM, et al. Fragile X-associated tremor/ataxia syndrome: clinical features, genetics, and testing guidelines. *Mov Disord*. 2007;22:2018–2030.
Bourgeois JA, Coffey SM, Rivera SM, et al. A review of fragile X premutation disorders: expanding the psychiatric perspective. *J Clin Psychiatry*. 2009;70:852–862.
Grigsby J, Brega AG, Jacquemont S, et al. Impairment in the cognitive functioning of men with fragile X-associated tremor/ataxia syndrome (FXTAS). *J Neurol Sci*. 2006;248:227–233.
Hunter JE, Abramowitz A, Rusin M, et al. Is there evidence for neuropsychological and neurobehavioral phenotypes among adults without FXTAS who carry FMR1 premutation? A review of current literature. *Genet Med*. 2009;11:79–89.
Jacquemont S, Hagerman RJ, Leehey MA, et al. Penetrance of the fragile X-associated tremor/ataxia syndrome in a premutation carrier population. *JAMA*. 2004;291:460–469.
Leehey MA, Berry-Kravis E, Goetz CG, et al. FMR1 CGG repeat length predicts motor dysfunction in premutation carriers. *Neurology*. 2008;70:1397–1402.
Leehey MA, Berry-Kravis E, Min SJ, et al. Progression of tremor and ataxia in male carriers of the FMR1 premutation. *Mov Disord*. 2007;22:203–206.
Rodriguez-Revenga L, Madrigal I, Pagonabarraga J, et al. Penetrance of FMR1 premutation associated pathologies in fragile X syndrome families. *Eur J Human Genet*. 2009;17:1359–1362.
Strom CM, Crossley B, Redman JB, et al. Molecular testing for fragile X syndrome: lessons learned from 119,232 tests performed in a clinical laboratory. *Genet Med*. 2007;9:46–51.

37

The Tremulous Driver Who Could Not Find His Way Home

Ignacio Rubio-Agusti and Kailash Bhatia

THE CASE

When I met Mr TD, he was 58 years old, and he had quit his job as a professional lorry driver roughly 4 years earlier because of "neurologic problems."

His symptoms had started approximately 7 years before with shaking of his arms, particularly bothering for him not only when he was using his hands but also at rest. His tremor had got progressively worse over the years, and he had developed additional symptoms. He felt that his balance was poor; he often tripped and had suffered several falls. He also felt stiff and slow, particularly when rising from a chair and when walking. After consulting a neurologist, he had been started on levodopa, up to 600 mg a day. Several tests had been arranged, including a brain MRI, which had just shown some nonspecific T2 hyperintense lesions in the pons. He himself felt that levodopa was not helping much, but his wife thought he had improved to some extent.

His symptoms had continued to worsen, and he had developed some autonomic symptoms. He had actually had erectile dysfunction from the very beginning and was also troubled by urinary urgency, nocturia, and occasional urinary incontinence. At that point, he was taking 800 mg of levodopa, with no marked benefit, and he had been referred to our clinic with the suspicion of multiple system atrophy (MSA).

When I first saw him, in the company of his wife, I confirmed the previous history of a long-standing tremor and balance problems, including several falls and autonomic symptoms, mainly involving the genitourinary system. He also remarked that he occasionally felt dizzy when standing up and had in fact fainted on a couple of occasions.

I questioned them about his sleep, and his wife mentioned that he was a heavy "snorer" and often seemed to stop breathing at night. He frequently talked and even shouted while asleep, and on occasions, he had even fallen down from bed. He was also very sleepy during the day and often dozed off while watching television.

I also enquired about his memory. They did not have any complaints in this regard initially, but on further questioning about the reasons that had forced him to quit his job, his wife got very excited and explained to us how he had become easily distracted. He had got lost on several occasions while driving and had also caused a minor car accident.

He had no relevant medical or family history.

When I examined him, I found he had a marked arm tremor, which was present not only both at rest and on posture but also with action, while performing the finger-to-nose maneuver. His rest tremor was not the typical pill-rolling tremor seen in Parkinson's disease, but rather involved flexion and extension of the fingers. His eye movements were normal apart from saccadic pursuit. He had mildly slurred speech, but without the quivering and strained quality so typical of MSA. When assessing his rapid repetitive movements, I felt that he was certainly slow, but I could not convince myself of true fatiguing. There was, however, clear rigidity and a component of cogwheeling in the upper limbs. He had hypoactive reflexes, and his plantars were down going. He walked with widened base and was unable to tandem walk. When testing his postural reflexes, he had clear retropulsion. I also performed a very short cognitive test, which showed difficulties in attention and concentration and in temporal orientation.

THE APPROACH

Summing up, we had a male patient in his late fifties with a longstanding history of bilateral rest and postural tremor, slowness of movement, balance and gait difficulties, autonomic dysfunction, dream enacting and possibly sleep apnea, and a poor response to levodopa. Indeed, MSA seemed to be a strong possibility, but I felt uneasy about his cognitive problems, and I was also intrigued about the reported nonspecific findings in his previous MRI. Could it be the so-called "hot cross bun sign," so typical of MSA?

With all this in mind, we decided to admit him to perform several investigations.

We repeated some blood tests, including liver and renal function, thyroid function, electrolytes, including calcium and magnesium and of course copper and ceruloplasmin, all of which came back normal.

We also arranged formal cardiovascular autonomic testing, which was unrevealing, and he was assessed by a neuro-urologist, who attributed his symptoms to an overactive bladder and prescribed tolterodine and yohimbine for his erectile dysfunction.

He underwent a sleep study, which confirmed nocturnal hypoventilation, and was shortly afterward started on nocturnal ventilatory support with a continuous positive airway pressure device.

Because his myotatic reflexes were difficult to elicit, we also arranged nerve conduction studies and electromyography, but they showed no evidence of associated large fiber peripheral neuropathy.

He had formal neuropsychological testing, which disclosed cognitive impairment, with focal deficits in naming skills and poor performance on tests of speed and attention, consistent with subcortical and to a lesser extent cortical dominant temporal involvement.

A DaT scan was performed, showing good transport of tracer to both striata, with a fairly symmetrical distribution in the caudate and putamen, therefore ruling out presynaptic denervation (Figure 37.1).

We had also sent some genetic tests at that point for complicated spinocerebellar ataxias (SCA), for example, SCA 2 and 3. A fresh MRI brain scan had also been undertaken, and when we saw the results, we knew that none of these would be positive, but that another genetic test that we had sent was likely to be positive.

The new MRI showed cerebral and cerebellar atrophy and symmetric T2 hyperintense lesions in the middle cerebellar peduncles very suggestive of the "MCP sign" (Figure 37.2).

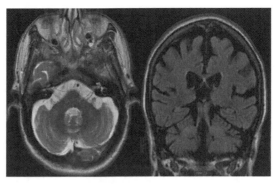

FIGURE 37.1
MRI scan showing cerebellar atrophy and symmetric hyperintense lesions in the middle cerebellar peduncles.

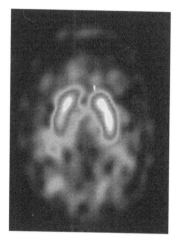

FIGURE 37.2
DAT scan showing symmetrical distribution of radio tracer.

A few weeks later, we received the report from the neurogenetic unit confirming the presence of 88 CGG repeats in the *FMR1* gene. Mr TD had the fragile X tremor ataxia syndrome (FXTAS).

THE LESSON

This patient had a longstanding history of tremor and slowness of movement resembling Parkinson's disease, but there were several atypical features, such as the poor response to levodopa, balance problems, and early autonomic dysfunction, which were suggesting MSA as an alternative diagnosis, and his sleeping problems also fitted very nicely with this (1,2). A more detailed history, however, revealed marked cognitive impairment, and that made us suspicious (1,2). Other conditions to keep in mind in this scenario included SCA 2 and 3 and FXTAS (3–5).

The presence of a normal DaT scan was very useful in this situation, making MSA, SCA2, and SCA3 unlikely (4–6).

FXTAS is a neurodegenerative disorder caused by a CGG repeat expansion in the premutation range (55–200) in the *FMR1* gene, whose mutation causes fragile X syndrome, the most common genetic cause for autism and mental retardation. It presents mainly in men with action tremor and gait ataxia, but the phenotype is very heterogeneous and may include parkinsonism, cognitive problems, mainly involving executive functions, autonomic symptoms, and peripheral neuropathy (3,7). Interestingly, these patients can have a normal DaT scan, even in the presence of clear parkinsonian signs (4). Imaging usually shows cerebral and cerebellar atrophy and white matter lesions, but the presence of symmetrical T2 hyperintensities in the middle cerebellar peduncles, a fairly frequent finding present in up to two thirds of male patients, is relatively specific (3,7). This case exemplifies the importance of reviewing previous scans yourself, whenever possible. A finding reported as nonspecific may turn out to be a relevant clue when placed in the adequate clinical context.

Nevertheless, the most important lesson to be learned from this case is to keep in mind what patients truly need: relief from their symptoms. Correctly diagnosing a genetic condition allows more accurate information regarding prognosis and genetic counseling, but in our case, it was much simpler things, such as prescribing tolterodine, yohimbine, and noninvasive ventilatory support, that actually improved Mr TD's quality of life, and none of these required any expensive or fancy genetic testing.

REFERENCES

1. Edwards M, Quinn N, Bhatia K. Multiple system atrophy. In: Edwards M, Quinn N, Bhatia K, eds. *Parkinson's Disease and Other Movement Disorders.* Oxford, UK: Oxford University Press, 2008:86–89.
2. Stefanova N, Bücke P, Duerr S, et al. Multiple system atrophy: an update. *Lancet Neurol.* 2009;8:1172–1178.
3. Leehey MA. Fragile X-associated tremor/ataxia syndrome: clinical phenotype, diagnosis, and treatment. *J Investig Med.* 2009;57:830–836.
4. Lastres-Becker I, Rüb U, Auburger G. Spinocerebellar ataxia 2 (SCA2). *Cerebellum.* 2008;7:115–124.
5. D'Abreu A, França MC Jr, Paulson HL, et al. Caring for Machado-Joseph disease: current understanding and how to help patients. *Parkinsonism Relat Disord.* 2010;16:2–7.
6. Kägi G, Bhatia KP, Tolosa E. The role of DAT-SPECT in movement disorders. *J Neurol Neurosurg Psychiatry* 2010;81:5–12
7. Edwards M, Quinn N, Bhatia K. Fragile X tremor-ataxia syndrome. In: Edwards M, Quinn N, Bhatia K, eds. *Parkinson's Disease and Other Movement Disorders.* Oxford, UK: Oxford University Press, 2008:246.

38

The Shaky Professor From India: A Tale of Tremors

AMANDA JANE THOMPSON

THE CASE

Our 63-year-old, right-handed university professor from northern India presented with an exacerbation of tremors originally diagnosed as benign essential tremor. His first symptom was shaky handwriting, which began 15 years ago. As his condition slowly worsened, he noticed a tremor of both the head and the hands, which was initially symmetric but, as years passed, became markedly worse in his left hand. The tremors were most notable with action or with activities requiring sustained posture. They made it difficult for him to perform fine motor tasks, including writing on the blackboard, typing, and correcting papers. Shortly thereafter, difficulties with cognition arose, including trouble with complex mathematics. He was diagnosed with mild cognitive impairment after a neuropsychological battery and decided to retire. After retirement, his gait became unstable, and he began having frequent falls. He reported a consistent feeling of imbalance and had difficulty moving from a sitting to a standing position without falling. He started using a cane or walker when he left his home. His most recent symptom was reported by his wife who complained that his speech was slurred in the evenings or when he was fatigued.

He had a medical history significant for ulcerative colitis, gastroesophageal reflux disease, hypertension, and diabetes mellitus. His medications included mesalamine, ranitidine, esomeprazole, olmesartan, and a multivitamin. He was married and lives with his wife. He had a PhD and master's degrees in mathematics and economics and retired as professor of environmental research. He drank alcohol three to four times weekly and reported that alcoholic beverages temporarily improved his tremors.

In the past, several medications were tried in an attempt to improve his tremors, including primidone, propranolol, clonazepam, carbidopa/levodopa, trihexyphenidyl, gabapentin, and levetiracetam. For a short while, he received some benefit from primidone but became intolerantly fatigued and discontinued it.

There was a strong family history of tremors and gait imbalance in his family, including his father and two paternal uncles who had resting and action tremors and frequent falling. His paternal grandfather was diagnosed with Parkinson's disease. His sister had mild gait instability.

Our general examination revealed no cardiopulmonary problems. He scored 27 of 30 on the Mini-Mental Status Examination, losing points for poor reversal and minimally impaired recall. He displayed re-emergence of primitive reflexes, showing a prominent suck reflex. Cranial nerve examination showed fragmented pursuit with saccadic intrusions. Strength testing was 5 out of 5 bilaterally, with no weakness, normal bulk, and mildly increased tone. He had brisk reflexes symmetrically and bilateral cross adductors and bilateral Babinski signs. A tremor rating scale was performed and showed a total motor score of 45. He did not have a face, tongue, or voice tremor. He had no right-arm tremor at rest but did have a moderate-amplitude postural and action tremor on the right side. On the left arm, he had a moderate-amplitude resting tremor and a marked postural tremor and moderate action tremor. He had no trunk or leg tremors. His handwriting was illegible. He had a great deal of difficulty tracing spirals and drawing straight lines. With both hands, he displayed a jagged and wild tremor, although he had considerably more difficulty with his left than his right hand. Cerebellar examination demonstrated marked dysmetria bilaterally on finger-to-nose testing. Rapid alternating movements were fairly regular but somewhat slow. His gait was mildly wide based, and he showed considerable staggering and difficulties with turning.

MRI of the brain showed punctate fluid-attenuated inversion recovery (FLAIR) hyperintensities consistent with small areas of microvascular ischemia and slight cerebral and cerebellar atrophy.

THE APPROACH

This pleasant, 63-year-old man of Indian descent had a long history of action tremors, much worse than postural tremors and gradual worsening of gait; examination confirmed resting and action tremor in addition to mild cerebellar signs. He also had slowly progressive cognitive impairment. He failed to see benefit from extensive pharmacologic treatment for his tremors, which included medications known to treat both essential tremor and Parkinson's disease.

The professor's strong family history of tremor and gait instability along with ataxia and marked tremor on his physical examination suggested an autosomal dominant tremor-ataxia syndrome. The constellation of clinical findings together with his South Asian descent led us to obtain a single genetic test: the one for a CAG expansion in the promoter sequence of the *PPP2R2B* gene. This revealed an expanded allele with 52 repeats and one normal allele. A diagnosis of spinocerebellar ataxia type 12 (SCA 12) was confirmed.

THE LESSON

SCA 12 is associated with a CAG repeat of the *PPP2R2B* gene on chromosome 5 (1). It is characterized by action and postural tremor of the upper extremities, which slowly progresses to include mild ataxia, hyperreflexia, parkinsonism, and dementia. The onset of symptoms ranges from childhood into the seventh decade but usually presents midlife. Brain imaging usually reveals mild global atrophy.

The action tremor is most prominent in the arms but can also be seen in the trunk, head, lips, and tongue (2). Cerebellar dysfunction is less prominent in SCA 12 than it is in the other SCAs, and individuals are usually able to remain employed throughout adulthood. SCA 12 does not impact longevity of life.

SCA 12 has been described in an American family of German descent (1) and several North Indian families. It is the second most common form of SCA in India behind SCA type 2 and is almost exclusively found in those of northern Indian descent (3,4). It should be considered in patients who develop action tremor of the hands in midlife who then go on to develop clinical symptoms of ataxia, hyperreflexia, parkinsonian features, and mild cerebellar dysfunction. The action tremor usually resembles an essential tremor, and some may respond to usual treatment with primidone or propranolol.

The differential diagnosis of SCA 12 is broad and should include essential tremor and the SCAs that are associated with an action tremor: SCA 2, SCA 3, SCA 6, and SCA 14. Multiple system atrophy could also mimic SCA 12, especially in those individuals with prominent parkinsonian symptoms such as bradykinesia and rigidity. The diagnosis is made by documenting the expansion of the CAG trinucleotide repeat in the *PPP2R2B* gene above the normal range of 32. Full penetrance is seen when the expansion reaches 51 repeats.

There are subtle differences between the American and Indian pedigrees. Individuals within the Indian pedigree have fewer parkinsonian features and more prominent cerebellar symptoms. American patients seem to have less severe cerebellar findings but are more prone to develop bradykinesia and cognitive impairment (5).

Our case of "The Shaky Professor" emphasizes the need for careful review of past medical records and reminds us that a longstanding diagnosis should be readdressed when conventional treatments have failed to improve symptoms.

REFERENCES

1. Holmes SE, O'Hearn EE, McInnis MG, et al. Expansion of a novel CAG trinucleotide repeat in the 5′ region of PPP2R2B is associated with SCA 12. *Nat Genet.* 1999;23:391–392.
2. Wadia NH, Sinha KK, Desai JD. Hereditary ataxia. In: Wadia NH, ed. *Neurological Practice: An Indian Perspective.* New Delhi: Elsevier, 2005:409–435.
3. Srivastava AK, Choudhry S, Gopinath MS, et al. Molecular and clinical correlation in five Indian families with spinocerebellar ataxia 12. *Ann Neurol.* 2001;50:796–800.
4. Bahl S, Virdi K, Mittal U, et al. Evidence of a common founder for SCA 12 in the Indian population. *Ann Hum Genet.* 2005;69:528–534.
5. Margolis RL, O'Hearn E, Holmes SE, et al. In: Pagon RA, Bird TC, Dolan CR, Stephens K, eds. *GeneReviews* [Internet]. Seattle, WA: University of Washington, 1993–2004. Accessed March 12, 2007.

Suggested Reading

Holmes SE, O'Hearn E, Brahmachari SK, et al. SCA 12. In: Pulst S, ed. *Genetics of Movement Disorders.* San Diego: Academic Press, 2002:121–132.
Holmes SE, O'Hearn E, Cortez-Apreza N, et al. Spinocerebellar ataxia 12 (SCA 12). In: Wells R, Azhizawa T, eds. *Genetic Instabilities and Neurologic Diseases.* San Diego: Academic Press, 2006.
Sinha KK. Spinocerebellar ataxia 12 (SCA 12). A tremor dominant disease, typically seen in India. In: *Medicine Update 2005.* Mumbai, India: Association of Physicians of India, 2005.

39

Early-Onset Hand Tremor and Later Adult Progression Without Speech Involvement: An Unusual DYT6 Presentation

JOSÉ C. CABASSA AND SUSAN B. BRESSMAN

THE CASE

This 63-year-old right-handed woman was first seen by us in 1984 at the age of 36 years for evaluation of dystonia. Her symptoms started at age 12 when she noted a mild tremor in her right hand, present with many activities. It did not interfere with daily activities, including writing, but was noted to worsen in certain positions, and she described a tight grip when holding a pen. She otherwise was in good health, and tremor was mild enough that she did not seek medical attention.

At age 34, she first noticed involuntary turning of her neck to the left, with associated neck, back, and left arm pain 6 months after she suffered a fall without head trauma, loss of consciousness, or other immediate sequelae. She was seen by a chiropractor and internist who considered her problems to be secondary to trauma and associated pain, and she received physical therapy and then propranolol and clorazepate with little improvement. By age 36, head turning progressed with a greater degree of turn and constant intensity and more disruption of her daily activities, such as reading and watching television; she was unable to drive. Because of continued pain, she consulted a neurosurgeon and was evaluated with a cervical computed tomography (CT) and electromyography and nerve conduction studies, which were unremarkable. She was treated with diazepam without any relief. Ultimately, she saw an orthopedist, who diagnosed a "basal ganglia disorder" and referred her to a neurologist.

After consulting a neurologist, she was diagnosed with cervical dystonia in 1984 and was tried on several medications with little success in symptom relief, including baclofen, amantadine, diazepam, and benztropine. When we evaluated her in late 1984, we noted that in addition to cervical dystonia, there was bibrachial, left leg, and lower face involvement. The patient did not notice the leg involvement because it did not seem to impair gait. She was then treated with botulinum toxin to the involved neck muscles with a good initial response, especially for pain. Over time, there was less benefit with shorter interval times of pain relief, and associated dystonic head tremor continued to cause significant pain and discomfort. In 1989, at age 39, she underwent a C1–6 posterior ramisectomy and denervation of the right sternocleidomastoid muscle, which produced an estimated 20% improvement of symptoms. She continued to receive botulinum toxin (onabotulinum toxin, type A) injections, and in 2001, at age 51, she was switched to rimabotulinum toxin, type B because of a decreased efficacy, likely from blocking antibody formation to type A. She had a moderate but variable response.

THE APPROACH

At the time of our initial evaluation, she had more extensive muscle involvement in both arms, lower face, and left leg, although subjectively was more focused on cervical dystonia and pain. On examination, she was noted to have severe left torticollis and laterocollis and milder anterocollis, with hypertrophy of involved muscles (left trapezius, left splenius, and right sternocleidomastoid). Holding her head upright with her hand would momentarily suppress the dystonia.

There was a bilateral but asymmetric irregular hand tremor (R>L) on sustention and finger-to-nose that was considered dystonic; she was clumsy with rapid alternating movements of hands and feet, and there was posturing of the arm with writing. She had a left leg "kick" on ambulation, which later developed into a left foot drag causing her to be unable to wear high heels anymore. Over the next decade, as symptoms progressed, there was additional muscle involvement because she developed a right trunk tilt while sitting, with pelvic thrusts while walking. There was also contraction of the platysma and risorius, and elevation of her left shoulder, but no voice or vocal cord involvement.

Our initial impression was that she had primary generalized dystonia, starting around 12 years of age, beginning in her right arm, and slowly progressing over 30 years without her recognizing the extent of involvement until reaching her 30s. Brain and spine imaging were unremarkable, and a secondary cause of dystonia or a dystonia-plus syndrome was not considered given the lack of any other associated signs or symptoms and negative imaging. Chemodenervation was continued, and several other medications were tried unsuccessfully, including trihexyphenidyl, topiramate, zonisamide pramipexole, and mexiletine (for refractory pain).

Her family was of Sicilian background, and there was no initial family history of dystonia or any other movement disorder. We initially suspected a genetic etiology for the primary dystonia given her early onset. During her care with us, she also described neck pain in her daughter, and in 1998, at age 29, her daughter was diagnosed with cervical dystonia with brachial involvement and writer's cramp. We obtained a DYT1 testing, which was negative. However, to our surprise, she tested positive for a DYT6 mutation when she was screened in 2009 as part of our clinical research protocol.

Since then, she has continued to receive local botulinum toxin injections with limited and temporary benefit; pain has continued to be a major symptom, and she is also followed up by a pain specialist. During her last visit, her medical regimen included diazepam, benztropine, trazodone, and zolpidem. Deep brain stimulation surgery was considered and discussed, but to date, the patient has not elected to pursue another surgical intervention.

THE LESSON

DYT6 dystonia is an autosomal dominant disorder with reduced penetrance (estimated at 60%); it is caused by heterozygous mutations in the *THAP1* gene on chromosome 8p21–p22. The gene was mapped in an Amish-Mennonite kindred in which a founder mutation was subsequently detected, but since discovery of the gene in 2009, more than 45 different heterozygous mutations have been described in families of diverse ancestry. DYT6 is now recognized as a cause of early-onset dystonia with a mean age of onset of 13 years, but with a broad range from early childhood to 50 years. Typically, onset is more often in an arm (58%), followed by cranial muscles (29%) and neck (17%), but more rarely in the leg (10%); this contrasts with DYT1 where about half the cases begin in a leg (with the other half starting in an arm). It spreads to a generalized distribution in about 50% of cases, and once generalized, the majority will have cranial muscle (77%) and speech (67%) involvement. In addition, although 50% of cases have leg involvement, disability ambulating is usually mild or moderate, and patients are rarely chair bound.

DYT6 dystonia frequently first develops in an arm. To have a long history of arm tremor alone preceding any other symptoms for many years is unusual, although this has been described in DYT1 (1). A neurologic examination in adolescence or early adult years might have helped differentiate tremor type and led to an earlier, more accurate diagnosis. Once our patient presented to us, it was clear that she had a generalized dystonia, and eventually, genetic testing confirmed the DYT6 diagnosis. However, it was unusual that there had been a delay of more than 20 years between development of arm dystonia and symptomatic cervical dystonia and subsequent worsening of dystonia in leg and axial muscles. The precise age onset of dystonia in leg and cervical muscles is unknown because she already had involvement when we first examined her, but there was clear worsening of dystonic contractions in her forth and fifth decades.

This progression later in life may occur in primary early-onset dystonia (2) but is not considered typical. Furthermore, although she developed typical features of DYT6 with neck, facial, limb, and trunk involvement, there was never speech involvement.

Our case illustrates how one needs to continually consider differential diagnoses, even in longstanding patients, when a definitive diagnosis is lacking. The identification of genetic causes for dystonia is an evolving story, and the availability of commercial testing for these genetic etiologies is also ever changing. Resources such as www.geneclinics.org can be very helpful in updating clinicians about clinical features, counseling, and genetic testing. Our case also emphasizes the need to consider diagnoses that may not "fit" perfectly into what is considered the typical phenotype associated with a genetic cause. This patient had onset with "tremor," late progression of symptoms and signs, and never developed speech involvement, all somewhat atypical for DYT6.

REFERENCES

1. Edwards M, Wood N, Bhatia K. Unusual phenotypes in DYT1 dystonia: A report of five cases and a review of literature. *Mov Disord.* 2003;18:706–711.
2. Elia AE, Filippini G, Bentivoglio AR, et al. Onset and progression of primary torsion dystonia in sporadic and familial cases. *Eur J Neurol.* 2006;13:1083–1088.

Suggested Reading

Bressman SB, Raymond D, Fuchs T, et al. Mutations in THAP1 (DYT6) in early-onset dystonia: a genetic screening study. *Lancet Neurol.* 2009;8:441–446.

Fuchs T, Gavarini S, Saunders-Pullman R, et al. Mutations in the THAP1 gene are responsible for DYT6 primary torsion dystonia. *Nat Genet.* 2009;41:286–288.

Houlden H, Schneider SA, Paudel R, et al. THAP1 mutations (DYT6) are an additional cause of early-onset dystonia. *Neurology.* 2010;74:846–850.

40

Untwisting a Double Twist: Severe Tremors in a Factory Worker With a Melanoma History

THIEN THIEN LIM, ILIA ITIN, STEPHEN HANTUS,
AND HUBERT H. FERNANDEZ

THE CASE

Mr FH is a 58-year-old left-handed man with history of hypertension and malignant melanoma who presented with a 2-year history of bilateral hand tremors. The tremors were high amplitude, low frequency and predominantly postural, absent at rest, and worse on the left compared with the right. The tremors were worse in the morning, during times of stress and cold temperature. The patient had difficulty eating, writing, dressing, and shaving. He volunteered that "peas would fly off the spoon when eating"; his handwriting has become larger and more scribbly, and it took more effort for him to button his shirt. He was unsure whether alcohol affected his tremors because he rarely consumed alcoholic beverages. Metoprolol and primidone prescribed by his primary care physician for tremor control did not improve tremor. The patient and his wife denied shuffling gait, softening voice, slowing down, and rigidity.

Interestingly, 4 months before presentation, in addition to tremor, he developed rapid cognitive decline, behavioral symptoms, and seizures. He could not remember children's names, dates, and later on was unable to remember and perform household chores. He was also unable to carry out his job at the Rubbermaid factory. He reported suicidal ideation.

In addition, he presented with paroxysmal episodes that were suggestive of seizures. He had acute and intermittent focal involuntary movements and other manifestations, including automatisms (such as sticking his lower lip out), hyperventilation, making squealing noises, staring off, sweating, and crying. He also would be agitated and confused after the event. He volunteered experiencing an aura before these episodes—having a headache, feeling anxious, nauseated, and jittery. Often, he was also intermittently confused. As an example, he often asked when his mother-in-law was coming to visit, although she died 13 years before; he attempted to eat a wax candle; he saw a reflection of a lamp shade in the window and thought it was going to attack the family; and he thought that he was going to be arrested for the Kent State University shooting in 1970.

He had a mole on the back that was excised in 2004, consistent with malignant melanoma. There was no history of smoking, head trauma, febrile seizures, meningitis or encephalitis, or family history of epilepsy. He had a strong family history of cancer: his father has lung cancer and his sister has breast cancer. He has another sister with pituitary tumor. His paternal grandmother had tremors.

On examination, he scored 24 out of 30 on the Mini Mental State Examination. He had bilateral postural hand tremors and "wing beating tremor." The tremor was absent at rest. He exhibited cerebellar signs on the left side, including poor rapid alternating movement and ataxia on finger-to-nose test. Archimedes spiral drawing was fairly impaired on the left and was abnormal, to a lesser extent, on the right. Rigidity and bradykinesia were not appreciated.

THE APPROACH

The patient presented with a prodrome of tremor, followed by rapid cognitive decline, psychiatric manifestations, and episodes suggestive of seizures. The initial extensive workup (which included full blood count, renal function, liver function test, alpha fetoprotein, beta-human chorionic gonadotropin, serum ceruloplasmin, 24-hour urine copper, B12 level, antimicrosomal and antithyroglobulin antibodies, metanephrine levels, thyroid function test, and toxicology screen and heavy metal screen) was unremarkable. Lumbar puncture was performed, including 14-3-3 protein in the cerebrospinal fluid (CSF), which was also unremarkable. However, the paraneoplastic antibody panel showed a high level of VGKC (voltage-gated potassium channel) antibody (4.22 nmol/L [normal ≤0.02 nmol/L]). Brain positron emission tomography (PET) scan was also performed showing hypermetabolism in the mesial temporal structures, which was consistent with limbic encephalitis.

He was followed up by the epilepsy service around this time, which initiated workup of possible seizures (MRI of the brain and a 48-hour video electroencephalography [EEG]). The MRI did not reveal a seizure focus, and no epileptiform discharges were seen on EEG. Nonetheless, because of the high clinical suspicion for seizures, he was given lamotrigine, clonazepam, and lacosamide with significant improvement. He was subsequently readmitted because of progressive clinical decline, and prolonged video EEG monitoring revealed seizure activity.

Because of his melanoma history, positive VGKC antibodies, and brain PET scan results, a thorough search for an underlying malignancy (complete skin examination; computed tomography [CT] scan of the chest, abdomen, and pelvis; PET scan of the neck, chest, and pelvis; ultrasound of the testicles) was performed with unremarkable findings. Two years after initial presentation, our patient has remained cancer free. Plasmapheresis was then performed. After five sessions of plasmapheresis, he improved cognitively and behaviorally, and his tremor was significantly reduced. He was able to write and sign his name, which he was not able to do before the treatment. His VGKC titers went down to 0.12 after a year, and he is now seizure free and continues to experience cognitive improvement, while maintained on lamotrigine, clonazepam, and lacosamide. To date, no underlying malignancy has been discovered that could account for this presentation. We conclude that it is probably a nonparaneoplastic limbic encephalitis presenting with tremor, autonomic seizures, psychiatric features, and rapidly progressive dementia and responding to immunosuppressive treatment.

THE LESSON

We illustrate a case of a factory worker with a rapidly progressive cognitive decline and behavioral dysfunction, accompanied by seizures, who initially presented with severe postural tremors 2 years before, in the setting of a malignant melanoma history, a positive paraneoplastic antibody titer, and a strong cancer family history. The seizures improved on antiepileptic medications but resolved after plasmapheresis. His tremors and cognitive and behavioral profile uniformly improved with plasmapheresis. No malignancy has been found to date.

There are several "twists" in this unique case: (1) despite his impressive episodic clinical presentation, most consistent with seizures, his brain MRI and video EEGs were unremarkable in the beginning; (2) although he had a positive VGKC antibody titer, and his brain PET scan was consistent with limbic encephalitis, our initial workup for new or recurrent malignancy had been unremarkable; and (3) his postural tremor predated the rapid cognitive and behavioral decline by almost 2 years, which challenged the notion that it was part of the subacute "paraneoplastic syndrome." These twists were "untwisted" by (1) his significant response to antiepileptic medications; (2) the significant improvement of his cognitive and behavioral dysfunction and resolution of his seizures with plasmapheresis, and the lack of any identified recurrence of malignant melanoma or new primary malignancy on subsequent workup, to date; and (3) the lack of tremor response to primidone and propranolol but with a significant tremor improvement to plasmapheresis.

To date, there was only one case report of tremor in VGKC-associated limbic encephalitis that presented with insomnia and hand tremor (1). Similar to our case, the authors also did not identify any neoplasm, and the patient's tremors improved with immunotherapy. The three major syndromes in anti-VGKC cases are neuromyotonia (NMT), limbic encephalitis (LE), and Morvan syndrome (MVS) (2), limbic encephalitis being by far the most common. The usual clinical features of limbic encephalitis include subacute memory impairment, a range of psychiatric features, including confusion, disorientation, and behavioral change, and seizures (which may be very difficult to control) (3). In most cases, VGKC antibodies have been associated with a nonparaneoplastic syndrome (4). This is, to our knowledge, the first case report of a nonparaneoplastic VGKC antibody–associated limbic encephalitis, preceded by a 2-year history of postural tremor. Ever since we encountered this case, we try our best to at least have a yearly follow-up for patients we suspect of having essential tremor, most especially for those who do not respond to conventional therapy.

REFERENCES

1. Takado Y, Shimohata T, Kawachi I, et al. Patient with limbic encephalitis associated with anti-voltage-gated potassium channel antibodies who presented with insomnia and hand tremor. *Rinsho Shinkeigaku.* 2008;48:338–342.
2. Merchut MP. Management of voltage-gated potassium channel antibody disorders. *Neurol Clin.* 2010;28:941–959.
3. Schott JM. Limbic encephalitis: a clinician's guide. *Pract Neurol.* 2006;6:143–153.
4. Vincent A, Buckley C, Schott JM, et al. Potassium channel antibody-associated encephalopathy: a potential immunotherapy-responsive form of limbic encephalitis. *Brain.* 2004;127:701–712.

41

Disabling Postural and Resting Tremor: What Should One Aim to Treat?

RAFAEL GONZALEZ-REDONDO, JORGE GURIDI, AND JOSÉ A. OBESO

THE CASE

Mr P is a 68-year-old right-handed lawyer who was sent to our movement disorders unit for surgical treatment of a disabling postural tremor. He presented with an 8-year history of upper limb, symmetrical postural tremor refractory to standard medical treatments (propranolol up to 120 mg/d, primidone 500 mg/d, zonisamide 300 mg/d, trihexyphenidyl 4 mg/d, and botulinum A-toxin 100 units in flexor–extensor muscles of the fingers and wrist). Eighteen months before the initial visit, a resting tremor of the left hand had become noticeable. There was no trace of any other neurologic illness. The patient also suffers from type II diabetes, mild hypercholesterolemia, and arterial hypertension, all properly controlled with oral drug treatments. He hunted, smoked, and drank alcohol moderately. Family history was positive for essential tremor (ET) through a maternal aunt and uncle.

The tremor began bilaterally in both upper limbs when maintaining a posture or holding objects such as a spoon, a cup, or a mobile. Over the next few years, the tremor severity gradually increased, particularly on the left upper limb, leading to major professional disability. Our initial physical examination revealed bilateral postural tremor in the arm with proximal predominance (3 points out of 4), which worsened during actions like the finger-to-nose test, and a rest tremor with involvement of hand and fingers, exclusively in the left upper limb (1 point out of 4). The outcome in the Archimedean spiral test evidenced the severity of the action tremor (Figure 41.1). Resting tremor clearly disappeared at the beginning of a voluntary movement with the left hand followed by a typical re-emergent phase. Froment's sign was present in both left limbs, and a Myerson's sign was observed. There was no evidence of bradykinesia, hypomimia, hypophonia, or micrography (Figure 41.2). Coordination, eye movements, gait, and balancing reflexes were all normal.

Electromyographic recording of tremor revealed alternating tremor in the left upper limb at 3.5 Hz ceasing with voluntary recruitment of the involved forearm and finger muscles. Postural tremor was recorded in both upper limbs during extension of the arms. On the right side, it revealed a rhythmic oscillatory frequency at 6.2 Hz, whereas in the left arm, there were two peaks at 5.4 and 3.8 Hz.

The response to apomorphine test was ascertained using several doses up to a maximal tolerated dose of 7 mg, with no improvement in the tremor. A cerebral 3 Tesla MRI showed some white matter hyperintensities, suggestive of diffuse mild microvascular encephalopathy; however, no lesion was observable in the midbrain (Figure 41.3). A complete battery of neuropsychological tests confirmed high cognitive achievement. Systemic causes of tremor were reasonably ruled out. A proton emission tomography scan with 6-[^{18}F]fluoro-L-DOPA (^{18}FDOPA-PET) demonstrated reduction of uptake, indicating a decreased dopaminergic innervation in the right striatum, mainly in the putamen and, to a lesser degree, in the caudate nucleus. There was a subtle rostrocaudal gradient (Figure 41.4). Uptake activity in the left striatum was within the standard normal ranges for his age.

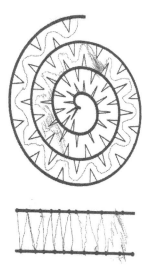

FIGURE 41.1

Archimedean spiral test performed by the patient with his left hand illustrating the severity of the action tremor.

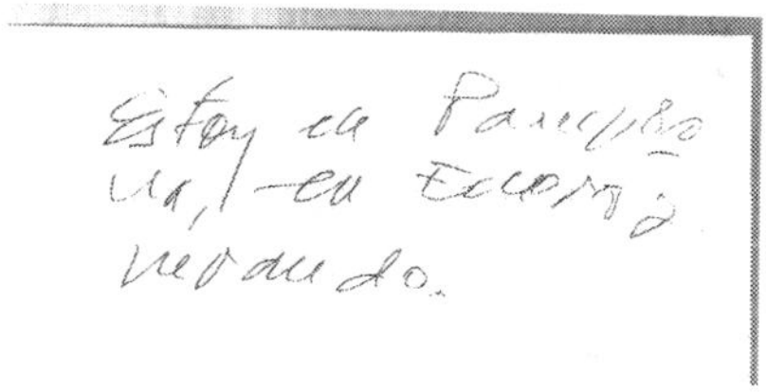

FIGURE 41.2

Sample of right-hand writing of the patient showing no signs of micrography or tremor in his letter performing.

THE APPROACH

This case posed a diagnostic dilemma and a therapeutic challenge. The clinical features of the left upper limb tremor were highly suggestive of a parkinsonian tremor. Thus, although there was tremor during a posture and action, there also was distal involvement of upper limb muscles at rest, which stopped at the onset of voluntary contraction with re-emergency subsequently. The diagnostic options include (1) ET associated later on with a focal lesion of the right nigrostriatal projection. This was considered unlikely because detailed assessment of 3 Tesla MRI showed no evidence of vascular, infectious, inflammatory, or tumoral lesion in the midbrain; (2) ET with an atypical resting tremor; and (3) ET evolving toward Parkinson's disease. Distinction between options 2 and 3 was difficult. ET may exhibit, when severe, what seems a tremor at rest, but it is much less likely that it will be associated with distal tremor of one hand only. The EMG

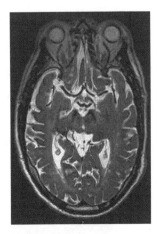

FIGURE 41.3
Brain MRI in a T2-weighted axial plane; there are no observable lesions in the midbrain.

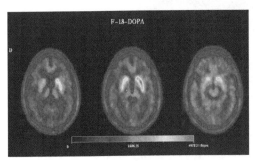

FIGURE 41.4
[18]FDOPA-PET scan revealing a functional depletion of dopamine in the right presynaptic nigrostriatal pathway, affecting putamen and caudate with a subtle rostrocaudal gradient. D means right.

recording also showed two main peaks of tremor activity in the left but not in the right upper limbs, suggestive of a different underlying mechanism. In addition, the [18]FDOPA-PET showed reduced uptake in one striatum, which is not a feature of ET. Thus, a more likely diagnosis would be a combination of ET evolving toward Parkinson's disease (i.e., option 3). However, dopaminergic depletion as revealed by DAT scan or [18]FDOPA-PET is asymmetrical but bilateral even in early Parkinson's disease, unlike the findings in our patient (1).

The therapeutic approach was not less challenging. Pharmacologic treatments of tremor had failed, and apomorphine had not induced benefit. Admittedly, we could have tried oral treatment with levodopa as a last pharmacologic resource. The patient was very anxious and in need for improvement and had already been advised and agreed to receive surgical treatment with deep brain stimulation (DBS).

What was then the right target?

In terms of quality of life, our patient's highest impairment on his professional activity derived from the left upper limb tremor, at rest and during action. In that sense, unilateral DBS of the ventral intermediate nucleus of the thalamus (Vim) was believed to be a better option than DBS of the subthalamic nucleus (STN) because the former provides a better control of the tremor, whereas the latter is better suited to improve akinesia and rigidity, with tremor also responding, but to a lesser extent (2). The possibility of double treatment by implanting electrodes in both Vim and STN was also contemplated but deemed too invasive and excessive for the disability of the patient at the time (3).

Thus, one electrode was inserted into the Vim of the right thalamus. DBS suppressed tremor in the left hand, and our patient recovered his normal professional and social activity. Over the consecutive follow-ups during the next 3 years, the patient started to complain of worsening of tremor in the right hand and slowness. Examination showed the appearance of facial hypomimia and cogwheel rigidity in the four limbs, more severe on the left side. He was started on treatment with a dopamine agonist (pramipexole, prolonged release up to 2.1 mg/d) with moderate improvement.

THE LESSON

Almost two centuries after James Parkinson wrote "An essay on the shaking palsy," tremor remains defiant today. Not only is its pathophysiology still incompletely understood, but current approaches to the diagnosis and treatment remain challenging today. We believe that understanding pathophysiologic basis of tremor in Parkinson's disease could provide substantial advancement in the origin and discriminative pathology of dopamine cells in the substantia nigra pars compacta, which is a formidable challenge for the upcoming generation of neurologists.

REFERENCES

1. Stoessl AJ, Brooks DJ, Eidelberg D. Milestones in neuroimaging. *Mov Disord.* 2011;26:868–978.
2. Limousin P, Speelman JD, Gielen F, et al. Multicentre European study of thalamic stimulation in parkinsonian and essential tremor. *JNNP.* 1999;66:289–296.
3. Reese R, Herzog J, Falk D, et al. Successful deep brain stimulation in a case of posttraumatic tremor and hemiparkinsonism. *Mov Disord.* 2011 26:1954–1955.

Suggested Reading

Hirai T, Miyazaki M, Nakajima H, et al. The correlation between tremor characteristics and the predicted volume of effective lesions in stereotaxic nucleus ventralis intermedius thalamotomy. *Brain.* 1983;106 (Pt 4):1001–1018.
Rodriguez MC, Guridi OJ, Alvarez L, et al. The subthalamic nucleus and tremor in Parkinson's disease. *Mov Disord.* 1998;13(Suppl 3): 111–118.
Watts RL, Standaert DG, Obeso JA, eds. *Movement Disorders.* McGraw-Hill, New York, 2011.

42

Pseudopsychogenic Tremors and Parkinsonism:
Two Presentations of Multiple Sclerosis That
Almost Fooled Us

THIEN THIEN LIM, ILIA ITIN, AND HUBERT H. FERNANDEZ

THE CASES

Case 1

JLS, a 31-year-old right-handed woman with history of migraines, bipolar disorder, post-traumatic stress disorder, and substance abuse was seen at our clinic in May 2011, accompanied by her mother, for abnormal involuntary movements. She was referred by her psychiatrist.

She presented rather acutely with bilateral resting and postural arm tremor, which was later accompanied by speech and gait difficulties. At one point, these tremors worsened and were accompanied by nausea and profuse sweating, prompting her to go to the emergency room. She was given only intravenous fluids, which lessened her tremors. She was discharged, but within a few hours, her tremors recurred. She could barely walk upon awakening the next day. In addition, she noticed difficulty using the computer, drinking from a cup, and performing her work and activities of daily living, prompting this consultation at our movement disorders center.

Ms JLS has a strong history of migraine with aura since her 20s. Her migraines were rather mild and relatively infrequent, not requiring any suppressive treatment. She was diagnosed in October 2010 with fibromyalgia when she complained of tingling sensation over the right hand, foot, and leg. She had a history of difficulty in emptying her bladder, but no formal diagnosis was given.

Moreover, she had been diagnosed with bipolar disorder recently. At the time of presentation, she was taking lithium and quetiapine. She was told that bipolar disorder could have been brought about by post-traumatic stress disorder due to possible childhood sexual abuse. She admitted to manic behavior with overspending and stealing her relatives' money. She has a history of substance abuse (Vicodin and Percocet) and admitted to illicit drug use (cocaine, marijuana, and Ecstasy) since she was 20 years old. However, she claims that she has been "clean" for the past year.

Furthermore, she had chronic abdominal pain due to endometriosis for years, but it improved with treatment recently.

On examination, our patient was somewhat disheveled but had good eye contact, and rapport was easy to establish. She appeared to be anxious with a pressured speech. She was cooperative throughout the examination. Her short- and long-term memory was intact. Cranial nerve examination was within normal with no evidence of optic neuritis or atrophy. Her reflexes were symmetrical and 2+ in all limbs. Sensory examination, including proprioception, was normal. Coordination and motor examination displayed normal tone and strength throughout. Our patient exhibited multifocal resting and action tremors of the arms, legs, and head from side to side with variable amplitude and frequency. The movements subsided when she was asked to perform simultaneous tasks such as opening and closing the right fist while spelling a long word. The movements also subsided when she was engrossed in a conversation. Her gait had features of astasia-abasia as she was lurching wildly when she walked. Despite such a gait, she did not fall, nor did she require any assistance to walk. Surprisingly, she could also perform tandem walking and able to hop on either foot without falling. She was steady in Romberg's position.

THE APPROACH

Her history and physical examination were more consistent with a psychogenic movement disorder. Her presentation was rather acute, and her features were variable, distractible, and did not correlate with a specific neurologic syndrome. Moreover, she had "risk factors" that made psychogenic disorders more likely, given her bipolar disorder and child abuse history.

Nonetheless, because psychogenic movement disorder is a diagnosis of exclusion, a full workup was still performed. It revealed normal full blood count, renal and liver function tests, negative hepatitis B and C, ANA, pANCA, cANCA, rheumatoid factor, and HIV serology, normal thyroid function tests, angiotensin-converting enzyme (ACE) level, and Wilson's disease screening. Testing for fragile X permutation was negative because female fragile X premutation carriers have a higher rate of anxiety disorder and other psychiatric manifestations. However, the MRI of the brain (Figures 42.1 and 42.2) showed areas of increased T2 and FLAIR signal within the deep and subcortical white matter. A few of the white matter abnormalities had an ovoid configuration and were perpendicular to the lateral ventricles. There was also mild increased signal within the body and splenium of the corpus callosum. In addition, the MRI of the cervical and thoracic spine showed an intramedullary lesion at C5 level. These findings prompted lumbar puncture, and cerebrospinal fluid (CSF) studies revealed evidence of intrathecal inflammation (i.e., positive for oligoclonal bands).

The patient was seen by our multiple sclerosis (MS) specialist who concurred with the diagnosis of MS. She is taking glatiramer acetate 20 mg daily subcutaneously (SQ) (Copaxone). She is continuing psychiatric follow-up. She continues to have abnormal movements but much less frequent and less severe.

Case 2
CCB is a 63-year-old right-handed woman who was seen in consultation for gait disorder. She was referred to our movement disorders center by another neurologist. She had previously seen two other neurologists before this evaluation.

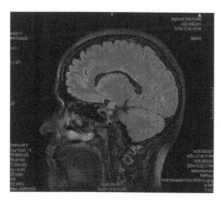

FIGURE 42.1
MRI brain FLAIR sagittal view showing periventricular white matter plaques typical of Dawson's fingers.

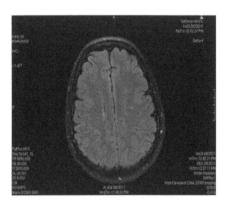

FIGURE 42.2
*MRI brain FLAIR axial view
showing white matter MS plaque.*

She had been feeling fatigued with left-sided "heaviness" for the past 3 years. The patient reported infrequent falls for the past 2 years, and she started ambulating with a cane over the past year. She also described multifocal "tremors," difficulty holding on to objects, and being "off balance." The patient admitted to having urinary frequency. She also denied depression or psychiatric history, but her demeanor and husband's reports did suggest psychological distress.

Of note, she was treated with oral steroids for the past 2 years for uveitis. The patient denied painful oral, genital, and skin lesions. She has history of migraines, which are well controlled by topiramate.

On examination, she had mild hypomimia, although it seemed more consistent with "depressive demeanor." There was no tremor at rest. Her fine motor movements were slower on the left-hand side. She was able to stand up from a chair after pushing herself up. At times, she was grinning with amusement without any reason. I noticed her exhibiting variable left-sided asymmetrical slowness and tremor while attempting to drink from a cup. She appeared clumsy with left finger tapping and had variable left-hand tremors when performing hand movements as though she was augmenting her symptoms. She had good postural stability, and yet when she walked, she had features of astasia-abasia and "gyrating gait," but she did not fall during testing. Muscle bulk and strength were within normal in all limbs. Coordination was normal. Other neurologic and systems examination was unremarkable.

THE APPROACH

Our second case had a history and examination findings that could suggest parkinsonism. She had asymmetrical "heaviness" on the left side, gait instability and falls (with no musculoskeletal defect, neuropathy, or vestibulopathy), hypomimia, resting tremors (by history only), and perhaps mild rigidity and bradykinesia. However, given the variability in her examination, unusual gait with features of astasia-abasia, and history of being evaluated now by two previous neurologists, our initial impression was that of psychogenic movement disorder. Nonetheless, a therapeutic trial of levodopa was initiated to assess her response to dopamine replacement and to provide the patient with some assurance that "something was being done" and that her case was not being taken for granted. Follow-up in 1 month showed that levodopa was not helpful and therefore discontinued.

However, the coexistence of uveitis with vague neurologic and psychiatric symptoms (although in the absence of painful genital and oral ulcers or skin lesions) raised the issue of possible Behcet's disease, which prompted us to perform some diagnostic tests. Brain MRI (Figure 42.3) revealed widespread demyelinating plaques throughout both hemispheres and

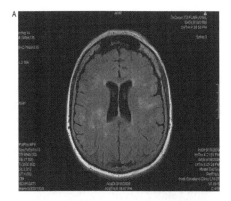

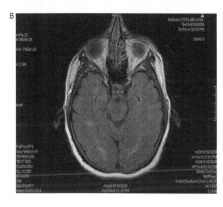

FIGURE 42.3

MRI brain FLAIR axial view showing multiple MS plaques over the periventricular, subcortical, and juxtacortical regions.

pons, which was typical for MS. Cervical spine MRI (Figure 42.4) showed multifocal cord signal hyperintensities involving C1, C2, C3, T3–T4, and maximally at C5-C6 consistent with transverse myelitis. CSF results were indeterminate for oligoclonal bands but showed increased IgG index of 0.58 (normal 0.06–0.17) and abnormal myelin basic protein level of 2.3 ng/mL (normal 0–1.6).

The patient's diagnosis of MS was confirmed by an MS specialist. She is being treated with low-dose oral methotrexate. She also started seeing a psychiatrist for her emotional issues, and currently, she is on mirtazapine. Unfortunately, her movement disorder symptoms have not significantly improved, and her tremors would worsen with anxiety.

THE LESSON

Both cases were initially thought to have had psychogenic movement disorders. The acute presentation and psychiatric history (in our first case), and the variability of the involuntary movements, distractibility, augmentation of symptoms, and accompanying seemingly unrelated symptoms (in our first and second case), were suggestive of a psychogenic disorder.

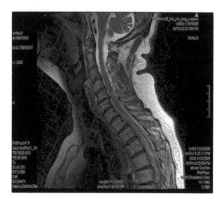

FIGURE 42.4
MRI cervical spine T2 showing MS plaque lesions over cervical region, prominent on C5–C6.

However, our workup (neuroimaging and lumbar puncture) established the diagnosis of MS in both cases. We used the term "pseudo-psychogenic" movement disorder in reference to the commonly used term "pseudo-pseudo seizures." This type of seizures is commonly seen in seizures of frontal lobe origin in which patients present with bizarre manifestations invoking clinical suspicion of pseudo seizures but turn out to have a true organic pathology. In our cases, we initially thought that our patients had psychogenic movement disorders, until our workup revealed the presence of multiple plaques in the central nervous system. It is certainly possible that the extensive MS plaques caused cognitive and psychiatric impairment and hence the abnormal movements. Moreover, the abnormal movements in our first case have significantly improved with immunomodulation therapy. The second patient could have embellished her symptoms (thereby looking psychogenic) in her effort for us to "listen to her case" because we were the fourth neurology practice to evaluate her.

MS remains a great mimicker. The diagnosis of MS has remained elusive in patients who have psychiatric problems or who have uncommon presentations of common diseases such as migraine, stroke, or neuropathies (1). It is not surprising that MS can also mimic psychogenic movement disorder. It is well known that MS can present with psychiatric manifestation. Therefore, it is also possible that MS lesions could also manifest themselves with psychogenic movement disorder. We have not found reports in the literature on MS causing psychogenic movement disorders. However, there have been several reports regarding parkinsonism as a manifestation of MS. Folgar et al. (2) described a 48-year-old patient with MS who presented with parkinsonism. At that time, there were eight patients in the literature with a similar presentation, which later on turned out to be MS (those presenting with conclusive imaging evidence and unequivocal response to corticosteroids). There were four others who had concomitant Parkinson disease and MS. However, none has explicitly stated in their report that they suspected psychogenic parkinsonism.

Psychogenic movement disorder diagnosis continues to be a diagnosis of exclusion. Therefore, it behooves a prudent clinician to consider possible organic conditions that may have bizarre psychiatric presentation before we definitely label the patient with a diagnosis of psychogenic movement disorder. And even if they did have psychogenic movement disorder, we are reminded by these two cases that "psychiatric patients can have organic medical and neurological problems too." The extent of workup should obviously be decided on a case-by-case basis. However, cost consciousness should be balanced against the danger of missing diagnosis of treatable neurologic disease and labeling the patient as "psychogenic." However, at a minimum, organic disorders known to present with bizarre manifestations, such as MS, should at least be entertained. We share two such cases where thoroughness helped to avoid this pitfall.

REFERENCES

1. Rolak LA, Fleming JO. The differential diagnosis of multiple sclerosis. *Neurologist.* 2007;13:57–72.
2. Folgar S, Gatto EM, Raina G, et al. Parkinsonism as a manifestation of multiple sclerosis. *Mov Disord.* 2003;18:108–113

IV

Chorea

43

The Clumsy Piano Teacher Unable to Play the Organ in Church

ANTHONY E. LANG

THE CASE

This 28-year-old piano teacher was first seen in March 1987. She was transferred from another hospital for investigation and management of involuntary movements. On March 17, she complained of "tiredness" in the right arm, and on the following day, she noted difficulty holding objects and involuntary movements in her right hand. On March 20, her husband noted involuntary movements of the right side of her face. The involuntary movements began to interfere with sleep. On March 21, she was unable to play the organ in church because of the abnormal movements. On March 24, she was admitted to hospital where a computed tomography (CT) scan with contrast and electroencephalography (EEG) were normal. Platelet count was slightly reduced at 119. On March 27, she began to have involuntary movements on the left side of the body; she had difficulty performing fine movements with both hands; she complained that her speech was "thick" and labored and that swallowing was more difficult.

She was transferred to the Toronto Western Hospital on March 27. In addition to the history above, her medical history included five spontaneous abortions over the previous 5 years; two of these were in the second trimester. In the fall of 1985, during one of these pregnancies, she was hospitalized for a depressive psychosis requiring haloperidol treatment. At that time, she also noted a rash over her back and face, which resolved after approximately 6 months. The medical history was otherwise unremarkable. Family history was negative for neurologic and psychiatric illness. Functional inquiry revealed urinary frequency for many years but no other problems. There was no history of thrombophlebitis or pulmonary emboli.

The general examination was unremarkable apart from a grade 2/6 systolic ejection murmur at the left sternal border. Higher cognitive function was normal apart from some impairment in concentration with poor immediate recall and easy distractibility. Speech was fluent but interrupted with occasional alterations of pitch and volume. She had generalized severe chorea, worse on the right. At times, the abnormal movements reached ballistic proportions, especially when she attended to mental or physical tasks. In addition to choreiform facial movements, she showed choreic movements of the eyes best appreciated under closed lids. There was impersistence of tongue protrusion and difficulty with rapid alternating movements of the tongue. The remainder of the neurologic examination was normal.

THE APPROACH

This young woman presented with relatively acute-onset hemichorea and then generalized chorea with an important medical history of repeated spontaneous abortions and an acute psychosis and skin rash during one of her pregnancies. This history is strongly suggestive of chorea associated with a lupus anticoagulant, possibly due to systemic lupus erythematosus (SLE). In fact, later when we were able to review previous records, we found that years earlier a lupus anticoagulant had been found after she was discovered to have an increased partial thromboplastin time (PTT).

Investigations in hospital included normal complete blood count, PT, thrombin time, fibrinogen, Venereal Disease Research Laboratory, routine blood and cerebrospinal fluid (CSF) chemistry, CSF cell count, rheumatoid factor, ASOT, antihyaluronidase, cryoglobulin, and serum beta–human chorionic gonadotropin. Erythrocyte sedimentation rate (ESR) was 30 and PTT was 50.7/30.9. No coagulation inhibitor was demonstrated. Serum protein immunoelectrophoresis showed increased polyclonal IgG and decreased C3 and C4. ANA was positive in a dilution of 1:1000 (pattern not specified), and anti-DNA antibodies were positive. CT scan was normal apart from moderate cerebral atrophy.

The patient was diagnosed as having chorea secondary to an antiphospholipid syndrome (APS) either as part of a lupus-like disorder or due to a primary APS. She was treated with prednisone 60 mg/d, ranitidine 150 mg/d, ASA 325 mg/d, and tetrabenazine 25 mg three times per day. Her chorea improved markedly, and she was discharged on April 16, 1987. When seen in follow-up on May 7 taking tetrabenazine 12.5 mg once daily and prednisone 60 mg/d, she had rare, low-amplitude choreic movements only when stressed. She had returned to a full load of teaching piano and was coping extremely well. Tetrabenazine was discontinued and prednisone tapered further. In early June on prednisone 25 mg/d, enteric-coated aspirin 350 mg/d, and ranitidine 150 mg/d, she continued to have occasional right-hand choreic movements that caused minimal clumsiness but no true functional disability. Prednisone was subsequently discontinued, and she remained only on one baby aspirin per day. She did well until July 1988 when she began noting occasional jerking movements in the left foot and involuntary movements of the left hand, most notably when playing the organ or when holding her new adopted son. She also described hearing her hand moving against his diapers as an indication that the abnormal movements were present. Examination demonstrated mild choreic movements in the left hand and fingers, which were particularly noticeable when she concentrated on tasks and while walking. Follow-up laboratory investigations continued to show low C3 and C4 and prolonged PTT. CBC was normal, sedimentation rate was 8, and anti-DNA antibodies were negative. She was followed up without change in medication, and in early October, the left side of chorea was slightly more prominent. Prednisone 15 mg/d provided no benefit. Subsequently, the dose is increased to 60 mg/d briefly. In late November on 30 mg/d prednisone, chorea was essentially unchanged, and she was beginning to develop a Cushingoid appearance, which she was quite unhappy with. In mid-December while taking prednisone 20 mg/d, abnormal movements gradually subsided. When reviewed in late January 1989, taking only one baby aspirin per day, she showed only slight chorea on the left and questionably brisker upper limb reflexes on the left compared with the right. In July 1989, neurologic examination was normal, and there was no chorea seen whatsoever. Over the following 8 years, she continued to do extremely well with no recurrences of chorea and no further need for prednisone therapy. She developed headaches compatible with migraine, and on last follow-up in 1997, she had developed hypertension requiring diuretic therapy. In November 1991, MRI scan showed several small foci of increased signal intensity in the white matter of the cerebral hemispheres bilaterally on T2-weighted images compatible with microangiography.

THE LESSON

Chorea is an uncommon but well-established manifestation of the APS associated with either full-blown SLE, a lupus-like syndrome when fewer than four classification criteria for SLE are met, or primary APS when no clinical symptoms or signs of SLE exist (1). The exact pathogenesis of chorea in these cases is probably mixed; only a minority has evidence of basal ganglia vascular pathology. The relationship to hormonal changes (chorea occurring in pregnancy or in response to oral contraceptive therapy) also supports nonvascular factors. Because the pathogenesis is uncertain or mixed, therapy is also not well established. As in my patient, treatment often includes steroids and antiaggregants, and in patients whose chorea interferes with function, symptomatic antichorea medication such as a dopamine antagonist is recommended. Management and long-term follow-up in my patient was very gratifying (although she did have a less severe recurrence of chorea); as in most patients, the chorea resolved without sequelae. Follow-up visits always included her husband and their new baby, which is an uncommon but pleasant change from the usual patient visits in movement disorders practices.

REFERENCE

1. Cervera R, Asherson RA, Font J, et al. Chorea in the antiphospholipid syndrome. Clinical, radiologic, and immunologic characteristics of 50 patients from our clinics and the recent literature. *Medicine* (Baltimore). 1997;76:203–212.

44

Chorea in a Man With Peripheral Neuropathy and Hepatomegaly: The Diagnosis Can Make a Difference!

RUTH H. WALKER

THE CASE

This patient was reported to have delayed walking until the age of 18 months and was evaluated by a pediatric neurologist at the age of 3 years for gait difficulties. He had one febrile seizure as a child. He was always hyperactive and clumsy and was noted to have mumbling speech, but he went on to college and obtained a Bachelor of Arts degree. There was no family history of neurologic disease. He was of Ashkenazi Jewish descent, and it was reported that his grandparents were first cousins. He was the only child. His mother had a sister who had two daughters, one of whom was his major caretaker. His mother died of a stroke at the age of 76, and his father died of myocardial infarction at the age of 66. He had no history of drug or alcohol use or psychiatric illness.

At the age of 37, on routine blood testing, he was found to have increased liver enzymes. He underwent evaluation for Wilson's disease, including a liver biopsy, but the results of these tests were negative. In the absence of pathology, he was given the diagnosis of Gilbert's syndrome (benign increase of liver enzymes). He was also told around this time of a "leak in his muscles." Abnormal involuntary movements and imbalance were noted to develop around this time.

At the age of 42, he was found to have peripheral neuropathy, for which he also underwent extensive investigations, including a bone marrow biopsy, which was essentially normal. In the following years, it was noted that he had increasing difficulty taking care of himself and performing tasks at work.

On examination, the patient was noted to be slow in processing information, to perseverate, and to inappropriately intrude into conversation. He has impaired attention but was cooperative with all testing. Eye movements were normal. Speech was dysarthric, and there were occasional tongue protrusions, although not particularly during eating. He was found to have chorea, affecting his neck and limbs and motor impersistence. Repetitive movements were slowed in all four limbs, but there was no dysdiadochokinesia. Deep tendon reflexes were absent throughout. Gait was wide based and lurching with bilateral foot drop. Neuroimaging showed atrophy of the caudate nuclei bilaterally.

THE APPROACH

In this patient, the exact age of onset was hard to determine, because there were symptoms of poor attention, hyperactivity, clumsiness, and dysarthria even in childhood. Consideration of pediatric metabolic disorders, particularly those potentially affecting the liver, would have been reasonable.

Exclusion of Wilson's disease was essential in a subject with increased liver enzymes and neurologic findings, particularly in the presence of abnormal movements or psychiatric features. Acquired hepatocerebral degeneration may result in chorea, especially orofacial, but is usually seen in patients with much more advanced liver disease, approaching hepatic failure.

Huntington's disease was considered as an explanation of his chorea even in the absence of family history, especially given the neuroimaging findings of caudate nucleus atrophy. However, the patient was found to have CAG repeat sizes of 15/18. In light of the patient's wide-based gait, he was tested for two of the autosomal dominantly inherited spinocerebellar ataxias (SCAs) and was found to have repeat sizes of 22 (both alleles) in the SCA2 gene and 23/33 in the SCA3 gene.

Serologic tests revealed markedly increased creatine kinase in addition to liver enzymes. Occasional acanthocytosis was reported on one peripheral smear but was reported as "2+ acanthocytosis" on repeat blood smear, suggesting the diagnosis of a neuroacanthocytosis syndrome. The two major neuroacanthocytosis disorders to be considered in this patient were chorea-acanthocytosis (autosomal recessive) and McLeod syndrome (X-linked) (1).

Erythrocyte antigen typing performed at the New York Blood Center demonstrated Kx−, and a weak expression of k, Kpb, and Jsb, indicative of McLeod phenotype. Genetic analysis of XK found 789 G→A in exon 3, predicted to result in a stop codon, confirming the diagnosis of McLeod syndrome.

THE LESSON

McLeod syndrome is an X-linked neuroacanthocytosis disorder, which tends to manifest neurologically in middle-aged men. However, the diagnosis may sometimes be made earlier, if blood typing is performed. As in this case, subjects may undergo extensive, invasive investigations for abnormal liver enzymes. Only very rarely does liver dysfunction become clinically problematic.

The diagnosis is made by sending blood to a regional blood center, and the laboratory should be asked to specifically "exclude McLeod phenotype." There are a number of Kell antigens, which should be tested for; thus, a report of "Kell negative" is not informative (1).

Increased creatine kinase, myopathy, and peripheral neuropathy are found in combination with a movement disorder in a limited number of conditions. In addition to McLeod syndrome, the other disorder to consider is autosomal recessive chorea-acanthocytosis (2). In both of these conditions, acanthocytes are an unreliable finding, although if present, they suggest the diagnosis. Some of the inherited cerebellar disorders, including Friedreich's ataxia and SCAs 1, 2, 3, and 6, may present with movement disorders and neuropathy, although routine laboratory testing should be normal in these disorders.

Acanthocytosis can also be seen in abetalipoproteinemia (Bassen-Kornzweig disease) and hypobetalipoproteinemia. However, the neurologic symptoms of these disorders are caused by vitamin E deficiency and consist of ataxia and peripheral neuropathy. Movement disorders are not associated with these conditions. Presentation is often during childhood, and the diagnosis may be suggested by steatorrhea as a result of fat malabsorption.

The diagnosis of McLeod syndrome is critical because of the implications for blood transfusions. If people with the McLeod phenotype (the presence of the diagnosis antigen profile on erythrocytes) are transfused with Kell+ blood, they may make anti-Kell antibodies. On subsequent transfusions with Kell+ blood, these antibodies will cause a hemolytic transfusion reaction, analogous to the Rhesus reaction in Rhesus-negative neonates.

This patient went on to have worsening balance, resulting in frequent falls and eventually a fractured hip. It was necessary to emergently identify appropriately matched blood for transfusion. In ideal circumstances, patients are encouraged to bank their own blood for autologous transfusion if required.

Another important, and potentially treatable, complication of McLeod syndrome is cardiac disease (3). Annual echocardiography is recommended to screen for cardiomyopathy, arrhythmias, and heart failure, which should be treated symptomatically.

The family history may be informative because any maternal uncles would have a 50% chance of being affected. This diagnosis has genetic counseling implications, because any daughters of affected men will be carriers, and their male children will have a 50% chance of inheriting the mutant X chromosome.

REFERENCES

1. Lee S, Russo D, Redman CM. The Kell blood group system: Kell and XK membrane proteins. *Semin Hematol.* 2000;37:113–121.
2. Walker RH, Jung HH, Dobson-Stone C, et al. Neurologic phenotypes associated with acanthocytosis. *Neurology.* 2007;68:92–98.
3. Oechslin E, Kaup D, Jenni R, et al. Cardiac abnormalities in McLeod syndrome. *Int J Cardiol.* 2009;132:130–132.

Suggested Reading
Jung HH, Danek A, Dobson-Stone C, et al. *McLeod Neuroacanthocytosis Syndrome.* http://www.ncbi.nlm.nih.gov/books/NBK1354/. Accessed March 26, 2007.

45

When the HD Gene Test Is "Negative": Our Memorable Case of a Nursing Assistant Fired From Her Job for Making Mistakes

DANIEL TARSY, ANDREW V. VARGA, AND PENNY GREENSTEIN

THE CASE

A 59-year-old Haitian woman presented with a 3-year history of subtle involuntary movements. She was largely unaware of them, but they had become increasingly noticeable to her daughter. These included fidgety movements of her hands and legs, rocking movements of her head, and shifting of weight while sitting. The patient also reported unexplained falls occurring about every 2 months. She was fired from her job as a nursing assistant a year previously because of a series of errors after which she became mildly depressed. Recent memory began to decline several months earlier. She remained at home showing little motivation to seek another job. Family history included her mother and brother with involuntary movements and sister with progressive motor deficits who became psychiatrically hospitalized. She had an unaffected son and daughter and two unaffected grandchildren. Examination showed mild frontal cognitive deficits, intermittant distal choreiform movements of her upper and lower extremities, weight shifting while seated, mild postural instability, and slow saccadic eye movements. There was no bradykinesia, rigidity, or tremor.

THE APPROACH

This middle-aged woman presented with chorea followed shortly afterward by a mild frontal dementia. Her family history was strongly positive for what sounded like chorea in her mother and brother and a chronic and progressive motor syndrome with psychiatric manifestations in her sister. Her medical history, examination, and family history were strongly suggestive of Huntington's disease (HD), but the HD gene testing was normal. The phenotypic features of this patient, namely frontal dysfunction, slow saccadic eye movements, and her Afro-Caribbean origin, were suggestive of HD-like 2 (HDL2) (1). Gene testing of the junctophilin gene demonstrated 46 CAG repeats in one allele, which is diagnostic for HDL2. The proband and her daughter were referred for genetic counseling where the implications of the diagnosis were discussed and the availability of genetic testing in unaffected adult family members was offered if desired. Because of the mild and nonintrusive nature of her involuntary movements, she was not treated with tetrabenazine for chorea. She was referred to psychiatry for evaluation and treatment of depression.

THE LESSON

HDL2 is an autosomal dominant disease caused by a trinucleotide CTG/CAG repeat expansion in the gene for junctophilin-3 located on chromosome 16q24.3. It was initially described in a large African American family in the southeastern United States. Subsequent studies have shown it to be a very rare cause of the HD phenotype occurring almost exclusively in individuals of African descent (2,3). Clinically, HDL2 closely resembles HD and causes chorea, dystonia, dysarthria, disturbed gait and balance, psychiatric symptoms, dementia, and weight loss. Onset is usually in the fourth decade with gradual progression to death within 20 years. Similar to juvenile HD, an akinetic rigid form without chorea has also been described with bradykinesia, rigidity, tremor, and a frontal lobe dementia. The neuropathology is similar to HD and is significant for ubiquitin-positive intracytoplasmic inclusion bodies with atrophy in the caudate nucleus, putamen, and frontal lobe. In some patients, there is additional neuronal loss in visual cortex and hippocampus. Diagnosis is made by gene testing. Normal CTG/CAG repeat length in the junctophilin-3 gene is up to 20 triplet repeats. Affected individuals with HDL2 have 41 to 58 triplet repeats. Similar to HD, brain MRI or computed tomography (CT) show caudate and cortical atrophy. Treatment is symptomatic. Tetrabenazine may ameliorate the chorea but carries the risk of aggravating bradykinesia and rigidity. Antianxiety, antidepressant, antimanic, and antipsychotic medications may be used when indicated.

REFERENCES

1. Margolis RL, O'Hearn E, Rosenblatt A, et al. A disorder similar to Huntington's disease is associated with a novel CAG repeat expansion. *Ann Neurol.* 2001;50:373–380.
2. Margolis RL, Holmes SE, Rosenblatt A, et al. Huntington's disease-like 2 (HDL2) in North America and Japan. *Ann Neurol.* 2004;56:670–674.
3. Greenstein PE, Vonsattel JG, Margolis RL, et al. Huntington's disease like-2 neuropathology. *Mov Disord.* 2007;22:1416–1423.

46

Late-Onset Sydenham's Chorea in a Middle-Aged Brazilian Woman

Francisco Cardoso and Débora Maia

THE CASE

At the age of 36 years, this woman noticed the gradual development of involuntary and continuous movements in the right side of her body. Initially, they were mild, but there was a gradual progression with increase of the severity and involvement of the left hemibody resulting in functional disability, which led her to look for medical assistance 1 year later. In other service, she was treated with diazepam with complete remission of the involuntary movements. Two years later, there was recurrence of the movements, which failed to improve with diazepam. At age 41, she was referred to the Movement Disorders Clinic of the Federal University of Minas Gerais. Her medical history was remarkable for the presence of an episode of arthralgia at age 12 years, which had been diagnosed as "rheumatism." Ten years before her first visit to our unit, she had pulmonary tuberculosis treated with the appropriate regimen of drugs for 6 months—at the end of which she was considered cured. The family history was unremarkable, and she had never been exposed to any hormone. Her neurologic examination was characterized by the presence of a continuous random flow of movements in all regions of her body with the exception of the right leg. The areas with choreic movements also displayed decreased muscle tone.

THE APPROACH

Once identified that chorea was the phenomenology of the movement disorder of the patient, we worked her up to identify possible underlying causes. Structural lesions, such as vascular disorder, and lesions suggestive of vasculitis, another common cause of chorea in adults, were ruled out by imaging studies. Tests to identify acute-phase reaction, such as C-reactive protein and sedimentation rate, were normal, and there was also no abnormality in the following tests: antistreptolysin test, thyroid function, glucose level, Venereal Disease Research Laboratory, antiphospholipid antibody, antinuclear factor, and spinal fluid analysis. Echocardiogram displayed double aortic lesion with stenosis greater than insufficiency and thickening and calcification of the valve leaflets. Using indirect immunofluorescence, enzyme-linked immunosorbent assay (ELISA), and western blot, we identified an increased titer of circulating antibasal ganglia antibodies. These findings were diagnostic of adult-onset Sydenham's chorea (SC) and valvar rheumatic disease in a patient with a previous history of rheumatic fever in childhood. She was treated with benzathine penicillin every 21 days, which as used irregularly, and pimozide. The latter suppressed the chorea and was withdrawn 18 months later. Five days after discontinuation of the neuroleptic, the patient developed recurrence of severe generalized chorea, leading to reintroduction of pimozide. However, this time, the patient failed to improve and developed mild parkinsonism. One month later, we discontinued the neuroleptic and started her on valproic acid. For the next 6 months, there was improvement of the choreic movements, although they never came into remission. At this stage, there was a new worsening of the severity of chorea. Thus, we decided to withdraw the valproic acid and treat her with intravenous methylprednisolone followed by oral prednisone to be gradually tapered off. Her chorea improved significantly during the steroid treatment. Two months later, she returned for a follow-up visit, describing recurrence of chorea after she discontinued the use of prednisone. A new methylprednisolone pulse therapy induced remarkable improvement of the patient's movement disorder. This time, she adhered to both penicillin prophylaxis and prednisone. Two years later, the steroid was discontinued, and she has remained without chorea since then. In 2002, at the time she underwent the second intravenous steroid treatment, the patient developed complex partial seizures, which remained under control with the use of carbamazepine. In 2010, there was a deterioration of the valvar lesion, which required surgical replacement by a biological prosthesis.

THE LESSON

The conventional concept of SC states that this is a condition restricted to children and teenagers. In fact, a review of a large cohort of patients in North America supports such a notion (1). Even in our own series of patients, the average age of onset was 8 years (2). The case of this patient teaches us, however, that it is possible to develop SC during adulthood. In a consecutive series of patients from Italy, the authors confirm that, although rare, SC may be the causative agent of sporadic chorea in adults (3). This is more common, although not exclusive, among patients with a previous history of rheumatic fever in childhood. Still related to the diagnosis of SC, this patient was one of the subjects studied in the collaborative investigation between the National Hospital of Neurology and our group, which led to a better understanding of the pathogenesis of SC. Using indirect immunofluorescence, ELISA, and western blot, we determined that there were circulating antibodies in the serum of this patient capable of recognizing basal ganglia and *Streptococcus* antigens (4). Although it remains to be determined whether these antibodies have a biological effect, accumulating evidence suggests that cross-reactive antibodies cause SC (5).

The second lesson this patient taught us is that in 25% to 50% of subjects, SC has a protracted course, lasting longer than 2 years. This is in contrast with the well-established notion that SC is always a self-limited condition (1). As a matter of fact, in a prospective study where we followed up a number of patients with SC, we demonstrated that remission does not occur in up to half of the patients. We have coined the term persistent SC to describe this situation (6). The underlying mechanism of the persistence of chorea in these patients remains unknown. We have shown that the majority of patients with persistent SC have circulating antibasal ganglia antibodies. However, because about 40% of patients with this condition do not test positive for these antibodies, one may speculate that nonhumoral mechanisms may also play a role in the persistence of SC (4).

The final lesson we learned with this patient was how to manage the chorea in patients with persistent SC. Although in many of these subjects the movement is so mild, it does not warrant treatment in others, including the patient herein reported, the chorea may be disabling. In some patients, treatment with valproic acid and neuroleptics, the mainstay of symptomatic management of chorea, is not effective and/or tolerated. In this circumstance, steroids are a useful alternative. The recommended regimen is intravenous methylprednisolone, 1 g a day for 5 days, followed by oral prednisone, which is gradually tapered off. Although the study was not controlled, we reported the positive results with this regimen in a series of patients with SC (7).

REFERENCES

1. Nausieda PA, Grossman BJ, Koller WC, et al. Sydenham chorea: an update. *Neurology.* 1980;30:331–334.
2. Cardoso F, Eduardo C, Silva AP, et al. Chorea in fifty consecutive patients with rheumatic fever. *Mov Disord.* 1997;12:701–703.
3. Piccolo I, Defanti CA, Soliveri P, et al. Cause and course in a series of patients with sporadic chorea. *J Neurol.* 2003;250:429–435.
4. Church AJ, Cardoso F, Dale RC, et al. Anti-basal ganglia antibodies in acute and persistent Sydenham's chorea. *Neurology.* 2002;59:227–231.
5. Cardoso F. Huntington disease and other choreas. *Neurol Clin.* 2009;27:719–736.
6. Cardoso F, Vargas AP, Oliveira LD, et al. Persistent Sydenham's chorea. *Mov Disord.* 1999;14:805–807.
7. Cardoso F, Maia D, Cunningham MC, et al. Treatment of Sydenham chorea with corticosteroids. *Mov Disord.* 2003;18:1374–1377.

47

A Case of Calcium-Induced Marital Stress

SHAWN F. SMYTH, LIANA ROSENTHAL, AND JOSEPH M. SAVITT

THE CASE

Our patient is a 71-year-old man with a 15-year neurologic history that first began with abnormal facial movements and subtle behavioral and cognitive changes that interfered with his occupation as a research toxicologist. Progressive motor impairment became more noticeable over the next 10 years and included upper kinetic limb tremor, micrographia, poor manual coordination, generalized stiffness, bradykinesia, and bulbar dysfunction with prominent drooling and dysphagia requiring a soft diet. In addition, he developed a shuffling and unsteady gait that led to falls. Over the last 3 to 4 years, there were new complaints of lightheadedness upon arising from a chair, urinary urgency, and constipation. Maintenance insomnia developed as well with bilateral leg jerking during sleep and episodic dream enactment with occasional episodes of falling out of bed.

Despite these numerous motor difficulties, his wife was most concerned about the cognitive and behavioral changes that began 15 years before. There was increasing irritability, apathy, anxiety, depression, paranoia, and disinhibition. The latter included episodes such as impulsively going off his soft mechanical diet, leading to aspiration and subsequent hospitalization. There were also frequent inappropriate comments that led to increasing social isolation and a new affinity for purchasing pornography. He was prone to occasional angry outbursts that included verbal threats. Such behavior was highly atypical for this previously gentle and caring man. Over the past decade, his wife also noticed progressive bradyphrenia, difficulty planning tasks, short-term memory loss, topographical disorientation, impaired judgment, perseveration, and lack of insight. Because his wife was his primary caretaker, she was becoming increasingly frustrated. She struggled most with his disinhibited behaviors, anger, apathy, and inability to organize routine daily activities. Her efforts to engage him and care for him were interpreted as nagging, and this led to his angry outbursts.

His previous medical problems included hypothyroidism, depression, and lumbar stenosis. Attempts at treatment, including low-dose duloxetine, donepezil, levodopa, and propranolol, were ineffective.

His family history included parkinsonism in his father; anxiety, depression, and late-life psychosis in his mother; and early-adult onset schizophrenia in his sister. He has two healthy children.

On our initial examination, 15 years after symptom onset, there was no orthostasis, and his general examination was unremarkable. On mental status examination, we found bradyphrenia, passivity, mild echolalia, stimulus-bound behaviors, and perseveration. He had difficulty mimicking Luria hand movements, had a positive glabellar reflex, and had no applause sign. His Montreal Cognitive Assessment (MoCA) total score was 24 out of 30, with deficits in clock drawing, naming, verbal fluency, and memory retrieval. Cranial nerve examination demonstrated saccadic pursuits, hypometric saccades, mild dysarthria, mild hearing loss bilaterally, and hypomimia. There were abnormal, nonrhythmic, and low-amplitude movements of the frontalis, tongue, and perioral muscles. His United Parkinson Disease Rating Scale (UPDRS) motor score was 20, including bilateral kinetic upper extremity tremors, mild rigidity of the neck and upper limbs, mild upper extremity bradykinesia that was more prominent on the right, a stooped posture, and mild retropulsion. There were intermittent bilateral choreoathetoid hand movements that were suppressible and that went largely unnoticed by our patient. On cerebellar testing, we found upper extremity dysmetria and impaired balance on tandem gait and stance. There was a mild length-dependent loss of sensation in the lower limbs. Tendon reflexes were present throughout, although diminished. He could walk independently, but he was mildly unsteady with a wide-based gait and reduced stride length.

THE APPROACH

Although our patient had many motor difficulties, the larger concern was his personality change and lack of motivation. Review of recent head computed tomography (CT) and brain MRI revealed extensive calcification of the bilateral basal ganglia, pulvinar, dentate cerebellar nuclei, and cerebellar white matter, with moderate to severe cerebellar and cerebral atrophy. Cerebral atrophy was most prominent on the left. Our first step was to evaluate for the etiology of these changes. Laboratory investigation ruled out abnormalities of calcium, phosphorus, parathyroid hormone, and metal intoxication and found no evidence of inflammatory or autoimmune processes. Imaging revealed no clear vascular etiology. Other laboratory tests were normal except for a mild iron deficiency anemia, a monoclonal gammopathy, and mild B12 deficiency. Electroencephalography (EEG) showed only slowing, and neurometric studies diagnosed a mixed axonal neuropathy. We initiated B12 repletion, hematologic referral, and more aggressive antidepressant therapy. Increases in duloxetine led to significantly less anxiety and improved social functioning. We referred him for speech, swallowing, physical, and occupational therapies. We did not start levodopa for his parkinsonism given his facial and limb dyskinesias and behavioral dysregulation. We encouraged him to attend a senior day program with structured activities not only for his benefit but also to provide a respite for his wife. We also highlighted the importance of dementia support groups for both to attend, provided caregiver resources regarding behavior management and preventing "burnout," and the future option of in-home behavioral management counseling. Finally, we instructed the patient and his wife that her reminders should be seen as her being his "spark" to get up and do things rather than as nagging because his initiative and insight were impaired. This was to be written on a page and hung on the refrigerator to continually remind our patient that his wife is his "spark." These latter nonpharmacologic interventions proved to be the most helpful.

THE LESSON

This case highlights the evaluation of cerebral calcification mainly affecting the motor system and the concomitant nonmotor symptoms that may be present. Although this clinical-radiographic picture is often referred to as "Fahr's disease," this term is nonspecific and likely leads to ambiguity. Alternatively, it has been proposed to anatomically name the sites of calcification, giving a more specific diagnosis. In our patient, his condition would be referred to as bilateral striopallidodentate calcinosis (BSPDC) [1,2]. This particular disorder might result from the abnormal leakage of plasma-derived fluids across the blood–brain barrier, leading to deposition of an acid mucopolysaccharide–alkali protein complex and ultimately calcium, iron, and other minerals [3,4]. Although the neurologic and psychiatric conditions in our patient's family history might suggest an autosomal dominant form of this calcinosis, we cannot rule out other familial or sporadic disease given the incomplete family records [1]. In a recent registry study of patients with striopallidodentate calcinosis, it was found that presentations of parkinsonism, hyperkinetic movement disorders, cognitive dysfunction, and cerebellar ataxia often coexist, as seen in our patient [3]. The pattern of significant behavioral dysregulation that occurred in our patient is not as often recognized in this disorder, and in this case, it overlaps with what is seen in behavioral variant frontotemporal dementia and in patients with Parkinson disease treated with dopaminergic agents [5,6]. Although strategies to address such cognitive and behavioral changes are often partially successful, structured approaches may improve the situation. Lessons learned from caring for our patient and the reports of others with similar disorders include:

1. Excessive calcification of the basal ganglia, dentate nucleus, thalamus, and connecting white matter tracts leads to a wide variety of neurologic and psychiatric symptoms (1–3).
2. The co-occurrence of hypokinetic and hyperkinetic movement disorders with behavioral dysregulation may limit pharmacologic interventions.
3. Treatment with an antidepressant can aid in behavioral symptoms.
4. Nonpharmacologic behavioral management strategies may be helpful in reducing disruptive behaviors. Building a collaborative relationship between the caregiver and patient is crucial for optimal management of troublesome behaviors.

REFERENCES

1. Manyam BV. Bilateral striopallidodentate calcinosis: a proposed classification of genetic and secondary causes. *Mov Disord.* 1990;5(Suppl 1):94.
2. Manyam BV. What is and is not "Fahr's disease". *Parkinsonism Relat Disord.* 2005;11:73–80.
3. Manyam BV, Walters AS, Narla KR. Bilateral striopallidodentate calcinosis: clinical characteristics of patients seen in a registry. *Mov Disord.* 2001;16:258–264.
4. Duckett S, Galle P, Escourolle R, et al. Presence of zinc, aluminum, magnesium in striopallidodentate (SPD) calcifications (Fahr's disease): electron probe study. *Acta Neuropathol (Berl).* 1977;38:7–10.
5. Piguet O, Hornberger M, Mioshi E, et al. Behavioural-variant frontotemporal dementia: diagnosis, clinical staging, and management. *Lancet Neurol.* 2011;10:162–172.
6. Ambermoon P, Carter A, Hall WD, et al. Impulse control disorders in patients with Parkinson's disease receiving dopamine replacement therapy: evidence and implications for the addictions field. *Addiction.* 2010;106:283–293.

Discrepancy in CAG Repeat Lengths in a Case of Clinically Manifest Huntington's Disease: The Psychological Ordeal of My 24-Year-Old Patient

JUAN SANCHEZ-RAMOS

THE CASE

A 24-year-old married woman with four very young children was referred to our Huntington's disease (HD) clinic for evaluation and possible genetic testing. Her chief complaints were increased clumsiness of the hands and forgetfulness. Her husband pointed out she was having difficulty taking care of her children and family. She denied involuntary movements, and in particular, she did not notice chorea or dystonia. She was very familiar with the motor manifestations in family members affected by HD.

She had a strong family history of HD. Both her father, still alive, and brother suffer from the illness. Her father first started showing the motor signs of HD when he was in his 20s and was diagnosed around the age of 25. In her family, she has met 23 people with HD. She first learned about her risk of inheriting the illness when she was 10 years old. She has had four children in the last 5 years, and this year decided to have a tubal ligation. Her medical history was unremarkable. She was not taking any medications other than sertraline, which was recently started by her local physician.

Her physical appearance was that of a pale, tired, depressed young woman, with a vacuous gaze. Examination of the cranial nerves II through XII revealed slightly slowed saccades. She needed to blink to initiate the saccades in both horizontal and vertical directions. She could protrude her tongue easily for 10 seconds. The motor examination revealed normal muscle tone and generalized bradykinesia. Finger tapping and hand movements were performed very slowly with small amplitude. Rapid alternating movements were performed with normal rhythm but slowly. She could not perform the Luria test even with cuing. No chorea or dystonia was noted throughout the visit. The deep tendon reflexes were markedly increased in upper and lower limbs with crossed adductor spread. Gait was slow and slightly awkward. Tandem gait was performed with three missteps out of 10 steps. Sensory examination was normal to all modalities.

Despite absence of chorea and dystonia, I was confident that her diagnosis was HD based on the presence of marked bradykinesia in all movements, especially finger taps, abnormal saccadic eye movements, and hyper-reflexia in the context of a strong family history of HD. She did not exhibit tremor or rigidity in the limbs that is often seen in young-onset HD. In addition, she exhibited cognitive deficits, especially in the realm of executive function, and she was depressed. At that initial visit, we provided psychological and genetic counseling for her and her husband. After our psychologist discussed her observations with the HD team, we decided not to perform the genetic test until we ascertained that her depression was improved and she was capable of handling news of positive or negative results.

In a follow-up visit 6 months later, she looked much better than she did in the past, with more color in her face. Her husband and newborn baby were present. She was very quiet and did not complain of anything. Her husband noted that she is irritable and becomes angry if she is interrupted while performing a household chore. We discussed the difficulty many patients with HD have in following through on tasks and the near impossibility to multitask. In general, although her antidepressant was working quite well to improve her mood, she did not sleep well and, according to her husband, was very tired during the day, partly because there were a lot of demands on her by the four little children. Her husband helps as much as he can, and her husband's family helps take care of the children.

On examination, she could not perform the Luria test, even with cuing. Cranial nerves revealed limited range in upward direction and full range downward and horizontally. Her saccades were very slow, and there is an increased latency to initiate the saccades. She could not keep her tongue protruded more than 8 seconds. Cranial nerves II through XII otherwise are normal. Motor examination revealed slight increase in tone with activation on the left arm. With arms extended, she exhibited dystonic posturing of her right hand and mild, intermittent chorea in her left hand. No chorea was noted in her face, toes, feet, head, or trunk. The sensory examination was normal, and deep tendon reflexes were markedly increased with spread. Gait was slow, wide based, and awkward. She missed steps three times in tandem gait testing and recovered spontaneously when tested for retropulsion.

THE APPROACH

After her last visit, there was little doubt about her diagnosis of clinically manifest HD. Nevertheless, she and her husband wanted to have a confirmatory genetic test. Because her depression seemed to be under control and her mood was stable, we drew a blood sample for genetic testing.

Two weeks later, we received an unexpected result. The CAG repeats numbered 18 on both alleles! We brought her and her husband into clinic for disclosure of the normal genetic test results. I explained that perhaps her illness was not HD, although I doubted this in light of her strong family history and clinical presentation. We suggested the possibility that she carried another gene or genes associated with HD-like clinical manifestations. We explained that several other distinct genetic disorders have been identified that can present with a clinical picture indistinguishable from HD. We offered, and she agreed, to send another blood sample to a laboratory at the University of Tennessee (UT) where testing for genetic mutations associated with HD look-alikes could be performed.

The results from the UT laboratory were even more surprising. The HD-2 results were negative, but the laboratory reran the HD CAG test and found positive results: CAG repeats of 48 and 19. I then asked for a repeat analysis of her sample in the Genetics Laboratory in All Children's Hospital in St. Petersburg where we send all of our routine HD samples for genetic testing.

This time, the test results were positive with alleles of 18 and 47 (+/−1) × CAG. However, the large alleles were very weak, much weaker than the large alleles of the 88 × CAG control that the laboratory normally uses. A primer site polymorphism resulting in poor amplification of the large allele was a possible explanation. The UT laboratory also had some problems detecting the larger allele. The primers that both laboratories used were from a published protocol and were identical in sequence. The two laboratories used different dye labels on the primers, but it is unlikely that dyes interfere with the polymerase chain reaction (PCR) amplification. The large discrepancy between the signal strength of our patient's normal allele and the larger one was about 200 to 1. The signal falls off in strength with increasing number of repeats, but even in the extreme case, i.e., the 88 × CAG control, the ratio is only 50 to 1. Therefore, it was difficult to explain this large degree of signal loss with only a moderate-size allele.

We sent a sample of DNA from the patient to a third site, Massachusetts General Hospital in Boston. The assay used the standard Huntington disease-cytosine adenine guanine (HD-CAG) assay (primers CAG1: 6FAM-ATG AAG GCC TTC GAG TCC CTC AAG TCC TTC and CAG2: GGC GGT GGC GGC TGT TGC TGC TGC TGC TGC), and both the normal (19 CAGs) and expanded HD (49 CAGs) alleles were detected.

Sequence analysis of this sample revealed an apparent juxtaposition of uninterrupted CAG and CCG repeats in one of the alleles: (CAG)n(CCG)n instead of the most common (CAG) nCAACAGCCGCCA(CCG)n repeat sequence. This region has already been reported as a mutation-prone region (1), and both CAA to CAG and CCA to CCG alterations described as polymorphisms in the single nucleotide polymorphism (SNP) databases (rs473915 and rs76533208, respectively). According to the laboratories' collected data, it seems that these uninterrupted repeats are not a rare event in HD chromosomes.

THE LESSON

Ninety-nine percent of HD phenotypes are caused by an expanded CAG allele (>37 units) (2). Several other distinct genetic disorders have been identified that can present with a clinical picture indistinguishable from HD, termed HD-like (HDL) syndromes. Four genes associated with HDL syndromes have been identified, including the prion protein gene (*HDL1*), the junctophilin 3 gene (*HDL2*), and the gene encoding the TATA box-binding protein (*HDL4*) (2). These disorders account for only a small proportion of HDL cases, and the list of HDL genes will very likely expand.

Although we initially concluded from the initial normal test results that our patient represented an HD look-alike, the explanation for our case was attributed to a polymorphism at the promoter site. The primers used for the initial testing were HD-1P: 5′ ATG AAG GCC TTC GAG TCC CTC AAG TCC TT-3′ and HD-C2: 5′ CGG CGG TGG CGG CTG TTG 3′. The reverse primer is designed to anneal exactly in this polymorphic region that bounds the CAG and CCG repeats. This likely accounted for the difficulty amplifying alleles with uninterrupted repeats.

Another question that arose during this exercise revolved around the fact that the original genetic test showed identical numbers of CAG repeats on both alleles and had missed the expanded allele. Should identical CAG repeats on both alleles be taken as a red flag for missing a very large expanded repeat or for failing to amplify the CAG because of a mutation in the promoter where the primers attach? DNA samples from 18 subjects who had undergone genetic testing and who were homozygous for CAG repeat (e.g., identical number of CAG repeats on each allele) were rerun to check for larger alleles that might have been missed. By doing an alternate detection protocol using Southern blotting, no larger CAG repeat was found in any of these cases. Hence, the finding of identical CAG repeats in both alleles need not raise alarms.

Acknowledgments
Grateful thanks to Dr Thomas Mueller (Director of Biochemical and Molecular Genetics, All Children's Hospital St. Petersburg, Florida); Dr Karla Matteson (Biochemical and Molecular Genetic Laboratories, University of Tennessee); and Dr Eliana Marisa Ramos and Dr Marci McDonald (Center for Human Genetic Research, Massachusetts General Hospital) for their help in solving this case.

REFERENCES

1. Williams LC, Hegde MR, Nagappan R, et al. Null alleles at the Huntington disease locus: implications for diagnostics and CAG repeat instability. *Genet Test.* 2000;4:55–60.
2. Schneider SA, Bhatia KP. Huntington's disease look-alikes. *Handb Clin Neurol.* 2011;100:101–112.

Suggested Reading
Persichetti F, Srinidhi J, Kanaley L, et al. Huntington's disease CAG trinucleotide repeats in pathologically confirmed post-mortem brains. *Neurobiol Dis.* 1994;1:159–166.
Wild EJ, Mudanohwo EE, Sweeney MG, et al. Huntington's disease phenocopies are clinically and genetically heterogeneous. *Mov Disord.* 2008;23:716–720.

49

Evolving Movement Disorder in a 13-Year-Old Girl From the Philippines Presenting Initially With Joint Pains

LILLIAN V. LEE, ROSALIA A. TELEG, JEANNIE AHORRO,
EDWIN MUNOZ, AND JOSE ROBLES

THE CASE

A fellow pediatric neurologist colleague referred a 13-year-old Filipino girl for involuntary movements in December 2004.

History revealed that 9 months before her first admission in October 2004, the patient had fever associated with joint pains, which resolved in a week after treatment with paracetamol and cotrimoxazole. In October, she developed choreiform movements of the right limbs, which progressed to involve the mouth with jaw opening and later the left lower extremity. She also had one episode of bowel incontinence, and this prompted the first admission to the Philippine Children's Medical Center. At admission, except for the involuntary movements, her physical and neurologic examinations were unremarkable. Complete blood count, C-reactive protein (CRP) and antistreptolysin (ASO) titers, serum electrolytes (sodium, potassium, chlorine, and calcium), serum creatinine and blood urea nitrogen (BUN), serum glutamic pyruvic transaminase (SGPT), chest x-ray, and routine qualitative and quantitative cerebrospinal fluid (CSF) analysis showed normal findings. Two-dimensional Echo/Doppler study was unremarkable. Notable were mildly increased erythrocyte sedimentation rate, epileptiform discharges on electroencephalography (EEG), and densities seen on bilateral basal ganglia on plain and contrast imaging of the brain. The working impression was Sydenham's chorea. She was treated with Benzathine Pen G Na 2 M units intramuscularly (IM) per day, and for the movements, she was given haloperidol and valproic acid. The patient was discharged improved. The involuntary movements were eventually controlled.

She was readmitted 3 days after discharge when she developed generalized papular rashes associated with fever and nonproductive cough. She was managed for viral exanthem and/or hypersensitivity reaction from either valproic acid or haloperidol. Her fever was controlled with paracetamol. Valproic acid was discontinued. Haloperidol was maintained at a lower dose. The patient was likewise given diphenhydramine and loratadine. The patient improved and was discharged after 4 days.

THE APPROACH

Our patient was initially treated as a case of Sydenham's chorea and treated with penicillin, haloperidol, and valproic acid. She apparently had hypersensitivity reaction to valproic acid and was maintained on haloperidol. A week after discharge, she had recurrence of the involuntary movements and increased sleepiness; therefore, she was readmitted for the third time. It was at this time that the case was referred to us for comanagement. On evaluation, the patient presented with dystonic movements of the right lower limb (hip flexion with knee extension). When made to walk, the patient was noted to have right foot equinovarus. There was also increased tone (rigidity and cogwheeling) noted, together with hypokinesia. No Kayser-Fleischer ring was seen. Viral encephalitis was the first consideration. Repeat EEG and routine CSF study showed normal results, and CSF studies on Japanese B and Herpes simplex encephalitides were negative. A repeat computed tomography (CT) scan showed hyperdense striatal areas. MRI showed increased signals in both striatum. Other possible causes of involuntary movements were investigated. Fasting blood sugar, renal and liver function tests, serum ceruloplasmin, 24-hour urine copper, serum iron, serum calcium, and phosphorus yielded normal or acceptable results. The patient was discharged partially improved.

While at home, episodic dystonic spasms of the right lower limb became more frequent and eventually generalized. Involuntary jaw opening and urinary incontinence followed, and these again prompted readmission for the fourth time because of possible acute dystonic reaction to haloperidol, although a postencephalitic movement disorder was still entertained. In the hospital, the patient became dysphonic and developed dysphagia requiring the insertion of a nasogastric feeding tube. Haloperidol was discontinued. The episodic spasms were controlled with diphenhydramine, and the patient was sent home on this medication.

In the next 3 months while at home, the patient had increased severity of generalized painful spasms involving mainly the lower extremities. Trihexyphenidyl (Artane) became available, and the patient was placed on an increasing dose of Artane till 30 mg/d in three divided doses was reached. The patient improved and the dystonia lessened. Unfortunately, 3 months later, commercial supplies of trihexyphenidyl HCl ran out in the market and therefore the patient had to be shifted to clonazepam. Anticipating that she might have an acute reaction with the withdrawal of trihexyphenidyl, she was readmitted (fifth time). At admission, the patient was conscious and was able to follow some commands but was dysphonic, perhaps part of the dystonia. There were no cranial nerves and sensory deficits. Motor grade was at least Medical Research Council (MRC) scale 3/5. She had generalized dystonia (jaw opening and closure, left elbow flexion, right elbow extension, bilateral wrist ulnar deviation and flexion, bilateral finger flexion, truncal lateral flexion to the right, bilateral hip flexion more prominent on the right, bilateral foot dorsiflexion, and inversion; see Figure 49.1). Dystonic postures would cease with sleep. Complete blood count (CBC), serum electrolytes, and liver and renal function tests were normal. Serum creatine kinase MM and creatine kinase MB were both mildly elevated (71 U/L). Repeat EEG was normal. Electromyography showed cocontractions of agonist and antagonist muscles consistent with dystonia. Muscle ultrasound was normal. By this time, spasms were fairly controlled with clonazepam 0.5 tab q8H and topiramate 50 mg/tab 1 tab q6H. The patient was discharged with some improvement of the generalized dystonia. She subsequently suffered from episodic painful dystonia of the legs, which became more frequent and appeared more like dystonic cramps. Clonazepam and topiramate offered some relief. Lidocaine injections were tried, but the effect did not last. Risperidone was added, which afforded some relief.

Despite the many drugs tried for the involuntary movements, there was no satisfactory response. The dystonic posturings became more frequent and soon she developed contractures (see Figure 49.1). Deep brain stimulation (DBS) was considered, hoping it might help. Therefore, in preparation, a repeat MRI of the brain was obtained. The second MRI, taken 8 months after the onset of dystonia, showed bilateral and symmetric signal abnormalities involving the caudate and lentiform nuclei with interval development of diffuse bilateral frontotemporal cerebral atrophy. A postinflammatory or infectious etiology was considered.

DBS as an option was abandoned, and the patient was followed up as an outpatient regularly.

While trying to look for other therapeutic options, 22 months after the onset of joint pains and 14 months after the onset of dystonic movements, we were informed that the child woke up in the middle of the night, screamed, became cyanotic, and died. Permit for a partial autopsy (brain) was granted. Pathology showed marked neuronal loss with reactive astrogliosis involving the caudate, putamen, globus pallidus, claustrum, portions of the basal forebrain, and substantia nigra. Also noted was white matter tract degeneration involving the anterior and posterior limbs of the internal capsule.

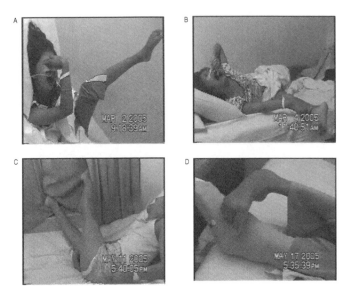

FIGURE 49.1
(A–C) The painful dystonic postures assumed by the patient during the fifth admission as described in the text. (D) The contracted ankle.

THE LESSON

Proper identification of the movement disorder is basic in the neurologic examination of a patient suspected of a movement disorder.

This patient initially presented with choreiform movements of the right limbs. Subsequently, there was chorei-dystonic overlap that eventually became predominantly dystonic. At one point, the presence of hypokinesia and rigidity suggested the presence of parkinsonian features. Afterward, dystonia progressed in severity, in frequency, and degree of painful contractions— and eventually, the dystonia generalized.

There were logical bases for the working diagnoses that were entertained: Sydenham's chorea, viral encephalitis, acute dystonic reaction, and postencephalitic movement disorder. There was no attempt, however, to look for the presence of a neoplasm or do a neuropsychological evaluation.

On review, after the pathology findings became evident and considering that all the neuroimaging tests performed kept pointing to abnormalities in the basal ganglia, the most apt consideration would have been a post-streptococcal acute disseminated encephalomyelitis with basal ganglia involvement or an autoimmune basal ganglia encephalitis. Demonstration of autoreactive anti–basal ganglia antibodies, if available, would have proven the diagnosis in this case. Perhaps, immunologic therapy such as the use of steroids, immune globulins (intravenous IgG) chemotherapy, or plasmapheresis could have helped.

Suggested Reading

Boyer WF, Bakalar NH, Lake CR. Anticholinergic prophylaxis of acute haloperidol-induced acute dystonic reactions. *J Clin Psychopharmacol.* 1987;7:164–166.

Ch'ien LT, Economides AN, Lemmi H. Sydenham's chorea and seizures. Clinical and electroencephalographic studies. *Arch Neurol.* 1978;35:382–385.

Church AJ, Cardoso F, Dale RC, et al. Anti-basal ganglia antibodies in acute and persistent Sydenham's chorea. *Neurol.* 2002;59:227–231.

Dale RC, Church AJ, Cardoso F, et al. Poststreptococcal acute disseminated encephalomyelitis with basal ganglia involvement in auto-reactive antibasal ganglia bodies. *Ann Neurol.* 2001;50:588–595.

Dale RC, Church AJ, Surtees AH, et al. Encephalitis lethargic syndrome: 20 new cases and evidence of basal ganglia autoimmunity. *Brain.* 2003;127:21–33.

Demiroren K, Yavuz H, Cam L, et al. Sydenham's chorea: a clinical follow-up of 65 patients. *J Child Neurol.* 2007;22:550–554.

Dure LS IV. Movement disorders in childhood. In: Watts RL, Koller WC, eds. *Movement Disorders: Neurologic Principles and Practice.* 2nd ed. New York: The McGraw-Hill Companies, Inc., 2003:826–832.

Florance RC, Davis RL, Lam C, et al. Anti-n-methyl-d-aspartate receptor (NMDAR) encephalitis in children and adolescents. *Ann Neurol.* 2009;66:11–18.

Palumbo E. Sydenham's chorea: diagnosis and management. *Recenti Prog Med.* 2008;99:39–41. [Abstract].

50

"Defiant and Rebellious" Behavior in a Canadian Teenager: Sarah's Difficult Journey

MARGUERITE WIELER AND W.R. WAYNE MARTIN

<hr>

THE CASE

Teenagers! Delightful, quarrelsome, defiant, irritable, confused, happy, sullen, talkative, rebellious, exuberant, oppositional, resistant, resentful, argumentative, moody, withdrawn, insolent, cranky, aggressive, depressed, witty, unpredictable, full of potential and promise, hostile, thrill seeking—teenagers!

Most people experience some emotional turmoil and relationship stress during their teenage years. Oftentimes, they are unable to explain why they do what they do or feel the way they feel. Many adolescents will get into trouble at one time or another. But when is "bad" behavior "just being a teenager" and when does it raise the index of suspicion of more serious underlying issues?

"Sarah" was a seemingly well-adjusted child living with her mother and adoptive father in a small, rural community. Shortly after entering her teenage years, she started to display disruptive and aggressive behaviors. Her relationship with her parents became tense and fractious. They were dismayed at her typical teenage "acting out" and the many arguments that ensued about everything. She exhibited some self-harming behaviors and had episodes of depression starting at age 15. She got involved with a boyfriend (of whom her parents disapproved) around that time and had a son at age 17. The relationship with her now ex-boyfriend and father of her child was virtually nonexistent. She dropped out of high school and was unemployed with no source of income and living with her parents.

In April 1999, at the age of 20, her depression required treatment. She was started on paroxetine and admitted for mental health counseling and day programs in her rural community.

She noted and grew concerned about the gradual onset of a strange "tic" in her shoulder and was admitted to her community hospital for investigation in August 1999. Serum ceruloplasmin at the time was normal. An MRI was reported to show "low signal intensity in the basal ganglia bilaterally." She was discharged, and shortly after discharge, she made a suicide attempt by cutting her left wrist with a butcher knife and overdosing on three bottles of paroxetine. This was followed in early October 1999 with an intentional or planned motor vehicle collision as a subsequent suicide attempt. She deliberately drove her parent's car through neighborhood gardens and fences, eventually colliding with a parked trailer. She was admitted to the inpatient psychiatric ward of a large urban hospital.

During this admission, she was noted to have the following depressive symptoms: unprovoked crying, immense sadness, sleep disturbances, derealization, hopelessness, poor concentration, worsening of short-term memory, anhedonia, and suicidal ideation with attempts. She denied any form of hallucination or delusions. There was no history of alcohol or substance abuse; she did admit to social smoking. The abnormal movement in her shoulder had increased and progressed to involve other body parts. She noted that she would sometimes trip and fall, spill cups of water, and had begun producing "weird" noises and chuckles. The attending psychiatrist felt she met criteria for borderline personality disorder superimposed on a primitive personality makeup with little insight and poor reasoning skills and judgment. Her medications at discharge were venlafaxine 150 mg every day before noon and zopiclone 7.5 mg every night at bedtime as needed.

THE APPROACH

She was referred to a general neurologist and the genetics clinic. The differential diagnosis while on the psychiatry unit was said to include pantothenate kinase–associated neurodegeneration, Huntington's disease (HD), a "striatal degenerative condition," and an ischemic episode. Liver function tests and hemoglobin were normal. Biochemical tests ruled out common metabolic and storage diseases. Electroencephalography (EEG) was normal. Single photon emission computed tomography scanning with ^{99m}Tc-HMPAO showed marked reduction in perfusion of the basal ganglia bilaterally and a small focal abnormality in the posterior right mesial temporal lobe. This was stated to be suggestive of HD. Neuropsychological testing revealed average verbal abilities, low average to borderline nonverbal abilities, mild to severe deficits of sustained attention, and right–left disorientation.

The general neurologist suggested low-dose haloperidol to treat the abnormal movements.

Sarah had no known family history of any neurologic disorders on her maternal side. However, her paternal family history was completely unknown because her biological father had not been involved since her birth.

The combination of behavioral symptoms, abnormal involuntary movements, and suspicious neuroimaging results led to genetic testing for HD. Sarah's result in December 1999 was positive (17 CAG repeats on one allele and 64 repeats on the other allele). Her mother's DNA test for HD was negative.

Sarah was referred to the Movement Disorders Program and seen in February 2000. On neurologic examination, she displayed typical eye movement abnormalities of early HD, motor impersistence, mild dysarthria, chorea in her trunk and limbs along with dystonic posturing in her neck, left upper limb, and both lower limbs. She had increased tone in all limbs, had mild bradykinesia, and walked with a wide base with preserved tandem gait.

She was unable to live independently and was not safe to leave the house unaccompanied, having lost her way in the neighborhood in the past. Noted at this time were impaired balance with frequent falls; difficulty with swallowing, particularly fluids, with occasional choking spells; impaired dexterity requiring help with dressing and cutting food; and some issues with speech. Her limitations with respect to motor function were not the main concern; rather her major disability was related to a depressed mood and being prone to compulsive, irresponsible, and disinhibited behavior. She required 24-hour supervision. She was unable to care for her 2-year-old son, and her parents were in the process of getting complete custody of him. The haloperidol that had been previously prescribed was discontinued, but venlafaxine and zopiclone were continued and risperidone 2 mg every day was prescribed.

Sarah was seen again 3 months later, in May 2000, and her stormy course continued unabated. Sarah required an in-home care worker for 60 hours per week with her parents supervising her for the remaining time. In April, she stabbed the care worker in the hand and spent 5 days in the remand center. At the time of the May visit, she was awaiting evaluation to determine her fitness to stand trial. Just days before this visit, she jumped out of her bedroom window and, without a license, drove the family truck into town. There had been multiple angry and physical outbursts particularly directed toward her mother who described Sarah as "defiant and rebellious."

THE LESSON

"Defiance and rebellion" are words used to describe Sarah's behavior for the next 9 years. Her behavior was so disruptive that by January 2001, she was unable to be cared for in her parent's home. Her mother, her greatest advocate, worked tirelessly to find appropriate accommodation.

She exhausted all avenues of financial support and venues to appropriately and adequately care for her only daughter. The next years were filled with frustration and exasperation for many people: Sarah, her mother, her father, her son, her siblings, the workers in various group homes, and the medical professionals who tried to ease the situation. Living in rural Canada presented challenges of access to suitable support, particularly mental health support for both Sarah and her family. The group homes in which Sarah lived were not geared to deal with people living with a neurodegenerative disorder and were often aggravated and annoyed by her inability to "get with the program." Despite education provided to the staff, it was an almost impossible task to divert them from an "improvement" model of behavior modification to a "maintenance" model, often resulting in frequent and vigorous disagreements between Sarah's mother and the group home staff regarding expectations of meeting milestones to improve independence. Sarah's mother was exhausted, angry, frustrated, and deeply sad, seemingly unable to take the time and effort necessary to "care for the care giver." Her frustration with "the system" and its inability to be flexible enough to meet the needs of her daughter was a major source of her anger.

As the years passed, there was the expected deterioration in Sarah's functional abilities with a significant decline starting in April 2008. She was placed in a rural long-term care facility in July 2008 where she was completely dependent on staff for the management of all aspects of her activities of daily living, unable to feed herself with significant swallowing issues and drooling resulting in weight loss of 35 to 40 pounds over a 2-year period. Involuntary dystonic arm and leg movements affected all attempts at voluntary movement. The disruptive and obsessive behaviors that had been so troublesome in the past were no longer an issue, in part because of Sarah's inability to function without substantial assistance. Sarah's mother was aware of the significant dysphagia but, based on previous discussions with her daughter, did not wish to consider the possibility of percutaneous endoscopic gastrostomy (PEG) feeding. In March 2009, Sarah passed away peacefully from complications of pneumonia.

A heart-wrenching conversation with Sarah's mother subsequently made a lasting impression—with tears in her eyes and an anguished look on her face, Sarah's mother said, "I am seeing things in my 12-year-old grandson that I saw in his mother. I just don't know how I am going to do it all over again...."

Suggested Reading

Ribai P, Nguyen K, Hahn-Barma V, et al. Psychiatric and cognitive difficulties as indicators of juvenile Huntington disease onset in 29 patients. *Arch Neurol.* 2007;64:813–819.

Siesling S, Vegter-van der Vlis M, Roos R. Juvenile Huntington disease in the Netherlands. *Pediatr Neurol.* 1997;17:37–43.

Juvenile Huntington Disease: A Resource for Families, Health Professionals and Caregivers. Huntington Society Canada, 2008. http://www.huntingtonsociety.ca/english/uploads/Juvenile_HD_2008.pdf.

The Juvenile HD Handbook: A Guide for Families and Caregivers. Huntington Disease Society of America, 2007. http://www.hdsa.org/images/content/1/1/11702.pdf.

51

The Challenging Case of Progressive Cognitive Decline in a Student: History in the Making?

DAVID J. BURN

THE CASE

A 19-year-old male student was referred to my neurology clinic by a local psychiatrist with a history of "atypical depression." Having previously been outgoing, fastidious, and interested in music, the patient had become withdrawn and untidy and had recently dropped out of his university course. The psychiatrist was worried, however, in that the affective disorder did not comfortably sit with a pattern she recognized, and moreover, she was concerned that there might be underlying cognitive decline.

When seen in my busy District General Hospital clinic (which I did on a weekly basis before subsequently retreating into my University Hospital "Ivory Tower"), it was difficult to get a clear feel of the situation from the patient. He made very little eye contact, and his responses to questions were brief, although appeared both appropriate and correct. His mother, who accompanied him, did feel that his short-term memory was less good than it was, that the whole problem had developed within the preceding 12 months, and that it was getting worse. There was no medical history of note, and he had received a full set of immunizations as a child, including measles. He had not traveled to exotic areas, and there was no known history of substance abuse or "high-risk" sexual activity. Examination at that stage revealed a possible mild gait ataxia but nil else. I simply did not have time to perform a formal cognitive assessment in clinic.

THE APPROACH

I initially thought that the patient was likely to be depressed and still wondered about illicit drug use (how many moms know exactly what their teenage children are getting up to, particularly when they live away from home?). But I was concerned, given the number of patients with depression my psychiatry colleagues see, that this patient's presentation had clearly raised alarm bells as being in some way "different." Furthermore, there was the unresolved question of a possible underlying cognitive decline and a mild gait ataxia. Therefore, I erred on the safe side and decided to admit him electively to my home base neurology ward for further investigations.

By the time of admission, 3 weeks later, the situation was essentially unchanged. Formal neuropsychometric assessment indicated mild global cognitive decline, compared with premorbid estimates, but with particularly severe impairments in verbal and visual memory. There was a mild gait ataxia, only evident on tandem walking. A host of routine blood tests, MRI brain scan, electroencephalography (EEG), and cerebrospinal fluid (CSF) analysis were all normal. His parents were frustrated by the lack of a diagnosis, and so was I. I looked up the literature for causes of cognitive decline in this age group, and we proceeded to a second wave of tests to exclude Wilson's and Huntington's diseases and Niemann-Pick type C, among others. Considering other rare storage and metabolic diseases such as hexosaminidase A deficiency and adrenoleukodystrophy as causes of cognitive decline in a young man, a battery of white cell enzymes and very long chain fatty acids were requested and were normal (1,2). Despite no history of high-risk sexual behavior, an HIV test was sent, with negative outcome. One of the main problems that we had at this stage was the absence of additional physical signs or "handles" to better inform the differential of a cognitive decline and mild gait ataxia.

Six weeks later, I decided to readmit the patient for further diagnostic workup, having been contacted by the parents who reported clear deterioration. Cognitively, the patient was worse and now needed help with several activities of daily living, although was continent and able to feed himself. In addition to worsening gait and limb ataxia, which made independent ambulation difficult, he had now developed mild but definite chorea. A repeat MRI brain scan indicated posterior thalamic high signal on T2-weighted images. Neither we nor the neuroradiologist had seen this subtle abnormality previously; it had not been reported in the literature and therefore we were unaware of its diagnostic significance. A repeat EEG was only nonspecifically abnormal and showed no evidence of subacute sclerosing panencephalitis or periodic lateralized discharges.

Ultimately, the patient was transferred to a long-care ward, where he became mute, akinetic, and incontinent. I had frequent meetings with the parents throughout this time and have never felt so helpless in my professional career. We considered but did not proceed to brain biopsy. He died of pneumonia 13 months after first being seen in my clinic. Toward the end of his illness, the possibility of an unusual form of prion disease was raised, given recent case reports that had begun to appear in the literature. A postmortem revealed pathologic features typical of new variant Creutzfeldt-Jakob disease (nvCJD). This case was one of 14 reported in a seminal publication describing the clinical presentation, natural history, and investigational findings of nvCJD (3). Post hoc genetic analysis revealed that our patient was homozygous for methionine at codon 129 of the PrP gene, in common with all other reported nvCJD cases.

THE LESSON

This was one of the most difficult cases that I have encountered as a consultant. Indeed, it came at a time when I had been in post for less than 2 years. The support from my neurologic consultant colleagues was invaluable during this patient's illness, particularly in terms of making diagnostic suggestions and general reassurance that my approach was comprehensive. There were several lessons to be learned from this case. First, always pay attention to your colleagues' doubts when a case clearly does not fit within their previous experience. In this case, it would have been easy to dismiss the psychiatrist's misgivings and simply label the patient as depressed. Although he would have undoubtedly presented sooner rather than later because of his rapid decline, such a dismissal would have got the whole journey and relationship with the parents off to a very poor start. Second, if you do not know what is going on, then be honest. The parents became increasingly and understandably frantic as their son deteriorated in front of their eyes and not uncommonly would come out with comments like: "Well, someone *must* have had an illness like this somewhere." Perhaps, the Movement Disorder Society (MDS) website for difficult cases now provides a forum to assist in such examples. However, what came across most clearly to me was the fact that if you have never seen something before and the literature is not there to help you, you are effectively breaking new ground—but that was not obvious to me at the time. I kept telling myself "I'm missing something here." How much we rely on pattern recognition? Therefore, when another case of nvCJD was admitted to our ward under the care of another consultant a few months later, I was asked to see her and was quite confident that this was the likely diagnosis, even though the clinical picture was not yet "full blown." From ignoramus to "expert" in two cases?! Reading this case vignette, many of you will have tuned in to the prion diagnosis at a very early stage and may find our lack of knowledge of the significance of the thalamic ("pulvinar") MRI sign surprising (4). But how would you react if nvCJD had not been previously well described, or the MRI signs that accompany it? We believe our case may actually have been the first where the thalamic signal changes were first noted (5). Historically, how many square pegs in our field, such as progressive supranuclear palsy and corticobasal degeneration, have been hammered into round holes because they did not fit previously recognized and described clinicopathologic entities?

REFERENCES

1. Forsyth RJ. Neurological and cognitive decline in adolescence. *J Neurol Neurosurg Psychiatry.* 2003;74 (Suppl I):i9–i16.
2. Kelley BJ, Boeve BF, Josephs KA. Young-onset dementia. *Arch Neurol.* 2008;65:1502–1508.
3. Zeidler M, Stewart GE, Barraclough CR, et al. New variant Creutzfeldt-Jakob disease: neurological features and diagnostic tests. *Lancet.* 1997;350:903–907.
4. Zeidler M, Sellar RJ, Collie DA, et al. The pulvinar sign on magnetic resonance imaging in variant Creutzfeldt-Jakob disease. *Lancet.* 2000;355:1412–1418.
5. Coulthard A, Hall K, English PT, et al. Quantitative analysis of MRI signal intensity in new variant Creutzfeldt-Jakob disease. *Br J Radiol.* 1999;72:742–748.

52

Multiple Involuntary Movements in a Young Male Patient With Nephrocalcinosis: A "Gold Medal" Story

Debabrata Ghosh

THE CASE

A 20-year-old young man presented to me at the Pediatric Movement Disorders Clinic in our institution with complaints of multiple disabling involuntary movements of the face and all extremities of several years' duration.

His birth history was unremarkable. At the age of 18 months, he was noted by his mother to be "fidgety" and to exhibit frequent jerking of the extremities and trunk. At the age of 3, he was noted to have hypotonia and cognitive delay. He subsequently developed spasticity and leg braces were required. His abnormal movements progressed over time; any voluntary movement would be interrupted by what was described as jerky movements that were forceful leading to pain. He also had frequent falls. The patient had a diagnosis of attention deficit hyperactivity disorder (ADHD), anxiety disorder, impulse control disorder, and depression with a history of suicidal ideation. There was no history of self-injurious behavior. He had an IQ of 71 on cognitive testing done at the age of 18. He had completed high school and was employed at a workshop.

He had short stature and evidence of delayed puberty, but otherwise his general physical examination was normal. On neurologic examination, his speech was dysarthric, and he had apraxia of articulating muscles combined with orofacial dyskinesias. He had forceful eye blinking and neck turning during the examination. Cranial nerve examination was unremarkable except the involuntary movements. Motor power was within normal in all extremities. Tone was variable. He had generalized chorea, ballism of upper limbs, athetosis, and dystonia of the fingers and toes. In addition, he had prominent action dystonia of both hands and arms. His gait was wide based, spastic with a lurching quality, and marked choreoathetosis of the feet led to gait instability.

THE APPROACH

His MRI of the brain was normal. Serum lactate, ammonia, creatine kinase, amino acid, carnitine, and urine organic acids were within normal values. At the age of 13, as part of the workup for short stature and delayed puberty, he was noted to have nephrocalcinosis. His blood uric acid was increased to 10.9 mg/dL. Increased uric acid accompanied by multiple different types of involuntary movements in a male child led to the suspicion of Lesch-Nyhan syndrome (LNS). Red blood cell hypoxanthine-guanine phosphoribosyltransferase (HPRT) enzyme analysis showed undetectable activity. HPRT gene sequencing revealed a hemizygous missense mutation causing an amino acid substitution of aspartic acid to valine at residue 80 (g.239A>T p.D80V).

At the time of presentation, the patient's medication regimen included one tablet of carbidopa 25 mg and levodopa 100 mg in the morning, two tablets at noon, and two tablets in the evening; clonidine 0.1 mg at bedtime; concerta 36 mg in the morning; paxil 30 mg daily; and allopurinol for his hyperuricemia. His abnormal movements had reportedly worsened, and multiple tics had emerged when his levodopa was increased. Carbidopa-levodopa was tapered to 1 tablet three times a day, with improvement but persistence of his abnormal movements. He was started on oral depakote 500 mg two times a day with improvement in all of his involuntary movements, including chorea, athetosis, tics, and dystonia. Significant improvement of gait was noted within 2 months of therapy. He was able to move into an assisted living community. Finally, he continued to do remarkably well and competed in the Special Olympics. He won three gold medals!

THE LESSON

LNS is caused by a mutation in the gene encoding HPRT, an enzyme which catalyzes conversion of the purine bases hypoxanthine and guanine into their nucleotides (1). In the absence of HPRT, the latter purine bases accumulate and are converted into uric acid, and the de novo pathway of purine synthesis is activated to compensate for the absence of purine base recycling (1). Clinically, LNS is marked by neurologic features with multiple movement disorders, developmental delay and other neuropsychiatric abnormalities, including self-mutilation, and nephrologic complications of hyperuricemia.

It is a common belief among neurologists that all cases of LNS must have self-mutilation. On extensive review of the literature, we noted that the clinical spectrum of HPRT deficiency is broad, and patients with HPRT deficiency have been categorized into four groups (2,3): (1) hyperuricemia/hyperuricosuria with normal development and without neurologic symptoms; (2) mild neurologic symptoms but with ability to independently perform most activities of daily living (ADLs); (3) severe neurologic symptoms, with confinement to a wheelchair, but without self-injurious behavior; and (4) classic LNS, marked by severe neurologic symptoms and self-injurious behavior. Mental retardation and self-injurious behavior may rarely be absent in patients with undetectable HPRT activity (2), as was the case in our patient who had no detectable enzyme activity and yet did not exhibit self-mutilation and was relatively higher functioning. We speculate that in vivo residual enzyme activity, undetected by the in vitro enzyme assay, is responsible for this. Our patient had a mutation not previously well described in the literature in an α-helix region predicted to be involved in the subunit A-B dimer interface.

A combination of nephrocalcinosis or renal stone in a patient with multiple involuntary movements and cognitive/behavioral/psychiatric abnormalities with or without associated self-mutilation (2) should help the clinician to suspect the diagnosis of LNS. Simple investigation of blood uric acid level in the clinical context will help in reaching that diagnosis.

Regarding the motor manifestations of LNS, dystonia is almost universally present and is the most severe (4). Other abnormal movements frequently observed include choreoathetosis and ballism. Corticospinal tract signs, including spasticity, clonus, and hyper-reflexia may be present (4).

Although structural and histologic changes have not been demonstrated in the basal ganglia of patients with LNS, the pathophysiology of LNS is related to neurochemical dysfunction in the basal ganglia. Decreased levels of dopamine have been demonstrated in various basal ganglia regions (1). The mechanism by which HPRT influences dopamine neurotransmission in LNS is not clear, but may include direct toxicity of accumulated metabolites on dopaminergic pathways, oxidative stress, and depletion of adenosine triphosphate (ATP) and/or guanosine triphosphate (GTP). The degree of dopamine depletion in the basal ganglia of patients with LNS is similar to that seen in Parkinson's disease (PD). It has been postulated that LNS is predominantly a hyperkinetic disorder in contrast to PD because of the age at which nigrostriatal dopaminergic neurons are damaged, leading to compensatory developmental changes (1).

In addition to a role for dopaminergic pathways in the pathophysiology of LNS, there is evidence to suggest dysfunction of GABAergic pathways related to the accumulation of hypoxanthine. It has been suggested that disruption of gamma-aminobutyric acid (GABA), dopamine, and acetylcholine neurons in the basal ganglia accounts for some of the abnormal movements observed in LNS (5).

The GABA-A receptor is a hetero-oligomeric protein complex composed of several subunits arranged to form a central pore permeable to ion channels (6). GABA-A receptors present several GABA recognition sites and binding sites for several modulatory compounds, including benzodiazepines. GABA-A receptor subunits are allosterically and functionally coupled to each other. For example, benzodiazepine agonism increases GABA-mediated neurotransmission (6). Hypoxanthine, which has been shown to be markedly increased in the cerebrospinal fluid (CSF) of patients with LNS, has been shown to competitively bind to rat and mammalian benzodiazepine-binding sites (7,8). It also binds to diazepam antibodies (7,8). A study of benzodiazepine receptor binding in the cerebral cortex of patients with LNS (deceased) has demonstrated increased sensitivity to hypoxanthine inhibition and reduced GABA stimulation of cortical benzodiazepine binding (9), suggesting that a high level of purines antagonizes the action of the endogenous benzodiazepine ligand at its receptor in LNS. Thus, hypoxanthine acting at the GABA-A receptor may decrease GABAergic neurotransmission in the basal ganglia of patients with LNS through inhibitory modulation of GABA.

Depakote was markedly effective in reducing my patient's involuntary movements. Perhaps, the mechanism of action of valproate in LNS is related to its GABAergic activity. In animal models, administration of valproate increases GABA levels in cortical and subcortical regions and particularly so in the substantia nigra (10). Valproate has been used to successfully treat Sydenham's chorea (11,12), but its use has not been reported in LNS (valproic acid has been reported to have been used once before in the literature in a patient with LNS, but further details of the rationale for use and its efficacy are not available) (4).

In summary, the "lessons" I learned from this case were the following:

1. Multiple types of involuntary movements with normal MRI brain in a male patient and presence of renal stone or nephrocalcinosis should alert the clinician to the possibility of LNS.
2. Self-mutilating behavior, although common, is not a must in all cases of LNS. My patient did not have any self-mutilating behavior despite undetectable HRPT enzyme activity. This phenomenon may be explained by the discrepancy between in vivo and in vitro assays.
3. The mechanism of genesis of involuntary movements in LNS is as yet unclear, but a GABAergic to a dopaminergic mechanism has been postulated.
4. In general, depakote should be considered in any patient with multiple types of involuntary movements after ruling out a mitochondrial dysfunction or polymerase gamma gene mutation. The excellent efficacy of depakote in our patient with LNS points to the early trial of depakote in patients with LNS.

REFERENCES

1. Visser JE, Bar PR, Jinnah HA. Lesch-Nyhan disease and the basal ganglia. *Brain Res Rev.* 2000;32:449–475.
2. Puig JG, Torres RJ, Mateos FA, et al. The spectrum of hypoxanthine-guanine phosphoribosyltransferase (HPRT) deficiency: clinical experience based on 22 patients from 18 Spanish families. *Medicine (Baltimore).* 2001;80:102–112.
3. Torres RJ, Puig JG. Hypoxanthine-guanine phosphoribosyltransferase (HPRT) deficiency: Lesch-Nyhan syndrome. *Orphanet J Rare Dis.* 2007;2:48.
4. Jinnah HA, Visser JE, Harris JC, et al. Delineation of the motor disorder of Lesch-Nyhan disease. *Brain.* 2006;129(Pt 5):1201–1217.
5. Lloyd KG, Hornykiewicz O, Davidson L, et al. Biochemical evidence of dysfunction of brain neurotransmitters in the Lesch-Nyhan syndrome. *N Engl J Med.* 1981;305:1106–1111.
6. Johnston GA. GABAA receptor pharmacology. *Pharmacol Ther.* 1996;69:173–198.
7. Daval JL, Barberis C, Vert P. In vitro and in vivo displacement of [3H]-diazepam binding by purine derivatives in developing rat brain. *Dev Pharmacol Ther.* 1984;7:169–176.

8. Asano T, Spector S. Identification of inosine and hypoxanthine as endogenous ligands for the brain ben-zodiazepine-binding sites. *Proc Natl Acad Sci USA.* 1979;76:977–981.
9. Kish SJ, Fox IH, Kapur BM, et al. Brain benzodiazepine receptor binding and purine concentration in Lesch-Nyhan syndrome. *Brain Res.* 1985;336:117–123.
10. Johannessen CU. Mechanisms of action of valproate: a commentary. *Neurochem Int.* 2000;37:103–110.
11. Daoud AS, Zaki M, Shakir R, et al. Effectiveness of sodium valproate in the treatment of Sydenham's chorea. *Neurology.* 1990;40:1140–1141.
12. Genel F, Arslanoglu S, Uran N, et al. Sydenham's chorea: clinical findings and comparison of the efficacies of sodium valproate and carbamazepine regimens. *Brain Dev.* 2002;24:73–76.

V
Dystonia

53

Seemingly "Progressive Postanoxic Dystonia"
Finally Diagnosed 26 Years After Symptom Onset

MAJA KOJOVIC AND KAILASH BHATIA

THE CASE

This 20-year-old woman, who was previously fit and well, underwent dental surgery for a routine wisdom tooth extraction on March 31, 1983. The procedure was performed under general anesthesia. During the induction of general anesthesia, she suffered a cardiorespiratory arrest, presumed secondary to misplacement of the nasotracheal tube in the esophagus. After resuscitation, she was treated in the intensive care unit for 48 hours but recovered quickly, to be discharged home a week later without residual deficit. When she was at home, her legs felt unsteady, but she did not note any other symptoms until 2 months later when she returned to work as a secretary. She then had difficulties with writing with her right hand, and her colleagues noticed that her speech had changed. She also had difficulties doing up buttons and knitting. Over the following 2 years, her symptoms continued to progress, and she had to resort to writing with her left hand. She had a tendency to shuffle her feet with her toes pointing inward and with posturing of her right foot. Five years into the illness, she developed severe speech and swallowing difficulties, and her mouth tended to remain open. There was further worsening of her gait with frequent falls. By 1999, a gastrostomy tube was inserted, and in 2007, an emergency tracheotomy was required after recurrent episodes of stridor. Before the anoxic episode, there were no symptoms to suggest dystonia or any other neurologic problems. There was no family history of neurologic or psychiatric illness. Her father died of hemochromatosis.

On examination, two and a half years after the hypoxic insult, the patient had a dystonic smile and blepharoclonus. In the limbs, there was a right dystonic writer's cramp, postural tremor of the right arm, mild bradykinesia, and micrographia. There was inversion and plantar flexion of her right foot on walking with her left sole shuffling along the ground. There were no sensory, pyramidal, or cerebellar signs. Six years after the initial event, she was dysarthric with a sardonic smile and suffered from emotional incontinence. She had severe lower limb dystonia and was using a stick for walking. Sixteen years after symptom onset, she was severely dysarthric and was using a communication device. She had a complete loss of postural reflexes and was wheelchair bound. Currently, 27 years after symptom onset, she has prominent oromandibular dystonia of 'jaw opening' type, and she is virtually anarthric. Her upper limbs are less affected than her lower limbs by dystonia and bradykinesia. She has a full range of normal eye movement, and there are no pyramidal or cerebellar features. One of the striking features is that she remains very bright intellectually with a good memory.

THE APPROACH

This woman developed a dystonic syndrome 2 months after a clear precipitating anoxic event and was initially diagnosed with postanoxic generalized dystonia. Two years after the disease onset, a medicolegal settlement was agreed on the assumption that further progression was unlikely. However, over the years, her symptoms continuously progressed, and this was considered atypical for postanoxic dystonia. Therefore, she was repeatedly investigated to exclude other secondary causes of dystonia or predisposition to the severity of the consequences of her hypoxia. Investigations included blood chemistry, serum ceruloplasmin and copper, 24-hour urinary copper, ophthalmologic examination to exclude Kayser-Fleisher rings, acanthocytes, plasma and urinary amino acids, white cell enzymes, pyruvate, and lactate. All the results were normal. Because of the family history, hemochromatosis was also excluded. The first brain MRI scan, 4 years after onset, showed bilateral hypointensity in the internal capsules, but the basal ganglia were reported as normal. In 1987, Professor Marsden, whose care she was under, wrote in one of his clinical letters "…I really am very unhappy with the continued progression of her illness so long after the original anoxic episode…It is certainly possible for the extrapyramidal effects of a period of cerebral anoxia to appear after a considerable delay of many months, and to progress for sometime afterwards. The question is for how long? Based on limited experience (thank heavens there aren't many such cases around) I would be comfortable with progression for a year, I would begin to worry if it goes on for two years, and I would be distinctly uncomfortable if it went on for three years or more. If it did, I would look aggressively for other causes…However, there is no other explanation that we can find…." The patient had no response to treatment with benzhexol, levodopa, diazepam, or baclofen. Fifteen years after the initial anoxic event, she underwent a second MRI scan, and this showed isolated bilateral T2 hypointensities in the globus pallidus, suggestive of mineral accumulation. A computed tomography (CT) scan to exclude calcification was normal, and the overall appearance was interpreted as consistent with anoxic injury, possibly related to hemorrhagic transformation associated with anoxia. Because of an unusually long clinical progression, we reported this patient in the literature as one of two cases of progressive postanoxic dystonia (1). But, continuing progression of her symptoms led us to the third MRI scan in 2007. This showed bilaterally abnormal low signal in globus pallidus with some foci of increased signal on T2 sequences, interpreted as an "eye of the tiger" sign (Figure 53.1). In retrospect, even the 1998 MRI scan did in fact show the "eye of the tiger" sign. When DNA sequencing of the *PANK 2* gene became available, the patient was found to be a compound heterozygote for mutations in exon 2 with c.498_499delITG and c.563T>A (p.Met188Lys) mutations. The diagnosis of pantothenate kinase–associated neurodegeneration (PKAN) was finally made 26 years after symptom onset (2).

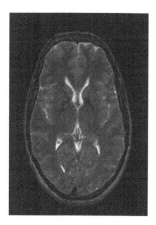

FIGURE 53.1

T2-weighted axial MRI performed 24 years after symptom onset shows typical "eye of the tiger" sign bilaterally.

THE LESSON

PKAN, formerly known as Hallervorden-Spatz disease, is an autosomal recessive disorder caused by mutations in the *PANK2* gene (3). It accounts for the majority of neurodegeneration with brain iron accumulation (NBIA) cases (4). Clinically, it is characterized by dystonia with prominent bulbar involvement and parkinsonism. Since the recognition of *PANK2* gene mutations, two main phenotypes have been described (3). Classic PKAN has an early onset (first decade) of gait and balance problems, rapid progression, and loss of ambulation over 10 to 15 years. Atypical PKAN starts in the second or third decade with speech difficulties; the progression is slower and loss of mobility occurs after 15 to 40 years. Basal ganglia iron accumulation giving the characteristic "eye of the tiger" sign is invariably present on MRI T2 sequences in both groups (3). Our patient clinically falls into the group of atypical PKAN.

One interesting aspect of this case is a clear temporal relationship between the anoxic event and symptom onset, thus suggesting the role of environmental factors in triggering clinical onset of genetic disease. A possible role of environmental factors in the genesis of dystonic symptoms has been reported in DYT1 mutation carriers who developed dystonia after exposure to neuroleptics or peripheral trauma (5). However, autosomal recessive diseases generally do not show reduced penetrance. Thus, it is likely that our patient would have developed the disease even in the absence of an anoxic event, but we cannot exclude that the anoxia somehow triggered the earlier expression of the underlying genetic defect.

Delayed onset of dystonia after hypoxic-ischemic events is a well-known phenomenon (6,7), especially in children and young adults. There are very few data in the literature concerning duration of disease progression. Bhatt et al. (6) described 10 cases of postanoxic generalized dystonia with latency to symptom onset of between 1 week and 3 years, and progression lasting up to 8 years. However, case 6 from their series is in fact our patient we herein describe; if she is excluded, then the longest period of progression in that series was 3 years. Similarly, in Burke's series, the progression was no longer than 3 years (7).

This illustrative case offers a few important teaching points. First, although periods of clinical worsening lasting up to several years are well recognized, postanoxic dystonia should ultimately be a static condition. Second, even in the presence of a clear precipitating factor, other causes of dystonia should be kept in mind, and the patient should be thoroughly investigated. Finally, in patients with progressive dystonia and MRI showing bilateral T2 hypointensities in globus pallidus, even without the classical "eye of the tiger" sign, NBIA should be suspected and genetic testing considered (8).

REFERENCES

1. Kuoppamäki M, Bhatia KP, Quinn N. Progressive delayed-onset dystonia after cerebral anoxic insult in adults. *Mov Disord.* 2002;17:1345–1349.
2. Kojovic M, Kuoppamäki M, Quinn N, et al. "Progressive delayed-onset postanoxic dystonia" diagnosed with PANK2 mutations 26 years after onset—an update. *Mov Disord.* 2010;25:2889–2891.
3. Hayflick SJ, Westaway SK, Levinson B, et al. Genetic, clinical, and radiographic delineation of Hallervorden-Spatz syndrome. *N Engl J Med.* 2003;348:33–40.
4. Gregory A, Polster BJ, Hayflick SJ. Clinical and genetic delineation of neurodegeneration with brain iron accumulation. *J Med Genet.* 2009;46:73–80.
5. Edwards M, Wood N, Bhatia K. Unusual phenotypes in DYT1 dystonia: a report of five cases and a review of the literature. *Mov Disord.* 2003;18:706–711.
6. Bhatt MH, Obeso JA, Marsden CD. Time course of postanoxic akinetic-rigid and dystonic syndromes. *Neurology.* 1993;43:314–317.
7. Burke RE, Fahn S, Gold AP. Delayed-onset dystonia in patients with "static" encephalopathy. *J Neurol Neurosurg Psychiatry.* 1980;43:789–797.
8. McNeill A, Birchall D, Hayflick SJ, et al. T2* and FSE MRI distinguishes four subtypes of neurodegeneration with brain iron accumulation. *Neurology.* 2008;70:1614–1619.

54

Dystonia, Ataxia, Dementia, and a Family History of "Huntington Disease"

JOSEPH JANKOVIC

THE CASE

This 40-year-old woman was initially referred to the Parkinson's Disease Center and Movement Disorders Clinic at Baylor College of Medicine in 1986 for an evaluation of right-hand stiffness, gross motor incoordination, and tremors of the right hand during handwriting. She claimed that since grade school she had had a tight grip when using a pen, but at the age of 28, the tightness began to increase, became more painful, and began to involve not only her hand but also her right arm. In addition, she noted incoordination of that hand and tremor, particularly at the end of day. The tremor was exacerbated by writing, steering, lifting heavy objects, and whenever her arm felt tired. She was diagnosed with writer's cramp and noted mild improvement of her tremor with baclofen.

On initial neurologic examination in 1986, there was no evidence of cognitive, memory, or language dysfunction. Furthermore, there was no evidence of Kayser-Fleischer ring or any oculomotor disturbances. The patient was able to rise from a chair and walk without any difficulties with normal arm swing. She had tight grip on the pen when writing with the right hand and dystonic flexion of the wrist and elevation of the right elbow. With persistent writing, she developed a rapid tremor of 6 to 7 Hz in the right hand and complained of painful stiffness in the right forearm and a tired feeling in the right shoulder. When arms were outstretched, she had a dystonic posture of the right hand with flexion at the wrist and extension at the metacarpalphalangeal joint and a mild flexion/extension tremor of 6 to 7 Hz of the right hand. There was no involvement of the left hand except slight "spooning" when the left arm was held in a wingbeating position. There was no evidence of cogwheel rigidity, bradykinesia, or spasticity. Deep tendon reflexes were normal, and plantar response was flexor bilaterally; there was no clonus. Sensory examination was unremarkable to all primary modalities. There was no evidence of cerebellar dysfunction.

Her subsequent course was slowly progressive. About 10 years after her initial evaluation, she complained of increasing difficulties with ambulation and uncontrollable movements in right more than left arm as a result of which she had increasing difficulties with writing and typing. She stopped working in March 1996 and stopped driving later in the same year. She had developed increasing difficulties with her balance as a result of which she fell frequently and required assistance with feeding. In addition, she had increasing word-finding difficulty, marked forgetfulness, and recurrent obsessions such as a persevering thought that both feet were broken.

She had rare generalized clonic-tonic seizures. In addition to distal and proximal dystonia, she had increasing worsening cerebellar dysfunction and axial and leg myoclonus.

The patient had no benefit from ethopropazine, primidone, and carbamazepine, but propranolol produced mild improvement in her tremor. Because she failed to respond to trihexyphenidyl, treatment with botulinum toxin about 120 units into forearm flexors of right hand was initiated in 1991 with moderate benefit in her handwriting. Initially, muscles injected consisted of forearm flexors and extensors, but subsequently, she required injections into the biceps, deltoids, pectoralis, and paraspinal muscles to control her dystonic spasms.

The family history indicates an autosomal dominant pattern of inheritance (Figure 54.1). The patient's mother had gait difficulties since age 47. She was in a nursing home and bedridden at the time of patient's initial evaluation but subsequently died without specific diagnosis. The maternal grandfather died at age 69 after a 10-year history of progressive gait disturbance and deafness. In 1996, the patient's younger brother died at age 36 after a 10-year history of "generalized" seizures and progressive gait difficulty. Gross examination of the brain apparently did not reveal any abnormalities in the basal ganglia, dentate, or cerebellum. No histologic examination was performed. The brain weighed 1300 g. Her older brother's symptoms began in the mid 20s with involuntary movements and gait problems. He has been diagnosed with "Huntington disease" (HD) and died at a nursing home without an autopsy. The patient is married but has no children.

THE APPROACH

Neuropsychological testing revealed mild early dementia with a combined IQ of 67 (verbal IQ 71; performance IQ 65) on the Wechsler Adult Intelligence Scale-Revised (WAIS-R). She also had findings consistent with clinical depression and exhibited delay in verbal learning and recall. There was evidence of impairment of visual recognition. Language function revealed defective fluency for category condition and lexical cues. She was unable to perform bimanual motor programming. There was also a decline in auditory comprehension and repetition. Thus, the neuropsychological testing was consistent with both a cortical and subcortical dysfunction. Given the patient's family history suggestive of an autosomal dominant inheritance, available genetic tests for spinocerebellar atrophy (SCA) were ordered but were all negative. Tests for HD, Wilson's disease, DYT1 dystonia, Refsum's disease, and vitamin E deficiency were also normal. Serum copper and ceruloplasmin levels were 36 mg/dL (normal 16–66 mg/dL); electromyography and nerve conduction studies were all normal. MRI in April 1998 revealed diffuse cerebral and cerebellar atrophy and T2 hyperintensity in the periventricular white matter. Dentatorubral-pallidoluysian atrophy (DRPLA) mutation with 60 CAG repeats (normal <35 CAG repeats) was detected by a DNA test.

THE LESSON

The patient's history and examination document a progressive disorder manifested by dystonic writer's cramp and dystonic tremor that gradually evolved into generalized dystonia over a course of several years. In addition, the patient developed seizures, cognitive decline, and ataxia. Because of a family history suggestive of an autosomal dominant pattern of inheritance, a variety of heredodegenerative disorders such as HD, SCA, and neurodegeneration with brain iron accumulation (NBIA) were initially considered in the differential diagnosis, but DNA tests were all negative, and MRI scans were not consistent with any of these disorders. Because chorea was not a prominent feature, DRPLA, often thought of as an HD-like disorder, was not initially considered, but the diagnosis was finally confirmed when the DNA test for DRPLA became available. The diagnosis was further supported by the typical white matter changes on brain MRI.

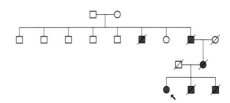

FIGURE 54.1
Pedigree of the DRPLA family.

DRPLA is an autosomal dominant neurodegenerative disorder that is particularly prevalent in Japan, but it has been also identified in Europe and in African American families ("Haw River syndrome") (1). Usually beginning in the fourth decade, the disorder may occur as an early-onset DRPLA (before 20 years of age)—manifested by a variable combination of myoclonus, epilepsy, and mental retardation—or as a late-onset DRPLA (after 20 years of age), manifested by cerebellar ataxia, choreoathetosis, dystonia, rest and postural tremor, parkinsonism, and dementia. Because of its overlap with HD, DRPLA should be considered as one of the most important HD phenocopies (2).

Unstable CAG expansion has been identified as the mutation in the *DRPLA* (or *ATN1*) gene on chromosome 12p13.31. The *DRPLA* gene codes for a protein that has been identified as a phosphoprotein, c-Jun NH(2)-terminal kinase, one of the major factors involved in its phosphorylation. In DRPLA, this protein seems to be slowly phosphorylated; thus, it may delay a process that is essential in keeping neurons alive. Similar to HD, there is an inverse correlation between the age at onset and the number of CAG repeats, and patients with high CAG repeats tend to have a more rapid progression and worse prognosis than those with CAG repeats in the low abnormal range (3). The early onset of DRPLA is associated with greater number of CAG repeats (62–79) compared with the late-onset type (54–67 repeats). As a result of the DNA test, the clinical spectrum of DRPLA has markedly expanded, and it now includes spastic paraplegia, a cerebellar syndrome, and many other phenotypes.

One lesson to be learned from this case is that a neurodegenerative disorder suggestive of HD but associated with evidence of widespread white matter changes should suggest the diagnosis of DRPLA. Involvement of oligodendrocytes and an increased number of affected glia have been believed to contribute to the widespread demyelination found not only in human brains of patients with DRPLA but also in brains of transgenic mice. Similar to HD, DRPLA has also been associated with the formation of perinuclear aggregates and intranuclear inclusions that stain intensely with ubiquitin. The DRPLA gene is expressed predominantly in neurons, but neurons vulnerable to degeneration in DRPLA do not selectively express the gene.

The age of onset of DRPLA is usually in the fourth decade (range: first to seventh decade). The early-onset subtype is usually manifested by a variable combination of myoclonus, epilepsy, and mental retardation, whereas the late-onset subtype is manifested by cerebellar ataxia, choreoathetosis, dystonia, rest and postural tremor, parkinsonism, and dementia. The early onset of DRPLA is associated with greater number of CAG repeats (62–79) compared with the late-onset type (54–67 repeats).

Although the representation in our case with dystonia and tremor is somewhat atypical, the age of symptom onset is characteristic for DRPLA. In addition, ataxia was not evident until 10 years into the course of her illness. After the onset of ataxia, her symptoms progressed rapidly, and she developed dementia, ataxia, dysarthria, myoclonus, and hemidystonia, and seizures. Although most patients with DRPLA present with an HD-like manifestation (chorea, cognitive decline, and psychiatric problems), some present with progressive ataxia, dystonia, and myoclonus. Clinical heterogeneity is typical for most neurodegenerative disorders associated with expanded trinucleotide repeats. There seems to be a correlation between the size of expanded alleles and the age of onset and phenotype. Thus, generally patients with progressive myoclonus and epilepsy have the earliest age of onset and largest expansions. Indeed, progressive myoclonus epilepsy of Unverricht-Lundborg type (EPM1) should be considered in the differential diagnosis of early-onset DRPLA.

Our patient is somewhat atypical in that she never exhibited chorea and her psychiatric disturbances developed later in the course of disease. In some cases of adult-onset DRPLA, patients manifest typical features of HD, and this may lead to misdiagnosis as in the case of our patient's brother who had been given a diagnosis of HD. Ataxia is a frequent feature of DRPLA, but because ataxia may also be the presenting symptom of HD, this clinical finding may not be used to differentiate between the two disorders. The presence of seizures in a patient with chorea is uncommon in adult-onset HD. Although this may help differentiate DRPLA from HD, other rare neurodegenerative diseases need to be considered, such as neuroacanthocytosis.

Of the SCAs, SCA3 (Machado-Joseph disease) and SCA17 are particularly important to consider because of overlapping clinical features.

Treatment of DRPLA is very difficult and should be directed to the most troublesome symptom. Thus, in this case, botulinum toxin injections were used in the treatment of focal and segmental dystonia. If chorea or other hyperkinetic movement disorder interferes with patient's functioning, antidopaminergic drugs, such as tetrabenazine, may be helpful (4). I am not aware of deep brain stimulation to be used in the treatment of DRPLA.

REFERENCES

1. Wardle M, Morris HR, Robertson NP. Clinical and genetic characteristics of non-Asian dentatorubral-pallidoluysian atrophy: a systematic review. *Mov Disord.* 2009;24:1636–1640.
2. Wild EJ, Mudanohwo EE, Sweeney MG, et al. Huntington's disease phenocopies are clinically and genetically heterogeneous. *Mov Disord.* 2008;23:716–720.
3. Hasegawa A, Ikeuchi T, Koike R, et al. Long-term disability and prognosis in dentatorubral-pallidoluysian atrophy: a correlation with CAG repeat length. *Mov Disord.* 2010;25:1694–1700.
4. Jankovic J. Treatment of hyperkinetic movement disorders. *Lancet Neurol.* 2009;8:844–856.

55

Friedreich's Ataxia Presenting With Childhood Onset Progressive Dystonia and Spasticity

JOSEPH JANKOVIC

THE CASE

This ambidextrous white man initially presented to the Movement Disorders Clinic at Baylor College of Medicine, Houston, Texas, in 1989 at the age of 24 years for evaluation of "dystonia." According to his mother, who brought him to the clinic, he was a product of a full-term pregnancy without any history of neonatal or perinatal complications. He was healthy until age 6 years when he started to limp. He subsequently developed progressive slurring of speech, which eventually became unintelligible. He was noted to have twisting movements of his legs, and because of gradual deformities, he required leg braces. The twisting movements later progressed to involve the trunk, cervical area, and, to a lesser degree, his arms. His gait and balance problems worsened to the extent that he became wheelchair bound by 12 years of age. Despite numerous evaluations by many physicians in highly prestigious institutions, no specific diagnosis was given, although some have attributed his neurologic deficit to cerebral palsy, and at 16 years, he was diagnosed with "Hallervorden-Spatz disease." In 1985, when he was 20 years old, he had a spinal cord stimulator placement, but without any relief of his leg and trunk spasms. In 1987, the spinal cord stimulator was removed for the purpose of brain MRI, which did not reveal any abnormalities suggesting Hallervorden-Spatz disease. He was maintained on high doses of diazepam for at least 13 years without much improvement. Since age 12, he underwent several surgical procedures to lengthen his Achilles tendons and correct his hammertoe deformities.

In 1989, he was gradually started on trihexyphenidyl, baclofen, dantrolene, clonazepam, and botulinum toxin injections with only modest improvement in his spastic dystonia and other involuntary movements. Baclofen pump was considered, but he was hesitant to pursue this interventional therapy. The patient continued to have progressive spasms and jerk-like movements involving his entire body. He could pull himself out of bed or wheelchair to crawl to the nearby bathroom.

He had extensive diagnostic evaluation, including MRI of his head and a variety of metabolic and other tests, without any specific abnormality found, except for factor VIII deficiency. His family history was negative except for hemophilia and Von Willebrand's disease in several family members.

Neurologic examination showed severe dysarthria, but he was able to communicate well using a computer. His extraocular movements were intact except for marked limitation of downward gaze, without any evidence of nystagmus. He had marked cervical dystonia with torticollis and laterocollis to the left, retrocollis, shoulder elevation, and opisthotonic posturing of the trunk. He had marked finger-to-nose ataxia, mild proximal arm weakness, and marked weakness in both legs (iliopsoas was only 2/5, and he had bilateral foot drop). His deep tendon reflexes were rated 4+ throughout, and he had a sustained ankle clonus bilaterally. He had a scissoring, spastic gait, but this was difficult to assess because he required assistance of two people due to severe leg and trunk weakness and ataxia.

THE APPROACH

Because of progressive dystonia, ataxia, spasticity, and vertical ophthalmoparesis, the possibility of Niemann-Pick type C was considered, but esterified long-chain fatty acids were normal. Despite his foot drop, he had no evidence of peripheral neuropathy on electromyography. A variety of other blood tests, including ceruloplasmin, alpha fetal globulin, blood smear for acanthocytes, creatine phosphokinase test (CPK), DNA tests for DYT1, Charcot-Marie-Tooth disease, and spinocerebellar ataxia panel were all negative except for mutation for Friedreich's ataxia (FA), which showed 12,500 GAA repeats (a second mutation on the other allele could not be found).

THE LESSON

The FA gene, discovered on a Saudi Arabian family initially evaluated at the Baylor College of Medicine, involves GAA trinucleotide repeat expansion mutation within the intron of X25 gene on chromosome 9q13, coding for the protein frataxin (1). Although normal gene expresses 8 to 33 GAA repeats, patients with FA have a GAA stretch ranging from 120 to 1700 repeats. It is possible that our case represents the small minority of patients with FA who are compound heterozygotes with a GAA repeat expansion in one allele and a point mutation in the other allele. The mutated frataxin presumably induces a deficiency of a mitochondrial iron-sulfur enzyme (aconitase) involved in iron homeostasis. Skeletal and cardiac muscles, fibroblasts, and possible neurons are affected by iron overload caused by this enzyme deficiency. Thus, it has been postulated that the clinical features of FA are primarily caused by mitochondrial dysfunction and free radical toxicity. Pathologically, demyelination is seen in large fibers in the posterior column of the spinal cord arising in the dorsal root ganglia. There is also marked involvement of Clarke's columns and the dentate nucleus. Degeneration also involves the lateral corticospinal tract. There is, however, only a mild neuronal loss in the cerebellar cortex. Functional impairments in patients with FA are largely attributed to a defect in afferent input from spinal cord to cerebellum.

Since the discovery of the gene mutation causing FA, the rich spectrum of clinical manifestations of this autosomal recessive disorder is being increasingly recognized (2–4). Traditionally considered an ataxia with hyporeflexia or areflexia, spastic FA variants, such as the case presented here, have not been well recognized. The most common of genetic spinocerebellar degenerations, FA is characterized clinically by progressive ataxia of the limbs and trunk, dysarthria, and sensory neuropathy, particularly involving the lower limbs, with or without pyramidal signs. Symptoms develop progressively and insidiously with onset usually before age 25 years, but onset as late as fifth decade has been described. The most common complaint in early stages is unsteadiness of gait, which is sometimes misinterpreted as a delay in the acquisition of motor developmental milestones, and the disorder is often wrongly attributed to cerebral palsy. Other related features include pes cavus, scoliosis, skeletal deformities, distal wasting, cardiomyopathy, dysarthria, and ophthalmoplegia.

In addition to ataxia, other movement disorders have been documented as either the presenting or accompanying feature of FA. These include tremor, dystonia, chorea, myoclonus, and spasticity. In addition to kinetic tremor, best demonstrated on finger-to-nose or toe-to-finger maneuver, patients with FA often exhibit low frequency (<1 Hz), large-amplitude omnidirectional postural truncal sway, termed "titubation." Dystonia, described in a variety of inherited spinocerebellar ataxias, often starts from FA in the legs, as in our patient, but the proband of the Saudi Arabian family from which the FA gene was cloned started with dystonic writer's cramp. In addition, his dystonic scoliosis was so severe that it required the placement of Harrington rods into the thoracic spinal column. Choreiform movements involving the face, arms, and legs that interfered with performing daily tasks have also been described in patients with FA. Slow chorea in patients with FA could also be a manifestation of pseudoathetosis associated with underlying proprioceptive deficit. Although Friedreich is credited for first defining myoclonus in a case of essential myoclonus, it has not been until quite recently that myoclonus with or without myoclonic epilepsy has become a recognized feature of FA. Finally, spastic paraparesis and hyper-reflexia, demonstrated by our patient, is now a well-established variant of FA.

Thus, the identification of specific genetic mutations in patients with FA has revolutionized the diagnosis of this disorder. Many cases, such as late-onset, hyper-reflexia, or other "atypical" patients with previously unrecognized clinical features can be diagnosed correctly by genetic analyses. Our case draws attention to the expanding clinical heterogeneity of FA.

There is no effective treatment for FA, although high-dose idebenone, a potent antioxidant, up to 3,000 mg or 45 mg/kg/d has been found to be well tolerated and provide modest improvement in neurologic function (5). I sometimes combine it with monoamine oxidase inhibitors (e.g., rasagiline or selegiline), but studies are needed to determine whether centrally acting iron chelators could also be useful in the treatment of FA (6).

REFERENCES

1. Campuzano V, Montermini L, Molto MD, et al. Friedreich's ataxia: autosomal recessive disease caused by an intronic GAA triplet repeat expansion. *Science.* 1996;271:1423–1427.
2. Hou J-G, Jankovic J. Movement disorders in Friedreich's ataxia. *J Neurol Sci.* 2003;206:59–64.
3. Pandolfo M. Friedreich ataxia. *Arch Neurol.* 2008;65:1296–1303.
4. Ribai P, Pousset F, Tanguy ML, et al. Neurological, cardiological, and oculomotor progression in 104 patients with Friedreich ataxia during long-term follow-up. *Arch Neurol.* 2007;64:558–564.
5. Di Prospero NA, Baker A, Jeffries N, et al. Neurological effects of high-dose idebenone in patients with Friedreich's ataxia: a randomised, placebo-controlled trial. *Lancet Neurol.* 2007;6:878–886.
6. Li X, Jankovic J, Le W. Iron chelation and neuroprotection in neurodegenerative diseases. *J Neural Transm.* 2011;118:473–477.

56

Dysarthria, Dystonia, and Cerebellar Ataxia: The Tale of Four Sisters

Marie Vidailhet, Mathieu Anheim, and Cécile Hubsch

THE CASE

Ten years ago, a speech therapist referred a 15-year-old girl to me. She had dysarthria since the age of 6 and had slowly developed oromandibular dystonia. When she was a teenager, she also complained of clumsiness, and at the time of my initial examination, I observed a writer's cramp (she is right handed). Neurologic examination was otherwise normal.

She was from a nonconsanguineous family; her parents were well, but her three sisters had similar history and similar troubles.

With time, she developed bilateral upper limb dystonia with abnormal postures of the hands and myoclonus. Because secondary dystonia was suspected, both on clinical presentation and from family history, extensive biological tests and MRI were performed but were normal. Although the girl (and her sisters) was disappointed by the unsuccessful treatment with levodopa and anticholinergic, she kept visiting me every year until she developed cerebellar ataxia and mild cerebellar atrophy (vermis + hemispheres) on MRI.

At the time, neurologic examination showed facial and upper limb dystonia, abnormal tandem gait, and brisk reflexes (plantar reflexes were normal). Eye movements were full, with hypermetric horizontal and vertical saccades (confirmed by eye movement recording, but velocity and amplitudes of the visually guided saccades were normal).

Because the sisters were anxious about genetic counseling (two of them were married and had children), new investigations were performed.

THE APPROACH

The patient was admitted to the hospital for further evaluation. Laboratory tests (nonexhaustive list) showed normal lysosomal enzymes and normal organic and amino acid dosages; lactate and pyruvate were normal (blood and cerebrospinal fluid [CSF]). Neurotransmitters in the CSF were normal. Genetic testing for DYT16, A0A1, and A0A2 were negative (albumin = 46 g/L, total cholesterol = 3.91 mmol/L; normal < 4).

Our eyes widened when we saw the following results: alpha-fetoprotein (AFP) 197.6 ng/mL (normal < 7).

The diagnosis of ataxia telangiectasia (AT) was suspected. Similar abnormalities of the AFP dosage were found in the three other sisters. The diagnosis of AT was confirmed by the identification of multiple DNA breaks of caryotype and by direct sequencing of ataxia telangiectasia mutated (ATM) gene.

The final diagnosis was AT with predominant facial and upper limb dystonia, without telangiectasia and with minor ataxia.

THE LESSON

The patient (and her sisters) has a rich and difficult semiology with a longstanding history of dystonia starting with dysarthria and oromandibular involvement (1). Initial repeated brain MRI and biological tests (including initial dosage of AFP) were normal.

This case emphasizes the interest of long-term follow-up of patients with atypical clinical presentations. In addition, it carries an important practical message for movement disorder neurologists: search for biomarkers of autosomal recessive cerebellar ataxia (including AOA1, AOA2, and AT) should be systematic in the assessment of unexplained movement disorders, including cerebellar ataxia (even though ataxia may not be the prominent sign).

AFP serum level is a very highly sensitive marker not only in AT but also in ataxia with oculomotor apraxia type 2 (AOA2) and to a lesser extent in ataxia with oculomotor apraxia type 1 (AOA1).

The AFP assay must be repeated because the increase appears sometimes during the course of the disease.

Although signs of AT often occur before the age of 3, neurologic features may appear later, including during the second decade.

Dystonia may be the prominent and/or the first sign of the disease (may be associated with chorea, parkinsonism, tremor, and/or myoclonus), and the lack of telangiectasia (auricular, buccal, conjunctival) and oculomotor apraxia (defined by increased saccade latencies) do not rule out AT (2).

In our patient (and her sisters), dystonia was the only symptom for years and cerebellar ataxia was only evident after the age of 20, and she (like her sisters) never had telangiectasias or oculomotor apraxia. She was still able to walk independently at the age of 24, whereas patients with AT usually become wheelchair bound and are prone to malignancies and to recurrent infections.

REFERENCES

1. Carrillo F, Schneider SA, Taylor AM, et al. Prominent oromandibular dystonia and pharyngeal telangiectasia in atypical ataxia telangiectasia. *Cerebellum.* 2009;8:22–27.
2. Le Ber I, Brice A, Dürr A. New autosomal recessive cerebellar ataxias with oculomotor apraxia. *Curr Neurol Neurosci Rep.* 2005;5:411–417.

57

Early-Onset Generalized Dystonia With Short Stature and Skeletal Dysplasia

MARIE VIDAILHET AND EMMANUEL ROZE

THE CASE

A 24-year-old woman with severe generalized dystonia was referred for bilateral pallidal stimulation. She had a normal life until the age of 16, when she had writer's cramp (right-handed). She subsequently developed progressive generalized dystonia including the face with a stiff smile, the neck (mild torticollis and laterocollis), and the upper limbs (abnormal posture of the hands and slow movements). On my initial examination, she had isolated dystonia (neurological examination was otherwise normal) predominately in the face, neck, and upper limbs. Mild dystonia was also observed in the trunk (mild back-arching and scoliosis) and lower limbs (claw-like posture of the toes). I also noticed general slowness of movements, stiff posture of the trunk and arms, and rigidity of the upper limbs. Neurological examination was otherwise normal and mental function was perfect (she worked full time as a secretary).

Secondary dystonia was suspected because of the rapid evolution, facial involvement with speech impairment, and associated dystonia and akinesia. At the time, brain MRI was considered normal.

She was tested for Wilson's disease and for hexosaminidase A and B and beta-galactosidase activity; organic acid and amino acids were normal and there were no elements in favor of mitochondrial disease. She was very badly disabled and eager for an operation. Considering her increasing disability, and despite some hesitation (unusual clinical features), she was put on the preoperative list. Results of the beta-galactosidase activity were obtained with some delay, and we were told that leukocyte-beta-galactosidase activity was only 5% of normal, just a few weeks before the time of deep brain stimulation (DBS). We decided to postpone the operation and to revise the diagnosis.

The full picture of adult-onset GM1 gangliosidosis was then unveiled.

THE APPROACH

Examinations showed a short stature (146 cm) and a scoliosis. Revision of brain MRI interpretation showed minor abnormalities with bilateral putaminal posterior hyperintensity on T2-weighted images. Single voxel spectroscopy showed increased myoinositol in the striatum (not in the white matter). The main clue was obtained by bone radiography and includes the following: (a) vertebral dysplasia with flattening and anterior beaking of the vertebral bodies with scoliosis and (b) hip dysplasia with flattening of femoral heads and acetabular hypoplasia. In addition, mild cardiac involvement was observed with mitral dysplasia and regurgitation.

Despite the fact that she had GM1 gangliosidosis secondary dystonia with potentially negative evolution (worsening of dystonia), she was operated (bilateral pallidal stimulation) with subsequent improvement (20% improvement on the Burke-Fahn-Marsden scale) as assessed by an evaluator blinded to the stimulation condition ("on" and "off" pallidal stimulation) with significant functional benefit (both subjectively and on Burke-Fahn-Marsden disability scale). There was no change in disease progression.

Two years later, she experienced a worsening of dystonia (facial grimacing, severe speech impairment with hypophonia), generalized dystonia, stiffness, and parkinsonism (she could barely drink from a glass or feed herself). Gait was severely impaired (with postural instability).

As she was badly disabled, while cognitively intact, she required additional surgery. Bilateral subthalamic nucleus (STN) stimulation was added to pallidal stimulation with subsequent functional improvement (she could stand up and walk on her own, slowly feed herself, and use a glass) (at 3 years follow-up of STN stimulation).

THE LESSON

Severe facial involvement, rapid progression, and association of dystonia and parkinsonism are highly evocative of secondary dystonia. Vertebral dysplasia and short stature are valuable diagnostic clues for GM1 gangliosidosis in patients with early onset secondary dystonia with severe facial and speech involvement and gait disturbances. As a consequence, these patients should undergo bone radiography in addition to blood tests [beta-galactosidosis activity—5% range (2%–11.3%)].

In addition to dystonia, patients may have parkinsonism, pyramidal signs, mental retardation, bone dysplasia (vertebral abnormalities), scoliosis, short stature, corneal opacities, and MRI abnormalities (putaminal hyperintensity).

Overall, clinical manifestations occur before the age of 20 in 83% of patients with a wide variation in severity and progression rate from severe disability in adolescence to mild symptoms with progressive worsening after the age of 40 (1).

To date there is no enzyme replacement treatment. Despite the potential poor functional prognosis of the disorder (evolutive disease), deep brain stimulation (DBS) may be considered in some carefully selected cases (provided the patient's functional objectives are perfectly clarified). A 20% motor impairment with functional relevance can be obtained with bilateral pallidal stimulation (2). Moreover, in the case of pallidal evolution of the disease, further benefit can be obtained from bilateral STN stimulation (akinesia, rigidity, although this remains a symptomatic treatment).

REFERENCES

1. Roze E, Navarro S, Cornu P, et al. Deep brain stimulation of the globus pallidus for generalized dystonia in GM1 Type 3 gangliosidosis: technical case report. *Neurosurgery.* 2006;59(6):E1340.
2. Roze E, Paschke E, Lopez N, et al. Dystonia and parkinsonism in GM1 type 3 gangliosidosis. *Mov Disord.* 2005;20(10):1366–1369.

58

The Highs and Lows of Deep Brain Stimulation in Dystonia: The Story of a Canadian Boy

W.R. WAYNE MARTIN AND MARGUERITE WIELER

THE CASE

A 12-year-old boy was referred for management of generalized dystonia. He was diagnosed to have this condition about 3 years previously, in 1990, when he had presented with involuntary inturning of the right foot. At that time, he was in grade 4 and described as an "excellent student." The family history was significant for two paternal second cousins previously diagnosed with dystonia, both of whom were severely affected. The patient had one sister, about 4 years younger, who was well. His parents, aged 31 and 35, were in good health with no history of a neurologic disorder. At his initial presentation in 1990, neurologic examination revealed correctible inversion and plantar flexion of the right foot and some increase in tone in the right arm. Investigations at that time were said to be negative and a presumptive diagnosis of idiopathic torsion dystonia was made. He was started on trihexyphenidyl, and the dose gradually increased to 75 mg daily.

Over the 3 years from diagnosis to presentation in our clinic, the motor symptoms gradually progressed. The left foot and right hand became involved about 2.5 years after the initial presentation. He began to use crutches to ambulate, using a wheelchair for going longer distances because of contractures in his feet. He continued to be an above average student.

When first seen in our clinic in 1993, neurologic examination revealed a pleasant, cooperative boy in no acute distress. There was unequivocal evidence of dystonic posturing affecting the neck with significant retrocollis, the back with scoliosis, and both lower limbs with plantar flexion and inversion. There was an apparent fixed flexion contracture of the right foot such that he was unable to stand on the right sole. The left foot was less severely affected. There were continuous dystonic movements affecting the toes of both feet. A postural/kinetic tremor was noted in the right upper limb. He was no longer able to ambulate with crutches but crawled either with both hands and legs or on his knees. His ability to use a manual wheelchair was impaired by his retrocollis, and he often got his fingers caught in the spokes of the wheels.

THE APPROACH

The characteristic clinical features, in conjunction with the family history, were believed to be indicative of a diagnosis of idiopathic torsion dystonia. The diagnosis was subsequently confirmed by DNA testing with the patient, his asymptomatic father, and his two second cousins all bearing the DYT1 mutation. Trihexyphenidyl was continued and a trial of levodopa recommended. Despite this, over the next few months, there was further progression particularly of the axial motor features with increased retrocollis and scoliosis. After extensive discussion with the patient, his parents, and a consulting child physiatrist, a trial of botulinum toxin injection was initiated with the objective of improving the retrocollis and the right foot deformity. The family was cautioned that if there was indeed a fixed contracture affecting the right foot, botulinum toxin was unlikely to be of significant benefit.

A total of 200 units of botulinum toxin was administered to the right posterior tibialis [75 units with electromyography (EMG) guidance] and to posterior neck muscles (125 units). These injections were continued about every 3 months over the next 9 months. Not surprisingly, the limb dystonia was unchanged, but there was significant improvement of the cervical dystonia component of his symptomatology with a reduction in the associated neck pain. The excessive trunk extension continued to be a significant source of disability.

Unfortunately, however, his other symptoms progressed, resulting in a significant increase in functional disability. By mid-1994, about 4 years after his initial presentation, he was unable to maintain a seated position because of involuntary extensor spasms of the spine. These spasms were marked; he "flopped around like a fish out of water" when attempting to lie on an examining table. Intermittent treatment with botulinum toxin injections continued with a total of 300 units administered to cervical and paraspinal sites. These injections were administered while the patient was lying on the floor because of the severity of the dystonic spasms. Throughout this time, he continued to use the sensory trick of holding an object in his right hand, usually a tennis ball or an old TV remote control, to attenuate the limb dystonia. He was pushed primarily in an adapted recumbent wheelchair, although he could independently move it for short distances when in a prone position. Despite this severe disability, he remained cheerful and optimistic about the future. When asked about potential careers, he replied that, while he loved the outdoors, he could not think of a job that he could do in the open air. If he thought about an "indoor" career, psychology would be a good option "because you don't have to sit in a chair" and because he had experiences that he believed could be useful to others.

The possibility of pursuing deep brain stimulation (DBS) for symptomatic management was raised with the patient and his parents. Although they found the concept to be intriguing, the parents were reluctant to commit to a surgical approach, preferring to wait until he had turned 18 and was able to make the decision for himself. On turning 18, he immediately chose to pursue this option, and a short time later, bilateral globus pallidus interna (GPi) electrodes were implanted using MRI guidance for DBS in 2000, about 10 years after the original onset of motor symptoms.

Once through the initial programming period, he responded extremely well to continuous bilateral GPi stimulation. The stimulator was kept on 24 hours per day even though the voltage, frequency, and pulse width requirements meant that the battery needed to be replaced approximately every 2 years. The stimulation parameters remained relatively stable, with adjustments in voltage typically made only after battery replacements.

He underwent surgical correction of the right foot deformity about 1 year after the DBS surgery, after which he was able to ambulate independently. He obtained his drivers' license in 2002 after a thorough evaluation demonstrated his ability to control a motor vehicle without adaptations. His once-voiced childhood dream was to go deer hunting with his father, and in the fall of 2002, not only was he now able to hunt but also, much to his delight, shot a five-point buck. He started college in September 2003, completing a diploma in the Natural Resource Technician Program and subsequently becoming involved in ecotourism. He had always considered himself an outdoorsman, and this was reflected in his work as a guide in a remote fishing camp. More recently, he worked as a manual laborer and started raising and racing sled dogs.

In early 2010, about 10 years after the original DBS surgery, and near the anticipated time for his fifth battery replacement, an unexpected increase in the impedance in the right lead was noted during a routine clinic visit. At that time, there was no change to his clinical status, but within about 2 weeks, he reported some "tightening" in his back reminiscent of his pre-DBS days. The back symptoms subsided, but about 1 month later, he experienced a sudden increase in dystonia while driving, resulting in his driving off the road. This sudden increase lasted for about 30 minutes before his body seemed to relax and everything returned to normal. Over the next 2 hours, there were several more transient episodes characterized by a marked increase in dystonia. Although he was not hurt and his vehicle was not damaged, he chose to stop driving until these problems are resolved. When seen in our clinic a few hours later, there was severe dystonic posturing in the trunk and the left upper and lower limbs. Interrogation of the implanted pulse generator (IPG) at 4 V (according to Medtronic protocol) again revealed high impedance of contacts on the right GPi lead. Interestingly, during the impedance check itself, the dystonia was almost completely suppressed. He was unable to get up off the floor of the clinic room unless the IPG was being interrogated.

The IPG was replaced, but postoperatively, the right brain contacts continued to show unusually high impedances. He continued to have episodes during which dystonic spasms were disabling in axial and left limb musculature. Because of the concern of a discontinuity in the circuitry between the IPG and the implanted right brain lead, a radiographic examination of the leads and extension wires was obtained. No discontinuity was evident on the examination. The response to stimulation became increasingly erratic to the degree that the stimulator was turned off pending further management decisions. During this time, he was significantly disabled, unable to pursue his previous activities, and unable to maintain an independent lifestyle. He is currently scheduled to undergo surgical evaluation of extension/lead integrity with detailed intraoperative impedance testing.

THE LESSON

Torsion dystonia can lead to a severe functional disability. Medical treatments in the past have been of benefit in some individuals, but many have remained severely disabled. The advent of DBS in these patients has been of tremendous symptomatic benefit, particularly in patients carrying the DYT1 mutation (1,2). In our patient, effective DBS resulted in the ability to pursue an independent and productive lifestyle in an individual who was previously dependent on others for much of his care even to the degree that he was unable to mobilize without assistance. Even after a sustained response that continued through multiple battery replacements, he experienced a reappearance of severe dystonic symptomatology with features suggesting a peripheral hardware malfunction most likely in the extension wires between the IPG itself and the brain electrodes.

These patients require close monitoring even after an apparent sustained symptomatic benefit. They are always at risk of complications because of untoward events such as lead fractures. This may be of particular relevance in the young, active individual who, quite naturally, wishes to live a normal lifestyle after having been trapped by severe dystonic features for years.

REFERENCES

1. Vidailhet M, Vercueil L, Houeto JL, et al. Bilateral deep-brain stimulation of the globus pallidus in primary generalized dystonia. *N Engl J Med*. 2005;352:459–467.
2. Andrews C, Aviles-Olmos I, Hariz M, et al. Which patients with dystonia benefit from deep brain stimulation? A metaregression of individual patient outcomes. *J Neurol Neurosurg Psychiatry*. 2010;81:1383–1389.

Suggested Reading

Albanese A, Asmus F, Bhatia KP, et al. EFNS guidelines on diagnosis and treatment of primary dystonias. *Eur J Neurol*. 2011;18:5–18.
Isaias IU, Alterman RL, Tagliati M. Deep brain stimulation for primary generalized dystonia: long-term outcomes. *Arch Neurol*. 2009;66:465–470.
Tarsy D, Simon DK. Dystonia. *N Engl J Med*. 2006;355:818–829.

The Opera Singer Who Cannot Hit the High Notes: Is It Always Spasmodic Dysphonia?

ILIA ITIN AND HESHAM ABBOUD

THE CASE

One of our most memorable cases is a 59-year-old college professor who used to be a professional opera singer. She started singing in high school and became a music education major in college. She worked for a while as a music teacher and obtained a master's degree in music education while teaching. She started her professional career as a singer locally and then moved to New York to join the Metropolitan Opera where she spent 11 years as a professional opera singer.

Her symptoms started while preparing for an upcoming show in 2001. She could not sing in high octaves during the rehearsals. She noticed that her lower jaw tended to shake and deviate to the right side when she opened her mouth widely to sing higher notes. In a short period of time, her abnormal jaw movement evolved into involuntary closure of the mouth, only when singing and not with other oral tasks. Initial evaluations by a number of neurologists and otorhinolaryngologists failed to give her a diagnosis or symptomatic relief. In 2003, she retired from opera singing because of her symptoms and moved to Ohio to become a voice professor. Despite this job change, her abnormal jaw movement persisted, interfering with teaching as it did with singing. In 2004, she was finally diagnosed with jaw dystonia but failed to respond to oral antidystonic medications, including tetrabenazine.

We saw her in 2009. At that time, she had already been experiencing difficulties with speaking and chewing for over a year. In addition to the history summarized above, she denoted a long history of nighttime bruxism and teeth grinding. She denied having any personal or family history of dystonia, dysphonia, or tremor other than her current problem. She also denied previous exposure to dopamine-blocking agents. She had no history of jaw trauma or excessive dental procedures preceding the onset of her symptoms.

When we examined her, we found no evidence of spasmodic dysphonia (SD) or dysarthria. Actually, she seemed quite normal while providing the history and during the general neurologic examination. She was able to hum and sing in a low pitch normally, but when we asked her to sing loudly, her lower jaw started to shake and deviate to the right side before it went into a complete closure. This abnormal jaw movement was reproduced when the patient was asked to speak or chew for sustained periods of time. We did not find any associated blepharospasm, facial grimacing, or lip pulling. Cranial nerve examination was normal when not singing, and the rest of her neurologic examination was unremarkable.

THE APPROACH

Despite the absence of clear voice abnormality in this patient, we decided to rule out laryngeal pathology given the patient's high risk for dysphonia. We referred the patient for videostroboscopy, which confirmed normal structure and function of the vocal cords, including normal mobility and absence of abductor or adductor spasms. The rest of her workup was essentially normal, including brain MRI and Wilson's disease workup. We diagnosed her with occupational jaw closure oromandibular dystonia (OMD) and associated jaw tremors. We decided to treat her with botulinum toxin injections to the masseter muscles on both sides. We escalated the dose gradually as we injected the patient every 3 months. She responded well to the injections and regained normal speaking and chewing abilities. She also reported a 40% improvement in her singing ability. Unfortunately, this partial improvement was insufficient for her to return to professional singing. However, she was able to keep her job as a voice professor.

THE LESSON

This case taught us to think outside the box and not pigeonhole each patient to known syndromes. Our patient's profession put her at risk for SD because of intense voice use (1,2) rather than jaw closure dystonia. Her complaint of inability to sing higher octaves strongly suggested a vocal cord problem and therefore most of her clinical evaluations were performed by ear, nose, and throat (ENT) doctors. Her ENT evaluations were repeatedly reported as normal, although the patient continued to suffer. Even when she was seen initially by neurologists, they kept sending her back to ENT specialists to look for SD. SD is a form of focal dystonia that has been linked to individuals who use their voice intensely like singers and teachers (3,4). Our patient seemed to be specifically prone to this problem because she is both a singer and a teacher. Unfortunately, this "red herring" delayed the accurate diagnosis of this patient's condition by obscuring her mandibular symptoms. It was not until 2004—1 year after her retirement—that "jaw dystonia" was proposed as a cause for her singing problem. Interestingly, it was an ENT doctor who made this diagnosis. Even after she was diagnosed, she resisted oral antidystonic medications and continued to suffer in her new job as a voice teacher. We do not know exactly why the use of botulinum toxin was not offered to the patient for the 5-year period between her diagnosis and her visit to our center. However, we assume that the documented poor response of embouchure dystonia to botulinum toxin injections may have played a role (5). Embouchure dystonia is the prototype of occupational OMD described in woodwind and brass musicians. Most cases of embouchure dystonia have lip involvement and are resistant to medical treatment. They mainly respond to professional retraining of the embouchure (changing the mouth piece or the musical instrument altogether) (5,6). Occupational OMD in nonmusicians is extremely rare. We believe that only four such cases have been reported at the time of this writing. All four cases involved a profession or a ritual that required repeated use of voice in a particular manner, namely auctioning, bingo calling, Islamic praying, and mantra recitation (7–10). We found that our case had a great resemblance to those case reports in terms of symptom spread, absence of sensory trick, and the responsiveness to botulinum toxin injections.

In conclusion, unlike other singers, this patient had an occupational OMD rather than SD; unlike most cases of occupational OMD, she was responsive to botulinum injections rather than professional retraining. Because of this, we decided to publish this interesting case (11) and share it with everyone. This case, albeit a case of one, reinforced to us that focal dystonias uncommonly respond in a meaningful way to anticholinergic and other oral pharmacologic agents. We also wondered, although botulinum toxin clearly helps with focal dystonias such as these, how often could this treatment be effective enough to save a patient's profession and whether a greater success would have been achieved with earlier intervention.

REFERENCES

1. Phyland DJ, Oates J, Greenwood KM. Self-reported voice problems among three groups of professional singers. *J Voice.* 1999;13:602–611.
2. Bellia S, Serafino L, Luca N, et al. Incidence of dysphonia in teaching staff of school. *G Ital Med Lav Ergon.* 2007;29:613–614.
3. Jankovic J, Ashoori A. Movement disorders in musicians. *Mov Disord.* 2008;23:1957–1965.
4. Tanner K, Roy N, Merrill RM, et al. Risk and protective factors for spasmodic dysphonia: a case–control investigation. *J Voice.* 2011;25:e35–e46.

5. Frucht SJ. Embouchure dystonia: portrait of a task-specific cranial dystonia. *Mov Disord.* 2009;24: 1752–1762.

6. Frucht SJ, Fahn S, Greene PE, et al. The natural history of embouchure dystonia. *Mov Disord.* 2001;16:899–906.

7. Scolding NJ, Smith SM, Sturman S, et al. Auctioneer's jaw: a case of occupational oromandibular hemidystonia. *Mov Disord.* 1995;10:508–509.

8. Diaz-Sanchez M, Martinez-Castrillo JC. Botulinum toxin in a task-specific oromandibular dystonia in a bingo caller. *J Neurol.* 2008;255:942–943.

9. Ilic TV, Potter M, Holler I, et al. Praying induced oromandibular dystonia. *Mov Disord.* 2005;20:385–386.

10. Bonanni L, Thomas A, Scorrano V, et al. Task-specific lower lip dystonia due to mantra recitation. *Mov Disord.* 2007;22:439–440.

11. Itin I, Abboud H, Fernandez HH. Occupational oromandibular dystonia in an opera singer mimicking spasmodic dysphonia. In press.

60

An 18-Year-Old Woman Who Attacked a
Policeman With a Knife: Our Memorable
Lesson on Treatable Causes of Dystonia

Shyamal H. Mehta and Kapil D. Sethi

THE CASE

An 18-year-old woman was extremely upset because her boyfriend had dumped her. She became very agitated and called him at inappropriate hours. One evening, she showed up at his house with a knife. Hearing the ruckus, the neighbors called the police, and when they arrived, this emotionally disturbed girl attacked one of the policemen with a knife. She was arrested and then subsequently sent to a psychiatric facility. She received low doses of haloperidol and a tricyclic antidepressant and after 2 weeks developed drooling, twisting of the neck to the right, and trouble walking. At that point, the psychiatrist consulted the movement disorders neurologist. Her medical history was significant for secondary amenorrhea. She had normal periods starting at age 14, but at age 16 she her periods stopped. She also noticed that she had a tendency to bleed a lot after minor cuts. There was no family history of a similar disorder. She denied illicit drug use.

THE APPROACH

The patient was examined while in the inpatient facility, and the pertinent findings are described as follows: during her examination, she was alert and cooperative. She had slurring of speech, and the eye movements were interrupted by saccadic intrusions, giving it the appearance of macro square wave jerks. She had drooling and cervical dystonia with laterocollis to the right with a mild rotational component. Mild bradykinesia was noticed bilaterally. Her gait was slow without shuffling or ataxia. The rest of the examination was normal apart from splenomegaly.

Preliminary hematologic investigations showed platelet count at 28,000. The computed tomography (CT) scan of her head was normal, and she refused to get an MRI. Ultrasound of the abdomen was done, which showed a nodular shrunken liver and splenomegaly. Given the constellation of her signs and symptoms, we also ordered some other labs and tests. Serum copper was normal. Serum ceruloplasmin was 20 with normal being 21–30. Her 24-hour urinary copper was normal. Eye examination revealed a golden brown pigment around the cornea, and the slit-lamp examination confirmed the presence of a Kayser-Fleischer ring (Figure 60.1).

This 18-year-old girl presented an interesting diagnostic and treatment challenge. At the outset, the differential diagnosis consisted of primary psychiatric disorder and a possibility of drug-induced movement disorder versus a spontaneous movement disorder with psychiatric manifestations as seen in Wilson's disease (WD). Thrombocytopenia and secondary amenorrhea were other features. Her tests confirmed the diagnosis of WD, and she was treated with penicillamine (250 mg thrice a day) with the knowledge that it can cause further drop in platelets.

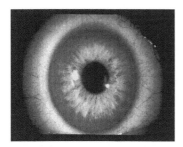

FIGURE 60.1
Slit lamp examination showing the process of a Kayser-Fleischer ring.

Fortunately, 2 months later, her platelets remained stable. The situation was further complicated by a car accident that resulted in a large splenic hematoma. She received platelet infusions and recovered without the need for surgical intervention. Over the next several months, her eye movement became normal and the cervical dystonia disappeared. The drooling improved, and the psychiatric problems also resolved after about 2 years.

THE LESSON

WD is an autosomal recessive disorder of copper metabolism resulting in protean manifestations, including hepatic, neurologic, and psychiatric symptoms to varying degrees. It was first described by Wilson (1) when he was still a resident in 1912. The *ATP7B* gene on chromosome 13 is involved in copper transport, and mutations in this gene are implicated in the pathogenesis of WD (2,3). Even though WD is rare with an estimated prevalence of 1/30,000 to 1/100,000 population, it should be suspected in any young individual with liver abnormalities of uncertain cause and a neuropsychiatric disorder. WD is a potentially treatable inborn error of metabolism and, if left untreated, leads to progressive neurologic deterioration and ultimately death (4).

In our young patient, new-onset psychiatric disturbances, cervical dystonia (confounded by antipsychotic exposure), and sequelae of liver dysfunction, i.e., thrombocytopenia and secondary amenorrhea, are all signs that necessitate a workup for WD. Common screening tests include serum ceruloplasmin (low in WD), 24-hour urinary copper (increased in WD), liver function tests, complete blood count, brain MRI, and ophthalmologic examination (Kayser-Fleischer rings on slit-lamp examination) (5). Although this represents a typical clinical and biochemical picture, patients may present with atypical clinical and laboratory findings. The dogma is that the eye movements are normal in WD, but as our patient demonstrates, these individuals can have significant eye movement abnormalities. Patients with neurologic WD and absent Kayser-Fleischer rings have also been reported (6). The initial screening tests such as ceruloplasmin and 24-hour urinary copper excretion may be normal as seen in our patient. If the clinical suspicion is high enough, a more diligent course needs to be pursued with genetic testing for the *ATP7B* mutations (if available) and liver biopsy for increased copper concentrations, which remains the best biochemical test.

Patients with WD, like our patient, if diagnosed early enough and treated appropriately with copper chelation therapy (penicillamine or trientine), prevention of intestinal copper absorption (with zinc or tetrathiomolybdate), or liver transplantation, do well and have a good prognosis.

Overall, this case illustrates that having a high index of suspicion regarding some of the rarer but potentially treatable disorders can have a significant impact in changing a patient's life for the better.

REFERENCES

1. Wilson SAK. Progressive lenticular degeneration: a familial nervous disease associated with cirrhosis of the liver. *Brain.* 1912;34:295–509.
2. Frydman M, Bonne-Tamir B, Farrer LA, et al. Assignment of the gene for Wilson disease to chromosome 13: linkage to the esterase D locus. *Proc Natl Acad Sci USA.* 1985;82:1819–1821.
3. Tanzi RE, Petrukhin K, Chernov I, et al. The Wilson disease gene is a copper transporting ATPase with homology to the Menkes disease gene. *Nat Genet.* 1993;5:344–350.
4. Ala A, Walker AP, Ashkan K, et al. Wilson's disease. *J Neurol Neurosurg Psychiatry.* 1999;67:195–198.
5. Gouider-Khouja N. Wilson's disease. *Parkinsonism Relat Disord.* 2009;15(Suppl 3):S126–S129.
6. Mehta SH, Parekh SM, Prakash R, et al. Predominant ataxia, low ceruloplasmin, and absent K-F rings: hypoceruloplasminemia or Wilson's disease. *Mov Disord.* 2010;25:2260–2261.

61

Rapidly Progressive Dystonia in a 52-Year-Old Thai Woman With SCA Type 2

ROONGROJ BHIDAYASIRI, WASAN AKARATHANAWAT,
AND PRIYA JAGOTA

THE CASE

A 52-year-old Thai woman was urgently referred to our movement disorders center because of progressive dystonia during the previous 4 months. Her symptoms began with blepharospasms when she was 39, and she responded well to botulinum toxin injections at that time. Last year, she began to complain of a stiff neck and difficulty with walking, which she attributed to a sprained neck and back. However, her stiffness progressed during the past 4 months to the point that she was unable to sit and required assistance with walking. She was seen by several neurologists and succeeding botulinum toxin injections were unsuccessful, although details of the dosage and muscle sections were unavailable. Her medical history included well-controlled diabetes and hypertension. She denied any history of neuroleptic exposure. She denied any family history of dystonia or other neurologic disorders.

When we saw her, the dystonia was intense in severity, affecting predominantly the cervical and truncal regions. She reported that it was increasingly difficult to breathe because of frequent severe spasms of her back muscles, resulting in intermittent episodes of opisthotonic posturing. Prominent retrocollis was seen, particularly when she attempted to sit upright or stand (Figure 61.1). She required two assistants to walk and managed only a few steps, limited by severe retrocollis and opisthotonic posturing of the back. Orofacial dystonia was observed, including blepharospasm and oromandibular dystonia. Her reflexes were brisk in all limbs but plantar responses were flexor bilaterally. A thorough examination was difficult, limited by the patient's symptoms. Less dystonia was observed in a supine position. On careful examination, we noticed that her saccades were slow with nonsustained gaze-evoked nystagmus. In addition, she had very mild finger-to-nose ataxia, but the dysmetria could be interpreted as a result of truncal spasm, which prevented a full range of upper limb movements. Finger taps revealed mild hypokinesia. Because of the severity of her dystonia, including her breathing difficulty, she was admitted to the hospital for immediate management of status dystonicus.

THE APPROACH

The traditional approach to dystonia focuses on the age at onset as the single most important feature in determining the outcome (1). The earlier the age at onset, the more likely it is that symptoms will be severe, with dystonia spreading to involve multiple regions. Dystonia that begins in adults usually involves the neck, cranial, or arm muscle symptoms first, and dystonia tends to remain localized (2,3). Therefore, in this case, the onset of blepharospasm 13 years ago, which initially remained localized, did not prompt the treating physicians to suspect anything unusual and concluded that she suffered from benign essential blepharospasm. However, there are several intriguing features about her dystonia that became evident when she later presented with rapidly progressive dystonia within a span of only 4 months. First, although it is common

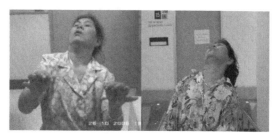

FIGURE 61.1
The patient showing retrocollis when she attempted to stand up.

for cranial dystonia to spread to adjacent regions, it is rather unusual for primary dystonia to progress rapidly or become generalized after reaching a plateau after more than 5 years since the initial onset. Indeed, the progression of her disorder was so severe that it became "status dystonicus," a term that describes frequent and severe episodes of generalized dystonia that necessitates urgent hospitalization (4). Moreover, the pattern of rostrocaudal progression of symptoms is unusual for primary dystonia. In addition, when the dystonia is severe, the extreme muscle contractions and abnormal postures could overshadow other physical signs. This case is a good example of this limitation—severe blepharospasm made the recognition of abnormal eye movements almost impossible to appreciate; the opisthotonic posture markedly limited the full range of movements of the upper limbs that are normally required during finger-to-nose examination; and the sustained contraction of the limbs inhibited the full response during reflex examination. Therefore, a combination of physical signs, including slow saccades, cerebellar and pyramidal signs, even though subtle apart from dystonia, and recent rapid progression of dystonia, made us consider that these are indicative of secondary or symptomatic causes (5).

The localization of mild cerebellar impairment, slow saccades, and brisk reflexes support the assumption that the lesion could be within the pontomesencephalic-cerebellar region. Because of the rapid progression of dystonia, the initial differential diagnosis included a mass lesion, demyelination, vascular lesions, or tardive dystonia. Alternatively, if we consider the first clinical presentation of blepharospasm to be part of the same manifestation, she could be suffering from a neurodegenerative disorder, which involves the cerebellum and the brainstem. However, the late progression of her dystonia is quite difficult to explain but is a recognized phenomenon. Despite a negative family history of neurologic disorders, there is still 8% to 15% possibility that she inherited a form of spinocerebellar ataxia (SCA), where the feature of slow saccades is suggestive of SCA2. Lesser possibilities include SCA3, Wilson's disease, or dentatorubral-pallidoluysian atrophy (DRPLA). Rapid-onset dystonia parkinsonism (RDP, *DYT12*) is another interesting disorder that should be considered in patients who have abrupt onset of bulbar and limb dystonia with parkinsonism, preceded by vague antecedent symptoms (6). However, the age at onset of RDP is usually before 20 years, and none of the cases with RDP reported signs of cerebellar dysfunction with slow saccades. Indeed, MRI of the brain of our patient did not reveal any focal lesions apart from mild cerebellar atrophy (Figure 61.2). Subsequent genetic tests confirmed the diagnosis of SCA2 with 36 CAG repeat expansion.

THE LESSON

The SCAs are a genetically and clinically heterogeneous group of autosomal dominantly inherited progressive ataxia. Recently, extrapyramidal signs are a well-recognized feature in almost

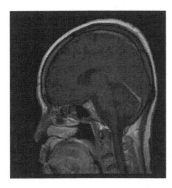

FIGURE 61.2
MRI scan displaying just mild cerebellar atrophy.

all types of ataxia, albeit with different frequencies (7). However, when they occur, these features are usually observed as a constellation of signs, including bradykinesia, slow alternating hand movements, flexed posture, reduced arm swing, and postural tremor. Dystonia is rare in all types of ataxia, but if present, dystonia strongly suggests the diagnosis of SCA3, observed mostly in early-onset patients before the age of 20 years. Indeed, extrapyramidal signs are more frequent in SCA3 than in other subtypes of SCAs. Therefore, rapidly progressive severe generalized dystonia in SCA2, as in this case, is rather unusual. However, a number of reports have recently described the association of SCA2 with cervical dystonia (8–10). In some cases, dystonia may precede the onset of ataxia by a few years (8). Why dystonia seems to be more common in SCA2 and SCA3 than other SCAs is unclear. Part of the explanation may be related to basal ganglia involvement in SCA2 as evidenced by a single photon emission tomographic study showing reduced striato-cerebellar ratios in the similar ranges as observed in patients with Parkinson's disease (11) and a postmortem study indicating a widespread degeneration affecting substantia nigra, pallidum, and neocortex (12). More interesting is why there is a predilection of dystonia to involve the cervical region in most patients with SCA2. Loher et al. (13) reported four patients with dystonia from pontomesencephalic lesions and all of them had craniocervical dystonia. A recent animal experiment using a special tracer indicated that the region of the red nucleus, which received input from basal ganglia, projected to the contralateral facial nucleus and upper segments of the cervical spinal cord (14). Therefore, disruption of this pathway may result in a variety of abnormal movements that involve the craniocervical region.

Traditional neurology emphasizes the basic approach based on a detailed history and a neurologic examination. This methodology continues to be the accepted procedure despite the era of modern diagnostic technologies. Although main neurologic signs should be focused, minor or even subtle physical signs should not be ignored because these features may reveal a clue leading to a final diagnosis. Moreover, when clinical manifestations progress out of the norm of the patient's underlying diagnosis, we should always challenge ourselves to consider a possible alternative disorder. With advanced molecular diagnostic techniques, we nowadays appreciate marked clinical heterogeneity of any specific disorder in which the main manifestation may not always reflect the underlying diagnosis. Our case provides a good example of this. Brisk reflexes and very mild finger-to-nose ataxia indicated multisystem involvement, not limited to basal ganglia, but suggestive of spinocerebellar degeneration. Slow saccades, which were difficult to elicit with marked blepharospasm, pointed toward the possibility of SCA2 even though the main manifestation of our patient was severe generalized dystonia, not ataxia. Hence, the more information that we are able to gain from a bedside approach will not only lead us to the correct diagnosis but may also limit unnecessary investigations. This is one case we will never forget.

REFERENCES

1. Marsden CD, Harrison MJ. Idiopathic torsion dystonia. *Brain.* 1974;97:793–810.
2. Greene P, Kang UJ, Fahn S. Spread of symptoms in idiopathic torsion dystonia. *Mov Disord.* 1995;10:143–152.
3. Bhidayasiri R. Dystonia: genetics and treatment update. *Neurologist.* 2006;12:74–85.
4. Jankovic J, Penn AS. Severe dystonia and myoglobinuria. *Neurology.* 1982;32:1195–1197.
5. Hartmann A, Pogarell O, Oertel WH. Secondary dystonias. *J Neurol.* 1998;245:511–518.
6. Brashear A, Dobyns WB, de Carvalho Aguiar P, et al. The phenotypic spectrum of rapid-onset dystonia-parkinsonism (RDP) and mutations in the ATP1A3 gene. *Brain.* 2007;130:828–835.
7. Schols L, Peters S, Szymanski S, et al. Extrapyramidal motor signs in degenerative ataxias. *Arch Neurol.* 2000;57:1495–1500.
8. Boesch SM, Muller J, Wenning GK, et al. Cervical dystonia in spinocerebellar ataxia type 2: clinical and polymyographic findings. *J Neurol Neurosurg Psychiatry.* 2007;78:520–522.
9. Kitahara M, Shimohata T, Tokunaga J, et al. Cervical dystonia associated with spinocerebellar ataxia type 2 successfully treated with levodopa: a case report. *Mov Disord.* 2009;24:2163–2164.
10. Walsh R, O'Dwyer JP, O'Riordan S, et al. Cervical dystonia presenting as a phenocopy in an Irish SCA2 family. *Mov Disord.* 2009;24:466–467.
11. Boesch SM, Donnemiller E, Muller J, et al. Abnormalities of dopaminergic neurotransmission in SCA2: a combined 123i-betacit and 123i-ibzm spect study. *Mov Disord.* 2004;19:1320–1325.
12. Estrada R, Galarraga J, Orozco G, et al. Spinocerebellar ataxia 2 (SCA2): morphometric analyses in 11 autopsies. *Acta Neuropathol.* 1999;97:306–310.
13. Loher TJ, Krauss JK. Dystonia associated with pontomesencephalic lesions. *Mov Disord.* 2009;24:157–167.
14. Pong M, Horn KM, Gibson AR. Pathways for control of face and neck musculature by the basal ganglia and cerebellum. *Brain Res Rev.* 2008;58:249–264.

62

A Young Girl With Presumed Cerebral Palsy and Her Grandfather With Depression, Dystonia, and Daytime Sleepiness: As Always, Family Is the Clue

Mark S. LeDoux

THE CASE

A general pediatrician referred a 5-year-old right-handed girl to me for evaluation of abnormal posturing in the lower extremities of approximately 1.5 years duration. The referral was prompted by the grandfather who had experienced similar manifestations as a child. This beautiful, joyful young girl had been examined by an experienced pediatric orthopedic surgeon and two pediatric neurologists. Unfortunately, she had not received an accurate diagnosis and had been exposed to unnecessary diagnostic procedures (brain MRI, lower extremity electromyography, and nerve conduction studies) and ineffective treatments (gabapentin and clonazepam). Moreover, the orthopedic surgeon had suggested that she could require bracing to treat her "cerebral palsy."

The young girl's first sign of neurologic dysfunction was inward turning of her left foot. The severity of this abnormality had progressed over the course of 1 year. Careful questioning indicated that there was significant diurnal variation to her signs with worsening of gait in the late afternoon and early evening. Reportedly, she exhibited a fine tremor in her distal upper extremities when fatigued. This patient was near normal in the morning upon arising from bed and improved after afternoon naps. Medical history was otherwise unremarkable, and all developmental milestones were met on time. Her father had shown evidence of a very mild gait abnormality during grade school with occasional inversion of the feet and "toe walking."

The grandfather presented to me at 47 years of age with a history of abnormal lower extremity posturing since the third grade. As a child, he had been treated by a prominent orthopedic surgeon with braces and corrective shoes for several years. He had been burdened by inversion of the right foot, and, to a lesser degree, the left foot, on almost a daily basis, since grade school. During the more immediate past, the grandfather had developed cramp-like sensations in his right arm while writing, particularly toward the end of the day. His wife indicated that her husband "moved slowly" and did not have "much energy." He had also been evaluated for anxiety and depression by a psychiatrist and had been treated with fluoxetine and clonazepam. On review of systems, the patient reported malaise and daytime sleepiness.

THE APPROACH

The young girl's general physical examination was totally normal with absolutely no evidence for cutaneous abnormalities or dysmorphic features. Neurologic examination was entirely normal except for action dystonia during ambulation and writing and a subtle postural tremor of the distal upper extremities.

Given the strong family history of dystonia and classic clinical presentation, this young girl was started on carbidopa/levodopa 25/100 mg, 1/2 orally twice a day for dopa-responsive dystonia, presumably due to a mutation in guanosine triphosphate (GTP) cyclohydrolase I. I was fairly confident about the clinical and etiological diagnoses but emphasized to the family (mother and maternal grandmother) that my opinion was purely clinical and confirmatory genetic testing could be performed in the girl's paternal grandfather. To limit the possibility of nausea, the patient was also prescribed carbidopa 25 mg and told to take 2 tablets before each dose of carbidopa/levodopa. Moreover, I told the young girl's mother, a pediatric nurse, to contact me within a few days regarding her daughter's clinical response to levodopa.

The next day, mid-morning, I received a page to call the young girl's home. Thankfully, she was running about the house without signs of dystonia and was not vomiting. Both the mother and grandmother were crying in tears of joy. She was cured, and I was a hero—that sort of status is usually reserved for surgeons! The young girl is now an active teenager and has continued to show a remarkably positive response to low-dose levodopa.

A definitive genetic diagnosis and management of the grandfather's case have been more challenging. At the time of initial evaluation, he had several comorbidities, including hypercholesterolemia, diabetes, hypertension, constipation, depression, and anxiety. He also reported daytime sleepiness and fatigue. Pertinent findings on neurologic examination included mild hypomimia, very mild bradykinesia, mild axial and appendicular rigidity without overt cogwheeling, mild postural instability with full recovery on the pull test, and difficulty with tandem gait. Intermittent mild lower extremity dystonia was noted with plantar flexion and inversion at the ankles. There was no rest or action tremor.

The grandfather was placed on carbidopa/levodopa 25/100 mg orally twice a day and responded with complete resolution of parkinsonism and dystonia. Unfortunately, his anxiety, depression, and daytime sleepiness actually worsened over the course of several years. Polysomnography and a multiple sleep latency test showed evidence of mild obstructive sleep apnea and excluded narcolepsy. Daytime sleepiness did not improve with continuous positive airway pressure.

The potential benefits of confirmatory genetic testing were discussed with the grandfather in the context of his positive family history and manifest dystonia in his granddaughter. We were able to get approval from his insurance company for GTP cyclohydrolase I sequence analysis. At that point in time, commercial laboratories were not offering analyses for detection of large deletion mutations, and the results of sequence analysis were interpreted as normal. Although I expounded, at great length, on the limitations of sequencing, the grandfather had obvious doubts regarding my diagnosis and did not understand why he was also struggling with anxiety, depression, and daytime sleepiness. I offered cerebrospinal fluid analysis of pterins (biopterin and neopterin), but the patient did not want to undergo lumbar puncture. The potential utility of a phenylalanine loading test was discussed with the patient but was not performed because of the very real possibility of a false-positive or false-negative result.

Given that the grandfather's depression and anxiety were not adequately controlled with several different selective serotonin reuptake inhibitors, including fluoxetine, sertraline, and escitalopram, I switched him to desvenlafaxine, a serotonin norepinephrine reuptake inhibitor. Within 2 months, the patient's depression and anxiety improved significantly. Regrettably, his daytime sleepiness remained a significant problem and did not improve notably with dextroamphetamine/amphetamine, modafinil, or armodafinil, all prescribed by a pulmonary sleep specialist. Because of his daytime sleepiness, the patient was struggling to get through the day at work and remained frustrated by the lack of a definitive etiologic diagnosis.

Determined to nail down the diagnosis, GTP cyclohydrolase I deletion analysis was obtained shortly after it was first offered by a CLIA (Clinical Laboratory Improvement Amendments)–certified commercial laboratory. With multiplex ligation-dependent probe amplification (MLPA), the grandfather was found to have a deletion mutation disrupting exon 1 of GTP cyclohydrolase I. Now, convinced of his family's diagnosis, we moved on to address the problem with daytime sleepiness. Fortunately, modest improvements in daytime sleepiness have been achieved with a combination of weight reduction, daily exercise, supplemental L-arginine, and satisfactory sleep hygiene.

THE LESSON

Diseases common to particular medical specialists may be quite rare and seem new to physicians in other disciplines. As apparent in this case, even experienced pediatric orthopedic surgeons and pediatric neurologists may fail to recognize dopa-responsive dystonia (1–3). Of utmost importance, all children with otherwise idiopathic dystonia deserve a trial of levodopa. In almost all patients with mutations in GTP cyclohydrolase I, the response to small doses of levodopa is marked and immediate. Furthermore, there is no need to delay treatment while waiting on genetic or biochemical testing. Biochemical analysis of cerebrospinal fluid requires lumbar puncture, and the phenylalanine loading test can be confounded by false-positive or false-negative results. In contrast, genetic testing is precise and provides the data, which is essential for genetic counseling.

An important percentage of causal mutations in GTP cyclohydrolase I, particularly large heterozygous deletions, will be missed by Sanger sequencing (4,5). Therefore, if clinical suspicion is high, and routine sequence analysis is normal, clinical testing for deletion mutations should be obtained. Quantitative polymerase chain reactions (PCR) or MLPA may be used to detect deletion mutations.

As apparent in this family, the motor and nonmotor phenotypes of autosomal dominant GTP cyclohydrolase I deficiency are broad and can lead to diagnostic confusion. Neurologic presentations include distal leg dystonia, cervical dystonia, tremor, tics, mild spasticity, and simple bradykinesia. In adults, mild parkinsonism with postural instability is not uncommon. Nonmotor manifestations include insomnia, frequent nightmares, obsessive-compulsive disorder, anxiety, depression, daytime sleepiness, and apathy (6).

Autosomal dominant GTP cyclohydrolase I deficiency often shows incomplete penetrance (1,2). Penetrance is higher in females than males. Therefore, is it not unusual that the young girl's father never sought medical attention for a relatively minor gait abnormality only apparent during his early grade school years. Although de novo mutations have been described, reduced penetrance in male family members is probably a more common cause for seemingly sporadic cases.

Although the differential diagnosis of childhood-onset dystonia is broad, the otherwise normal general physical and neurologic examinations, family history, and marked positive response to low-dose levodopa were virtually diagnostic of GTP cyclohydrolase I deficiency in my young patient. *TOR1A* and *THAP1* dystonia do not improve markedly with levodopa. Tyrosine hydroxylase deficiency is a recessive disorder, whereas sepiapterin reductase deficiency typically presents within the first 2 years of life and is commonly associated with cognitive impairment, oculogyric crises, and early parkinsonism (7).

GTP cyclohydrolase I synthesizes tetrahydrobiopterin (BH4), a cofactor for tyrosine hydroxylase, tryptophan hydroxylase, phenylalanine hydroxylase, nitric oxide synthase, and alkylglycerol monooxygenase. Therefore, deficiency of BH4 is predicted to cause deficiency of dopamine, serotonin, norepinephrine, epinephrine, melatonin, and nitric oxide. Although the focus of treatment in movement disorder clinics is on correction of dopamine deficiency with levodopa, deficiency of other transmitters may contribute to nonmotor manifestations such as anxiety, depression, and sleep disturbances.

In summary, the clinical and genetic features of this family with an autosomal dominant heterozygous deletion of GTP cyclohydrolase I (exon 1) point out many of the key issues related to the diagnosis and management of dopa-responsive dystonia:

◈ Dopa-responsive dystonia must be distinguished from dopa-responsive dystonia-plus syndromes.
◈ Penetrance is incomplete and higher in females.
◈ Clinicians must recognize the possibility of substantial intra- and interfamilial phenotypic heterogeneity.
◈ The motor features respond markedly to low-dose levodopa.

● Nonmotor features can exert significant contributions to overall morbidity.
● Genetic testing must include assays for deletion mutations when Sanger sequencing is nonrevealing.

REFERENCES

1. Segawa M. Hereditary progressive dystonia with marked diurnal fluctuation. *Brain Development.* 2011;33:195–201.
2. Furukawa Y. GTP Cyclohydrolase 1-deficient dopa-responsive dystonia. In: Pagon RA, Bird TD, Dolan CR, Stephens K, eds. *Gene Reviews* [Internet]. Seattle, WA: University of Washington; 2002. Accessed August 4, 2009.
3. Jan MM. Misdiagnoses in children with dopa-responsive dystonia. *Pediatr Neurol.* 2004;31:298–303.
4. Hagenah J, Saunders-Pullman R, Hedrich K, et al. High mutation rate in dopa-responsive dystonia: detection with comprehensive GCHI screening. *Neurology.* 2005;64:908–911.
5. Zirn B, Steinberger D, Troidl C, et al. Frequency of GCH1 deletions in dopa-responsive dystonia. *J Neurol Neurosurg Psychiatry.* 2008;79:183–186.
6. Van Hove JL, Steyaert J, Matthijs G, et al. Expanded motor and psychiatric phenotype in autosomal dominant Segawa syndrome due to GTP cyclohydrolase deficiency. *J Neurol Neurosurg Psychiatry.* 2006;77:18–23.
7. Clot F, Grabli D, Cazeneuve C, et al. Exhaustive analysis of BH4 and dopamine biosynthesis genes in patients with dopa-responsive dystonia. *Brain.* 2009;132:1753–1763.

Suggested Reading

Nagatsu T, Ichinose H. Regulation of pteridine-requiring enzymes by the cofactor tetrahydrobiopterin. *Mol Neurobiol.* 1999;19:79–96.
Opladen T, Okun JG, Burgard P, et al. Phenylalanine loading in pediatric patients with dopa-responsive dystonia: revised test protocol and pediatric cutoff values. *J Inherit Metab Dis.* 2010;33:697–703.

63

I Cannot Eat, Even Though I Want To: An Illustrative Case From Mr A on the Consequences of Dystonia

Mwiza Ushe and Joel Perlmutter

THE CASE

Mr A, a 67-year-old man with no medical problems, was admitted to the hospital by his primary medical doctor with a few days of severe anxiety associated with involuntary tongue movements. He had a 10- to 20-pound weight loss over the previous 4 months because of these involuntary tongue movements that impaired eating despite a good appetite.

Mr A's difficulty with involuntary movements may have begun 45 years ago with increased eye blinking and intermittent episodes of sustained closure. Fifteen years ago, he developed excessive right-hand tightness when he wrote. About 5 months ago, he started having occasional tongue involuntary movements predominantly to the roof of his mouth. These could occur at any time, including at rest, but were most prominent while eating or talking. About a month later, he developed occasional involuntary tongue thrusting with sustained thrusts lasting several seconds. These tongue movements gradually worsened over the next 4 months to the point that they interfered with socialization and eating. He had to place his tongue back into his mouth using his fingers. He denied difficulty with swallowing but stated that it felt as if his tongue was in the way, causing food and drink to dribble down his chin. He had been unable to complete a meal for at least 3 months. When the movements were at their worst, he had episodes of sustained tongue protrusions associated with shortness of breath and anxiety. These symptoms improved mildly with large doses of clonazepam and diphenhydramine, but sedation from the medications impaired his function. He denied vocal problems, other involuntary movements, or stiffness and cramping except for the right hand with writing. He was not exposed to any relevant medications. He had no family history of movement disorders. He was a retired mail carrier and never used illegal drugs.

Mr A had a normal general medical examination. His mental status was normal except poor attention, and he described his mood as "mellow." His language was normal, but speech was dysarthric. He had no Kayser-Fleischer rings, normal pupils, full extraocular movements, and bilateral horizontal nystagmus. He had bilateral blepharospasm, mild lower facial dystonia with sustained grimaces, and occasional tongue thrusting not increased by talking. The tongue thrusting pushed crackers out of his mouth when trying to chew them. The remainder of the cranial nerve examination was normal. He had moderate writer's cramp of the right hand; otherwise, there was no evidence of dystonia in his other limbs or neck. His strength was normal and had normal muscular tone and bulk. Mr A's gait was wide based and unsteady (but taking benzodiazepines at the time of the examination), although finger-nose-finger and heel-knee-shin were normal. His sensation was also normal.

THE APPROACH

Mr A had a cranial dystonia with lingual dystonia and blepharospasm with lower facial involvement (Meige syndrome) and right-hand writer's cramp. The differential diagnosis included idiopathic multifocal dystonia, neuroacanthocytosis, Wilson's disease, or brainstem lesions.

The evaluation included a normal complete blood count with a normal peripheral smear. Acanthocytes were not seen on a thick peripheral smear. A basic metabolic panel and hepatic function tests were normal, and the ceruloplasmin level was also normal. An MRI scan of the brain was normal. These studies made neuroacanthocytosis, Wilson's disease, and brainstem lesions very unlikely.

Mr A was diagnosed with a primary multifocal dystonia, including cranial dystonia with blepharospasm, lower facial involvement, and lingual dystonia and simple typewriter's cramp of the right hand. Although these manifestations could be consistent with a tardive syndrome, careful review of records and repeated questioning of the patient and family found no hints of potential relevant drug use. The recent weight loss was likely secondary to the difficulty in eating with tongue thrusting. Oral medications were marginally effective but required such large doses, which led to undesirable side effects like the wide-based, unsteady gait. We decided to inject botulinum toxin A directly into the anterior-inferior aspect of the genioglossus muscle. He had good response to treatment and regained the lost weight over the next several months. Each botulinum toxin treatment provided benefit that lasted about 6 months with minimal side effects (initial slowness of chewing). The blepharospasm and writer's cramp did not bother him enough to require treatment.

THE LESSON

Dysfunctional eating patterns may complicate the course of oromandibular dystonia or lingual dystonia in up to 15% of patients (1). This can be a problem for people with oromandibular dystonia with either jaw opening or jaw closing difficulty. Excessive opening of the jaw can impair ability to keep solids or liquids in the mouth and may respond to injection of the jaw opening muscles like the lateral pterygoids and sometimes the digastrics. Excessive jaw closing can impair the ability to put solids or liquids into the mouth and may respond to injections of botulinum into the jaw closing muscles like masseters and sometimes the temporalis or medial pterygoids. Our patient had trouble with eating because of direct pushing of solids or liquids from the mouth with the forward and upward involuntary tongue protrusions. Injections near the front of the genioglossus muscle approaching from below the jaw and injecting upward or injecting directly into the base of the upthrusting tongue may be useful; however, excessive doses or misplacement of botulinum can impair swallowing or eating further. Difficulty eating from any of these forms of dystonia may be the symptom that interferes most with patients' lives. Each interaction with a patient with either oromandibular dystonia (jaw opening or closing dystonia) or lingual dystonia should include a general evaluation of nutritional status, a history of dysfunctional eating, and strategies to improve the dysfunction. Botulinum toxin injection and tetrabenazine and other specific antidystonia medications may be effective in improving eating and may result in weight gain (1,2).

REFERENCES

1. Papapetropoulos S, Singer C. Eating dysfunction associated with oromandibular dystonia: clinical characteristics and treatment considerations. *Head Face Med.* 2006;2:47–50.
2. Esper CD, Freeman A, Factor SA. Lingual protrusion dystonia: frequency, etiology and botulinum toxin therapy. *Parkinsonism Relat Disord.* 2010;16:438–441.

64

Painful Muscle Spasms, Twisting, and Loose Stools: What a Combination in an Adolescent Girl!

RAYMOND L. ROSALES AND JACQUELINE E. BANZON

THE CASE

Born preterm at 32 weeks of gestation, this female Filipino patient's obstetrician mother noted that since birth, the girl has been experiencing watery stools three to five times a day. There were also episodes of vomiting occurring at least twice a month. Radiologic abdominal studies performed at that time, including hemograms, blood chemistries, and serial electrolyte studies, were not yielding. Thus, esophagogastroduodenoscopy followed by colonoscopy was performed and revealed normal findings except for flattened mucosal folds. Despite being put on lactose- and gluten-free diets, the loose stools persisted. It seemed like the patient went on with her normal childhood and schooling, having the loose stools as part of her daily life and nuances. There were no other pertinent historical abnormal records since then.

At 16 years of age, she stepped into our neuromuscular and movement disorders clinic on referral by the fifth pediatric neurologist who took care of her. It was because they needed to sort out why this patient developed recent generalized muscle spasms of 3-month duration. The spasms initially started as isolated, brief painful contraction of the distal legs, which were earlier precipitated by physical activity. Within a week, the episodes recurred even at rest and had become generalized, eventually leading to stiffness of the trunk and painful contractions of the distal extremities. The intermittent spasms last for minutes, occurring as frequently as more than 10 attacks per day. Search for "hot spots" ("sensory tricks") were not yielding. Specialists initially tried, but in vain, phenytoin and carbamazepine. Prednisolone oral treatment was likewise not helpful after a 4-week trial. Tests performed elsewhere yielded normal results for serial electrolytes (i.e., Na, K, Ca, and Mg), chemistries, electroencephalogram, and brain computed tomography (CT) scan followed by brain and spine MRI. On our evaluation, we took notice that in her family, the two male siblings and her parents have not been remarked to have a similar clinical profile. However, her mother had a recent diagnosis of breast cancer; a 72-year-old maternal great-grandfather died of gastric cancer, and a maternal aunt was diagnosed with Crohn's disease when she was in her 30s because of frequent loose stools.

On physical examination, vital signs were normal. Her height and weight fell within normal ranges for her age (p50), and body mass index (BMI) was 20. She had thick hair, and the eyebrows, eyelashes, and body hair were present on initial examination. There seemed to be no dysmorphism in the head, but she had a slight dextroscoliosis, without other accompanying bone deformities. She had a pubertal stage according to Tanner (P3 B3). Menarche was at 11 years of age. There was no history of "red urine" (myoglobinuria). The skin was not edematous, had a normal turgor, with no complaints of hypersweating or dryness. The liver was not enlarged, and cardiac examination was normal.

Neurologic examination revealed no signs of cognitive dysfunction (indeed an honor student!) or cranial nerve deficits in that her eye movements, facial muscles, swallowing, neck, and tongue muscles were strong. Funduscopic eye evaluation was also normal. There was slight atrophy of the anterior and posterior distal leg compartments, sparing the intrinsic foot and hand muscles. Fasciculations and myokymia were not evident and neither were there grip nor percussion myotonia. We found no muscle hypertrophy, and on manual muscle testing, the muscles were neither tender and rigid nor spastic. Her arm and hand muscles were strong [Medical Research Council (MRC) 5/5], whereas her proximal/distal leg muscles were slightly weak (MRC 4/5). Deep tendon reflexes were symmetrically hyper-reflexic, but she had plantar flexor responses.

During the examination, the patient had an attack of generalized muscle spasms, which started initially at the distal legs, followed by the hands and then the trunk. The spasms were evidently painful, causing stiffness and abnormal posturing of the hands and feet (Figure 64.1). Because spasms were movement induced, she was afraid to ambulate, preferring to be in wheelchair, and assisted in aspects of daily living activities.

THE APPROACH

Muscle diseases (especially channelopathies and metabolic disorders, including periodic paralysis and disorders with continuous muscle fiber activity) had to be on the top differential diagnostic considerations (1). The first test performed was a total creatine kinase that showed normal results on two occasions (before and after a bout of painful muscle spasms). Electrolyte and thyroid function tests, including antithyroid antibodies and antinuclear antibodies, were not yielding. Blood samples sent to a UK laboratory (courtesy of Professor Angela Vincent of Oxford) yielded no other abnormal muscle-related antibodies that included voltage-gated potassium channel antibody, glutamic acid decarboxylase (GAD) antibody, and acetylcholine receptor/muscle-specific kinase antibodies. The ischemic forearm exercise test (IFET), comparing lactate, pyruvate, and ammonia levels, was not indicative of a metabolic muscle disease (i.e., myoadenylate deficiency, glycogen storage, lipid storage, and mitochondrial disorders). Dystonia occurring in the young typically led us to do slit-lamp eye examination, including serum ceruloplasmin, which, from results, effectively ruled out Wilson's disease.

Routine nerve conduction studies (NCS) showed normal latencies, conduction velocities, and amplitudes of the compound muscle potentials/sensory nerve action potentials (i.e., motor tests: median, ulnar, peroneal, and tibial nerves, including F-responses and H-reflexes; sensory nerves: median, ulnar, radial, and superficial peroneal and sural nerves). Neither were there significant decrements nor increments on repetitive 3-Hz ulnar and axillary nerve stimulations. Electrophysiologic short and prolonged exercise tests (SET and PET), testing for periodic paralysis, were tried but did not yield significant decrements from baseline. Interestingly, the painful muscle spasms were induced by a 3-Hz repetitive ulnar nerve stimulation. Hence, even as we planned voluntary and stimulated single-fiber electromyography (SFEMG), these procedures were deemed difficult for the patient. In addition, during the painful muscle spasms, the concentric needle electromyography (EMG) revealed synchronized motor unit discharges of fast

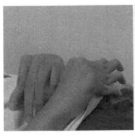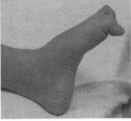

FIGURE 64.1
Painful muscle spasms and posturing of the hands and feet in Satoyoshi syndrome

frequencies, mimicking voluntary muscle contractions in the right triceps, first dorsal interossei, and vastus lateralis. The right vastus lateralis had low-amplitude polyphasic potentials. There were scarce fibrillations over the right first dorsal hand interossei; however, there were no fasciculations and myokymic or myotonic discharges.

Diagnosis

A syndromic combination in the young of chronic painful muscle spasms, twisting/posturing, and loose stools led to a clinical diagnosis of Satoyoshi syndrome (2). First reported in 1967 by Eijiro Satoyoshi, Satoyoshi syndrome is a rare postnatal disorder characterized by recurrent muscle spasms associated with multisystem involvements, including alopecia, gastrointestinal, endocrinologic, and joint deformities (2–6). The present account led to about 60 cases diagnosed worldwide, with two-thirds of the cases coming from Japan (3). This sporadic condition has an age of onset of 5 to 19 years (mean 10.9 years) and is almost twice as common in females (7). The intermittent painful muscle spasms are so severe that the affected body part is twisted into a sustained abnormal position (8) and induced by repetitive nerve stimulation, alleviated by sleep or general anesthesia (9). EMG recordings reveal synchronized motor unit discharges of 40 to 50 Hz and of 4 to 10 mV amplitude. It is believed that the muscle spasms are likely generated because of massive hyperactivity or disinhibition at the alpha motor neuron level (9). Presumed to have autoimmune origin, overlapping antinuclear antibody positivity and evidence of deposition of GAD or other immune complexes have been reported (10).

Therapy

Hinged on a presumed autoimmune mechanism, and on the basis of previous intravenous gamma globulin (IVIgG) and glucocorticoid treatment effects (6,11–13), our recommendation was to initiate IVIgG at 0.4 kg/d for five doses, combined with symptomatic dantrolene sodium oral maintenance therapy. With the regimen, the painful muscle spasms gradually reduced and abated after 5 days of IVIgG. There were no recurrences of the generalized spasms, but she remained hesitant to move the limbs for another 2 days after the last IV dose was given. Since then, she was maintained on oral dantrolene sodium (50 mg/d) for muscle spasms. Although she continued to have loose stools (averaging three times a day), 6 months after the administration of IVIgG, the patient could ambulate independently without any recurrences of the spasms. She had returned to school, ambulating alone. Two other occasions were reported 2 years henceforth with painful muscle spasms, both of which were attributed to failure to comply with dantrolene daily doses. IVIgG was recommended but could not be performed for financial constraints, and hence, pulse methylprednisolone (1 g/d for 3 days) was instituted. Relief of muscle spasms occurred after 1 week, whereas dantrolene was instructed to be taken religiously. On another clinical note, 2 years later, alopecia became evident, which completed the Satoyoshi syndrome of painful muscle spasms, loose stools, alopecia, and joint abnormalities. Botulinum toxin therapy has been prepared for this patient for symptomatic relief of painful spasms after a report of relief in masticatory spasms of Satoyoshi syndrome (14).

THE LESSONS

Three lessons can be derived from this present case:

1. Episodic painful muscle spasms/cramps: Although Satoyoshi syndrome does have painful muscle spasms, neuromuscular junction (NMJ) and muscle disorders ought to be initially ruled out (1). Episodic weakness with exercise intolerance and fatigue are common in postsynaptic NMJ disorders e.g., myasthenia gravis: ruled out by Tensilon test, repetitive nerve stimulation (RNSS), single fiber electromyography (SFEMG), and AchR/MuSK

antibodies] and in metabolic disorders in glycogen, lipid, adenine nucleotide, and mitochondria (e.g., glycogen storage disease types II [Pompe's], V [McArdle's], and VII [Tarui's]; Carnitine palmitoyl deficiency; myoadenylate deaminase deficiency). These fatigue-related muscle disorders are ruled out by absence of myoglobinuria, hepatic-cardiac abnormalities, dysmorphism, and abnormalities in the IFET, muscle biopsy and glycogen, fatty acid, and oxidative/mitochondrial enzyme activities. Muscle channelopathies (e.g., chloride, potassium, sodium, and calcium, including thyrotoxic periodic paralysis) also figure as a differential diagnosis in this constellation of symptoms and may be ruled out by thyroid hormone, electrophysiologic SET/PET, and channel antibodies. Clinical myotonia, not only the sole domain of myotonic dystrophies but also a common finding in channelopathies, is defined as a delayed relaxation after forceful muscle contraction (as in a grip) and can be elicited by direct percussion of the muscles (percussion myotonia). EMG in true myotonia will show prolonged waxing and waning electrical discharges with gradually declining amplitude and the characteristic "dive bomber's" sound.

Key point: The muscle spasms of Satoyoshi syndrome is not associated with increased muscle enzymes and certainly not clinical or EMG myotonia.

2. Muscle stiffness with continuous muscle fiber activity corroborated by EMG: These features are typical of Isaac's syndrome and stiff person syndrome. Isaac's syndrome (also called neuromyotonia) is associated with antibodies to voltage-gated potassium channels along nerve terminals. The main presentation is usually in the limbs with stiffness plus myokymia, fasciculations, and pseudomyotonia (i.e., differs clinically from true myotonia because delayed muscular relaxation increases instead of decreases with repetitive activity, and percussion myotonia is absent). Myokymia is a clinically visible and continuous muscle twitching (like ripples) and best distinguished from vigorous fasciculations by EMG. Stiff person syndrome is usually associated with GAD antibodies in the spinal cord and presents mainly with the stiffness of truncal muscles (i.e., lumbar lordosis and paraspinal hypertrophy). Interestingly, because of the shared autoimmune background (i.e., presence of target antibodies and response to immunotherapy), Satoyoshi syndrome may be considered as an "atypical stiff person syndrome." The accompanying severe pains in Satoyoshi syndrome should be an important clinical clue, apart from the syndromic presence of loose stools and alopecia.

Key point: The muscle stiffness of Satoyoshi syndrome is painful, involving the limbs and the trunk, and certainly not associated with myokymia, fasciculations, and continuous muscle fiber activity.

3. Muscle stiffness and twisting/posturing and pain: Before Satoyoshi syndrome is even considered because of this symptom cluster, the phenomena of spasticity and dystonia should also be on the clinician's platter. Spasticity is a movement disorder because of the disordered sensorimotor control resulting from an upper motor neuron lesion, presenting as intermittent or sustained unwanted activation of muscles in addition to restrictive passive and active mobilities (15). Sustained muscle contractions causing stereotyped twisting or turning/directional movement or abnormal postures, often with changing patterns, typify dystonia (16). What could be shared by dystonia and spasticity are the sustained, unwanted movements with posturing, overflow of muscle movements, and pain (17). Although spasticity is typically velocity dependent, with an "end catch" on passive limb movement, dystonia is distinguished by the presence of "geste antagoniste" ("sensory trick") that abolishes the abnormal movement as one touches certain skin "hotspots" or through proprioceptive maneuvers (18). Pseudodystonia are neurologic syndromes in which abnormal postures may be present but are not considered true dystonia. In this regard, Satoyoshi syndrome is a pseudodystonia,

together with movement disorders such as Sandifer syndrome, inflammatory myopathy, Arnold-Chiari malformation, and Syrinx, among others (19).

Key point: The twisting/posturing of Satoyoshi syndrome is intermittent, not velocity dependent, and certainly not abolished by "sensory tricks."

REFERENCES

1. Rosales RL. Muscle cramps. In: Lisak RP, Truong DD, Carroll W, Bhidayasiri R, eds. *International Neurology: A Clinical Approach.* United Kingdom: Wiley and Blackwell; 2009:461–464.
2. Satoyoshi E. A syndrome of progressive muscle spasm, alopecia, and diarrhea. *Neurology.* 1978;28: 458–471.
3. Ikeda K, Satoyoshi E, Kinoshita M, et al. Satoyoshi's syndrome in an adult: a review of the literature of adult onset cases. *Intern Med.* 1998;37:784–787.
4. Haymon M, Willis R, Ehlayel MS, et al. Radiologic and orthopaedic abnormalities in Satoyoshi syndrome. *Pediatr Radiol.* 1997;21:415–418.
5. Wisuthsarewong W, Likitmaskul S, Manonukul J. Satoyoshi syndrome. *Pediatr Dermatol.* 2001;18:406–410.
6. Asheron R, Glampaolo D, Strimling M. A case of adult-onset Satoyoshi syndrome with gastric ulceration and eosinophilic enteritis. *Nat Clin Pract Rheumatol.* 2008;4:439–444.
7. Hegar S, Kuester R. Satoyoshi syndrome: A rare multisystemic disorder requiring systemic and symptomatic treatment. *Brain Dev.* 2006;28:300–304.
8. Fung V, Thompson P. Rigidity and spasticity. In: Jankovic J, Tolosa E, eds. *Parkinson's Disease and Movement Disorders.* Philadelphia, PA: Lippincott Williams and Wilkins; 2007:506–509.
9. Drost G, Verrips A, van Engelen BG, et al. Involuntary painful muscle contractions in Satoyoshi syndrome: a surface electromyographic study. *Mov Disord.* 2006;21:2015–1018.
10. Drost G, Verrips A, Hooijkaas H, et al. Glutamic acid decarboxylase antibodies in Satoyoshi syndrome. *Ann Neurol.* 2004;55:450–451.
11. Cecchin C, Felix T, Magalhaes RB, et al. Satoyoshi syndrome in a Caucasian girl improved with glucocorticoids. *Am J Med Genet.* 2003;118:52–54.
12. Endo K, Yamamoto T, Nakamura K, et al. Improvement of Satoyoshi syndrome with tacrolimus and corticosteroids. *Neurology.* 2003;60:2014.
13. Arito J, Amano S, et al. Intravenous gammaglobulin therapy of Satoyoshi syndrome. *Brain Dev.* 1996;18:409–411.
14. Merello M, Garcia H, Nogues M, et al. Masticatory muscle spasm in non-Japanese patient with Satoyoshi syndrome, successfully treated with botulinum toxin. *Mov Disord.* 1994;9:104–105.
15. Pandyan AD, Gregoric M, Barnes MP, et al. Clinical perceptions, neurological realities and meaningful measurement. *Disabil Rehabil.* 2005;27:2–6.
16. Fernandez HH, Rodriguez R, Skidmore F, et al. The twisted patient. In: *A Practical Approach to Movement Disorders: Diagnosis, Medical and Surgical Management.* United States: Demos Medical Publishing; 2007:117.
17. Rosales RL, Kanovsky P, Fernandez HH. What's the "catch" in upper-limb post-stroke spasticity: expanding the role of botulinum toxin applications. *Parkinsonism and Relat Disord.* 2011;17:S3–S10.
18. Rosales RL, Dressler D. On muscle spindles, dystonia and botulinum toxin. *Eur J Neurol.* 2010;17(Suppl 1):71–80.
19. Fahn S, Jankovic J. Dystonia: phenomenology, classification, etiology, pathology, biochemistry, and genetics. In: *Principles and Practice of Movement Disorders.* Philadelphia, PA: Churchill Livingstone (Elsevier); 2007:307–343.

65

Why Did a Competitive Rower Lose His Skill?
An Unusual Case of Task-Specific Action Dystonia

Jed Barash, Michael Ronthal, and Daniel Tarsy

THE CASE

After 3 years of intense training (year-round, six sessions weekly), a 22-year-old competitive rower experienced a persistent feeling of right-sided incoordination, which significantly compromised his performance. Specifically, he noted a "hitch" in his right arm and difficulty planting his right foot while pulling back on his oar with each stroke. No involuntary movements or abnormal postures were observed while performing a variety of other routine activities. His history was notable for Lyme disease, which was diagnosed when he developed a truncal rash 6 months after the onset of his presenting motor symptoms. There were no neurologic complications, and he was treated with doxycycline for 3 weeks. There was a history of multiple mild concussions sustained during sporting events, the most recent of which occurred 5 years previously. No family member was known to have a movement disorder of any kind. Physiotherapy and chiropractic treatment were unhelpful. Initial neurologic consultation suggested mild right shoulder girdle weakness. He was referred for a movement disorders consultation.

THE APPROACH

The day before his visit, his mother, who is a nurse, called to ask whether he could bring his rowing machine to the clinic! Discussion with her indicated the problem was limited to rowing and did not seem to be a problem of muscle weakness. This circumscribed and apparently task-specific motor deficit raised the possibility of dystonia even before he was seen. There was no family history of dystonia. Neurologic examination was normal with no signs of dystonia at rest. However, when observed on his rowing machine, he displayed immediate and persistent hyperabduction of his right arm only while pulling back on his oar (Figures 65.1 and 65.2) and inability to fully plant his right heel during the forward drive of each stroke. Serum ceruloplasmin, MRI of the brain, cervical, thoracic, and lumbar spine, and electromyography were all normal. There was no improvement in his stroke during a 3-week trial of levodopa 25/100 mg three times a day. He declined botulinum toxin because of his concern that it would cause arm and shoulder weakness.

THE LESSON

Task-specific action dystonia is a form of focal dystonia precipitated by the performance of repetitive, highly skilled movements. The most common task-specific dystonias are writer's cramp and musician's dystonia. The condition has also been described with several recreational sports, including pistol shooting, dart throwing, long-distance running, table tennis, and golf. These are uncommon disorders that often go undiagnosed for long periods of time. Here, we describe a case of task-specific action dystonia in the context of rowing, which does not seem to have been previously described. This seemed to be a task-specific action dystonia because

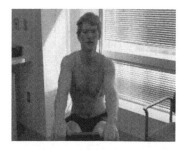

FIGURE 65.1
Rower in forward position with arms in normal position.

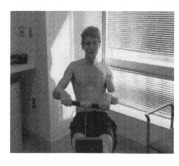

FIGURE 65.2
Rower pulling back on oars with right-arm abducted posture.

of its exclusive occurrence during performance of a skilled motor task, its occurrence after a prolonged period of intensive training, and the absence of any other contributory neurologic or orthopedic abnormalities. Although the cause of task-specific action dystonia is unknown, environmental factors together with abnormal cortical mechanisms of inhibition and plasticity possibly play a role in its pathogenesis.

Suggested Reading
Le Floch A, Vildailhet M, Flamand-Rouviere C, et al. Table tennis dystonia. *Mov Disord.* 2010;25:394–397.
Torres-Russotto D, Perlmutter JS. Task-specific dystonias: a review. *Ann NY Acad Sci.* 2008;1142:179–199.

66

"Tremors" and Gait Difficulties in an 18-Year-Old Hispanic Teenager: An Illustrative Case on the Power of Levodopa

Daniel A. Roque and Carlos Singer

THE CASE

An 18-year-old right-handed Hispanic teenager presented to our clinic with complaints of "hands shaking" and gait difficulties. She had a normal development throughout childhood. At the age of 12 years, she began to experience a tremor of both hands, worse with action but still present at rest. The onset was insidious and progression was slow, with transient worsening of her symptoms at times of increased anxiety. Furthermore, every time she attempted to write out schoolwork or homework, her hand would cramp up and writing would become difficult to perform, awkward in appearance, and mildly painful. She also started to avoid social situations, believing that the tremor or cramps might appear while holding other objects and create embarrassing situations.

Approximately 5 years later, she began to experience right lower limb cramping. She first noted the episodes while sitting in class, and she was unable to relax the extremity from "tensing up." Within days, both lower extremities were affected albeit asymmetrically (right greater than left), but this eventually worsened enough to impair her ability to ambulate. Her father described her gait as "walking like a robot" when this occurred. The greater the degree of activity she performed, the tenser her legs became and the more likely she would have to rest to let her pain and cramping subside.

When reviewing additional symptoms, she admitted to only a few additional symptoms such as experiencing vivid dreams and nocturnal limb movements during sleep witnessed by her parents. She and her family denied acting out her dreams or episodes of sleep walking. They also denied mood abnormalities, autonomic dysfunction (e.g., palpitations, bowel/bladder dysfunction, diaphoresis), or endocrine complaints (e.g., menstrual abnormalities, weight changes).

Our patient's family history revealed that her father, now 55 years old, had begun suffering from tremors of his hands at an early age as well. He admitted that his hand tremors were similar in character to his daughter's, except that she had developed them earlier in life, and he denied abnormal posturing of the hands while writing. The patient's mother also reported having a tremor of her hands as a teenager, but that it was present only when she was "nervous." Two older brothers (24 and 23 years old) had no history of adventitious movements or posturing. Our patient denied smoking, use of alcohol, or use of illicit drugs.

Developmentally, the patient was born from a normal, uncomplicated gestation, although her delivery was pitocin induced with an abrupt delivery and cord wrapping around the neck with rapidly recovering Apgar scores. She reached her developmental milestones as expected.

On physical examination, the patient demonstrated exclusively motor-related abnormalities, sparing cognitive, autonomic, brainstem, and other appreciable higher cortical functions. Blood pressure (BP) and pulse were recorded sitting and standing without a significant difference (sitting BP 133/85, heart rate [HR] 66; standing after 3 minutes BP 135/98, HR 95). Cranial nerve examination was unremarkable, as was sensory examination to pinprick, light touch, vibration, and joint-position testing.

Our motor examination revealed a mild postural tremor in the palms-in position and an intention tremor during finger-to-nose testing. While writing with her right hand, she continuously flexed and extended the right thumb while concomitantly hyperflexing the fingers of the left hand. Attempting to write with her left hand produced a worsening tremor on the left, with tensing of the right hand and tremors of the right fingers. Examination of her lower extremities revealed she was capable of hyperflexing her knees and ankles and hyperinverting her feet bilaterally. The patient's deep tendon reflexes were hard to elicit in the upper extremities and 2+ in the lower extremities, with symmetric flexor plantar responses. She had no notable gait abnormality.

Review of her laboratory studies from her course onset, obtained by her pediatrician, revealed a complete blood count with differential and complete metabolic panel, all within normal limits. Her serum ceruloplasmin was minimally decreased at 16.7 mg/dL (normal 17.9–53.3 mg/dL), but her serum copper of 79 mcg/dL (normal 80–180 mcg/dL) and, particularly, urine copper of 6 mcg/24 hour (normal 15–60 mcg/24 hour) were normal. Thyroid function tests were normal. Serum iron levels were reported at 137 mcg/dL (normal 35–155 mcg/dL).

THE APPROACH

Our clinical impression was that her hand tremors were dystonic in nature and that her stiffness of lower extremities was probably dystonic because we could find no evidence of upper motor neuron signs or stiffness or rigidity.

An MRI of the brain with and without contrast demonstrated no structural abnormalities. Her ventricular system was normal in size and shape, and the grey-white junction seemed to be unaltered. Contrast injection did not reveal areas of abnormal enhancement. The only notable finding was within the choroidal fissure on the right, an unenhancing 8-mm rounded area of low signal intensity on the T1-weighted study, with high signal intensity on T2-weighted images, favored to be a cyst and believed to have no clinical significance.

Given the minimal decrease in serum ceruloplasmin, we repeated the laboratory workup in trying to definitely rule out Wilson's disease. An ophthalmologic examination performed by a senior neurophthalmologist disclosed no Kayser-Fleisher rings or sunflower cataracts, with normal eye movements and optic discs. New laboratory draws reported a normal ceruloplasmin level of 24.3 mg/dL (normal 21.0–53.0 mg/dL) and low urine copper level. At this point, Wilson's disease had fallen out of favor as a likely diagnosis, and considering the presence of dystonia in the setting of postural tremor, the possibility of a genetically driven familial dystonia was considered. It was at this time that a levodopa trial with carbidopa/levodopa was initiated to assess for responsiveness, with counseling to both the patient and parents on potential adverse effects.

On the patient's return to clinic after 2 months on levodopa 200 mg daily, she reported a marked improvement in her tremor and writer's dystonia and complete resolution of her lower extremity stiffness. With further increase to levodopa 300 mg daily, the patient noted a 90% subjective improvement in her handwriting and still further control of her tremors. When we compared her Archimedes spiral before and after treatment with carbidopa/levodopa, which clearly demonstrated much smoother lines with less tremulousness and significantly better target accuracy, we concluded the patient had dopa-responsive dystonia (also known as Segawa disease) with a somewhat atypical presentation but unquestionable response to treatment with carbidopa/levodopa.

THE LESSON

Our patient's history illustrates an atypical evolution of symptoms in a well-documented genetic disorder, with correct diagnosis identified in her case only once the disease manifested itself over the course of time. As reported by Dr Segawa (1) in 1976, the typical manifestation begins with an asymmetric lower extremity dystonic posturing, with preservation of locomotion. Only in their 20s and 30s do patients begin to typically manifest additional movement disorders, including postural tremor. Even in cases of action-dystonia type Segawa disease, patients presenting with writer's cramp at onset do not usually present with symptoms until their adulthood (1).

Our patient presented with a complaint that both she and her parents labeled as "hand tremors." Careful examination of the actual performance during handwriting, looking for abnormal posturing, and mirror dystonia were the critical clues that directed us to the phenomenological conclusion that this was a dystonic process (2). Her peculiar stiffness of lower extremities was not associated with upper motor neuron signs or with findings of stiffness or rigidity of lower extremities while seated. We therefore hypothesized that perhaps this "stiffness" was underlied by a dystonic mechanism, even despite no clinical evidence of dystonic posturing while ambulating. It is of interest to point out again that her asymmetric involvement of lower extremities followed the "hand tremors" by 5 years.

We recognize that diagnosing "dopa-responsive dystonia" does not necessarily stop the diagnostic process because additional testing may reveal the specific gene affected. For example, it has been observed that patients with tyrosine hydroxylase deficiency have a far poorer and incomplete response to levodopa compared with their *GCH1* mutation counterparts with dystonia (where both genetic mutations present with a dystonic phenotype). Thus, it is recommended to attempt a levodopa trial, starting with low doses and slow titration, for both diagnostic and potentially therapeutic reasons. As long as patients and parents are counseled on potential side effects of the medication, we believe this is an appropriate first treatment option once dystonia-plus syndromes are suspected.

An additional clinical point that can be made includes the degree to which the type of presentation and the sequence of symptoms deviated from the classic prototype described by Segawa. In a typical case, the disorder starts in children with action dystonia of the legs and only later do dystonias of the upper extremities—especially writer's cramp—and postural tremor of the same appear in adulthood. She developed involvement of upper and lower extremities during the course of her teens (not yet adult) and in a sequence opposite to the one described by Segawa.

REFERENCES

1. Segawa M. Hereditary progressive dystonia with marked diurnal fluctuation. *Brain Dev.* 2011;33:195–201.
2. Asmus F, Gasser T. Dystonia-plus syndromes. *Eur J Neurol.* 2010;17(Suppl 1):37–45.

67

A Tendon Transfer That Could Have Been Avoided: My Memorable Case of a College Student With Dopa-Responsive Dystonia

Robert L. Rodnitzky

THE CASE

I received a consultation from an emergency room physician who had just sutured facial lacerations on a 22-year-old man who had tripped over his own feet and fallen, striking the ground face forward. Because he had attributed his fall to involuntary downward and inward movements of his feet, the emergency room physician appropriately referred him to the neurology movement disorder clinic after suturing his lacerations.

When I first saw him, he gave a history of periodic and progressively worsened inward and downward foot cramps since age 16. Now a university student, what seemed most unusual to him was the fact that this problem was seldom present when walking to class in the morning but often appeared when returning from class in the late afternoon or evening. At age 18, he had been evaluated for this problem by an orthopedic surgeon who treated him by performing bilateral tendon transfers on his feet. No neurologic consultation was obtained at that time. The tendon transfers improved the involuntary foot postures minimally, but they continued to occur, almost like clockwork, late in the day. The medical history was negative aside from his lower extremity symptoms. His parents were alive and healthy. He had two siblings who were also healthy. There was no family history of neurologic symptoms similar to his.

On examination, late in the day, the patient exhibited bilateral dystonic posturing of the feet while walking. There was slight, symmetrical hyperreflexia in the lower extremities. The remainder of his neurologic examination was normal. Specifically, there was no bradykinesia, rigidity, or tremor. He was normally alert and cognitively intact, consistent with his record of being a successful university student.

THE APPROACH

His brain MRI was normal. On the basis of the history of regular appearance of lower extremity dystonia occurring in a distinct diurnal pattern, a presumptive diagnosis of dopa-responsive dystonia (DRD) was made (1). I undertook a "diagnostic administration" of carbidopa/levodopa because patients with this condition are typically markedly improved by this treatment. After the first dosage of a 25/100 tablet, there was considerable improvement and virtual complete disappearance of his dystonic symptoms. He reported that he could now engage in activities such as jogging or recreational basketball at any time of the day without fear of falling. On the basis of this remarkable response, I did not consider it necessary to test him for the presence of a mutation of the GCH1 gene, the most common known cause of DRD.

THE LESSON

DRD can result from a variety of different genetically determined conditions. The most common of these is a dominantly inherited syndrome caused by mutations in the guanosine triphosphate (GTP) cyclohydrolase 1 gene (2). In autosomal recessive conditions resulting in DRD, including tyrosine hydroxylase deficiency and autosomal recessive GTP-CH1 deficiency, there are similar dystonic symptoms, but they are most often associated with cognitive abnormalities as well, which were not seen in this case. Accordingly, a clinical diagnosis of autosomal dominant DRD secondary to a mutation in the GTP cyclohydrolase gene was made. GTP cyclohydrolase catalyzes the first step in the biosynthesis of tetrahydrobiopterin, which is an essential cofactor for tyrosine hydroxylase, the rate-limiting enzyme in the production of dopamine. The administration of levodopa, a precursor of dopamine, bypasses this metabolic blockage of dopamine production, restoring normal neurologic function, and in this case, relieving the patient's bilateral lower extremity dystonia. Other associated findings such as hyperreflexia may also improve after levodopa therapy. With aging, however, some patients with DRD develop signs and symptoms of parkinsonism that is also responsive to levodopa (3). Penetrance of the *GTP-CH 1* gene has been determined to be approximately 87% in women and 38% in men, accounting for the higher incidence of the full clinical syndrome in women. Because the genetic abnormality has variable penetrance, there may not be a definite family history of the condition as was the case with this patient, but the clinical story alone should suffice to strongly suggest the diagnosis.

Although the genetic abnormality has been identified and the causative gene for this form of DRD can be commercially tested, the assay is expensive and the cost is often not covered by medical insurance. Accordingly, the presence of a brisk response of levodopa can render genetic testing unnecessary except in cases where genetic consulting is critical to other family members. There are no bridges burned by not obtaining immediate genetic consulting because it could be done at any time and the results will still be the same.

One last lesson for all of us is not to rely entirely on the evaluative and diagnostic skills of our own, sometimes narrow, subspecialty expertise when evaluating unusual symptoms involving other organ systems. This seems to have been the mistake made by the orthopedic surgeon who performed the tendon transfer in this patient. A referral by the orthopedist to a neurologist, especially a movement disorder specialist, would likely have yielded the correct diagnosis at an earlier date and saved the patient from what we now know was an unnecessary tendon transfer operation.

REFERENCES

1. Cheyette BN, Cheyette SN, Cusmano-Ozog K, et al. Dopa-responsive dystonia presenting as delayed and awkward gait. *Pediatr Neurol.* 2008;38:273–275.
2. Trender-Gerhard I, Sweeney MG, Schwingenschuh P, et al. Autosomal-dominant GTPCH1-deficient DRD: clinical characteristics and long-term outcome of 34 patients. *J Neurol Neurosurg Psychiatry.* 2009;80:839–845.
3. Segawa M. Hereditary progressive dystonia with marked diurnal fluctuation. *Brain Dev.* 2011;33:195–201.

68

The Serendipitous Discovery of the Beneficial Effect of Zolpidem on Dystonia

Virgilio Gerald H. Evidente

THE CASE

I had just arrived back in the Philippines after 7 years of residency and fellowship training in the United States, which culminated in my training in movement disorders. During my training, I had read about Lubag or X-linked dystonia-parkinsonism, although I did not see a singular case in the United States. I knew that with my return to the Philippines in 1998, I would eventually see those cases. And true enough, within a week of opening a movement disorders clinic in Manila, one morning, I found camped out in my office a Filipino man in his mid 30s who had developed involuntary twisting of his neck and opening of the jaw 2 years before. He apparently was a farmer from the southern Philippine Island of Panay who was desperate for help because the local doctors could neither confirm his diagnosis nor give him the right medicines to relieve his symptoms. He had sold one of his cows, packed his bags along with a blanket, foldable straw mattress, and pillow, and took a 2-day journey by boat to Manila. And there he was one morning in front of my office door, asleep on the floor awaiting my arrival. From his account, he had symptoms for a couple of years, which started with involuntary twisting of his head to the right, followed later on by involuntary opening of his jaw, drooling, bending forward of his trunk, slurring of his speech, difficulty swallowing, and some slowness in walking. He was initially tried on haloperidol, which did not alleviate his symptoms. He was also given clonazepam and biperiden at separate times, which only helped minimally.

THE APPROACH

When I first saw him, I appreciated on neurologic examination involuntary jaw opening, dysarthria, severe drooling, cervical dystonia (with his head turning to the right and flexing forward), and flexion dystonia of his trunk. He also had breakdown of rapid alternating movements of all four extremities, shuffling gait, and significant retropulsion on pull test. I then prescribed him a combination of trihexyphenidyl and clonazepam at maximum tolerated doses with no benefit. I also tried him on clozapine, which resulted in severe sleepiness and minimal improvement of his movements. I then decided to put him on a trial of levodopa to see whether his dystonia is levodopa responsive and because he had some parkinsonism. Given that he was having trouble sleeping because of his severe dystonia, he also asked for a sleeping pill. I, thus, ended up prescribing him zolpidem 10 mg at bedtime and carbidopa/levodopa 25/100 mg half tablet three times a day. A few days later, on follow-up, he informed me that the carbidopa/levodopa had no effect on his movements. He noticed, however, that the zolpidem he took after dinner almost immediately improved his dystonia. I was dubious of his claims, because I have never heard of zolpidem having any antidystonia effect. I then proceeded to give him a test dose of 10 mg in my office on follow-up, and within 20 minutes, he had remarkable improvement of his jaw, neck, and truncal dystonia. His shuffling gait and bradykinesia also improved, although not as remarkably as his dystonia. The effect lasted about 8 hours. He experienced mild sleepiness with the 10 mg zolpidem dose. Given the remarkable improvement that I witnessed in my office,

I decided to prescribe him zolpidem 10 mg three times a day. He had almost complete resolution of his dystonia for the next 2 to 3 months, although he related to me that the duration of effect became progressively shorter with time. On follow-up 6 months after initially prescribing him zolpidem, his dose of zolpidem had stabilized at 5 mg every 4 hours with good results and with no daytime sleepiness.

THE LESSON

This case highlights the role of serendipity in the discovery of medical breakthroughs. Lubag is poorly responsive to medications, especially when the dystonia becomes multifocal or generalized (1,2). In severe cases of Lubag, pallidal deep brain stimulation may benefit their dystonia and parkinsonism (3). The zolpidem that I had prescribed this patient with Lubag and generalized dystonia was meant to help his insomnia but, unexpectedly, had a tremendous impact on his dystonia. I then proceeded to test zolpidem on other patients with Lubag and confirmed the same results. This led to a publication in 2002 of a series of patients with Lubag whom I had prescribed zolpidem with significant improvement of their dystonia and less impressive improvement of their parkinsonism (4).

Zolpidem's beneficial effect on movement disorders was first discovered in a serendipitous fashion as well. Daniele et al. (5) reported a 61-year-old woman with Parkinson's disease (PD) who received zolpidem for insomnia. After the first 10 mg dose, she showed no drowsiness but had significant improvement of her akinesia and rigidity. She eventually received zolpidem 10 mg four times a day without dopaminergic drugs for 5 years with sufficient relief of her parkinsonism. This case inspired Daniele et al. (5) to conduct a double-blind, placebo-controlled crossover study of zolpidem in 10 patients with PD. Six of the 10 patients showed motor improvement within 45 to 60 minutes after administration, with duration of benefit lasting 2 to 4 hours. Drowsiness was reported by four patients, which was mild to moderate in two and severe in two others. Levodopa-associated dyskinesias in a patient with advanced PD were also reported to improve for around 2 hours with 2.5 to 5 mg dose of zolpidem (6). Daniele et al. (7) also performed a double-blind, placebo-controlled crossover study in 10 patients with probable progressive supranuclear palsy (PSP). They reported not only improvement of motor function in some patients with PSP but also voluntary saccadic eye movements. Side effects were drowsiness and increased postural instability. Farver and Kahn (8) also reported a case of antipsychotic-induced parkinsonism and tremor that improved with zolpidem at a dose of 5 to 10 mg four times a day.

After the initial report of zolpidem on dystonia in patients with Lubag, Garretto et al. further described the beneficial effect of zolpidem in one patient with blepharospasm and two patients with Meige syndrome (9). Improvement was noted within 20 to 30 minutes and was maximal by 1 to 3 hours. Park et al. (10) also described a case of dystonia-myoclonus involving the neck that responded favorably to zolpidem. The patient had near complete resolution of symptoms with 10 mg zolpidem for around 6 hours per dose. Chen et al. (11) reported a patient with advanced PD with severe jaw and neck dystonia who responded markedly to 10 mg zolpidem. With a maintenance dose of 5 mg zolpidem three times a day, the patient exhibited more pronounced and prolonged improvement of dystonia and dyskinesias compared with his parkinsonism.

Zolpidem has also been described to benefit patients with spinocerebellar ataxia (SCA) (12). Clauss et al. described a family of five patients with SCA-2, four of whom had clinical improvement of ataxia, intention tremor, and titubation within an hour after taking 10 mg of zolpidem. All five patients had single photon emission computed tomography with technetium-99m labeling that showed subnormal tracer concentrations in the cerebellum; one had decreased uptake not only in the cerebellum but also in the thalamus, which interestingly normalized after treatment with zolpidem.

The mechanism of action of zolpidem for movement disorders remains speculative. Zolpidem is a short-acting hypnotic gamma-aminobutyric acid (GABA)-ergic drug that is a selective agonist of the benzodiazepine subtype receptor BZ1 (13). The highest density of this receptor in the human brain has been noted autoradiographically in the globus pallidus, ventral thalamic complex, subthalamic nucleus, substantia nigra, and cerebellum (14), which are the same structures that are often pathologically affected in movement disorders. By binding to these sites, zolpidem may perhaps help restore the basal ganglia output influence on the thalamus and motor cortex, leading to improvement of the abnormal movements (15).

In summary, the current case report highlights two things. First, zolpidem can be a pharmacologic option in patients with certain movement disorders, particularly those with dystonia and parkinsonism. Second, the clinician needs to be vigilant in recognizing unintended benefits from medications or medical interventions, because an astute observation even in one patient may lead to important discoveries or medical breakthroughs.

REFERENCES

1. Evidente VG, Advincula J, Esteban R, et al. Phenomenology of "Lubag" or X-linked dystonia-parkinsonism. *Mov Disord.* 2002;6:1271–1277.
2. Evidente VGH. In: Pagon RA, Bird TD, Dolan CR, Stephens K, eds. *GeneReviews* [Internet]. Seattle, WA: University of Washington; 1993–2005. Accessed June 22, 2010.
3. Evidente VG, Lyons MK, Wheeler M, et al. First case of X-lined dystonia-parkinsonism ("Kuba") to demonstrate a response to bilateral pallidal stimulation. *Mov Disord.* 2007;22:1790–1793.
4. Evidente VG. Zolpidem improves dystonia in "Lubag" or X-linked dystonia-parkinsonism syndrome. *Neurology.* 2002;58:662–663.
5. Daniele A, Albanese A, Gainotti G, et al. Zolpidem in Parkinson's disease. *Lancet.* 1997;349:1222–1223.
6. Ruzicka E, Roth J, Jech R, et al. Subhypnotic doses of zolpidem oppose dopaminergic-induced dyskinesia in Parkinson's disease. *Mov Disord.* 2000;15:734–735.
7. Daniele A, Moro E, Bentivoglio AR. Zolpidem in progressive supranuclear palsy. *N Engl J Med.* 1999;341:1632.
8. Farver DK, Khan MH. Zolpidem for antipsychotic-induced parkinsonism. *Ann Pharmacother.* 2001;35:435–437.
9. Garretto NS, Bueri JA, Rey RD, et al. Improvement of blepharospasm with zolpidem. *Mov Disord.* 2004;19:55–70.
10. Park IS, Kim JS, An JY, et al. Excellent response to oral zolpidem in a sporadic case of the myoclonus dystonia syndrome. *Mov Disord.* 2009;24:2172–2173.
11. Chen YY, Sy HN, Wu SL. Zolpidem improves akinesia, dystonia, and dyskinesia in advanced Parkinson's disease. *J Clin Neurosci.* 2008;15:955–956.
12. Clauss R, Sathekge M, Nel W. Transient improvement of spinocerebellar ataxia with zolpidem. *N Engl J Med.* 2004;351:511.
13. Langtry HD, Benfield P. Zolpidem. A review of its pharmacodynamic and pharmacokinetic properties and therapeutic potential. *Drugs.* 1990;40:291–313.
14. Dennis T, Dubois A, Benavides J, et al. Distribution of central omega 1 (benzodiazepine1) and omega2 (benzodiazepine2) receptor subtypes in the monkey and human brain. An autoradiographic study with [3H] flunitrazepam and the omega 1 selective ligand [3H]zolpidem. *J Pharmacol Exp Ther.* 1988;247:309–322.
15. Abe K. Zolpidem therapy for movement disorders. *Recent Pat CNS Drug Discov.* 2008;3:55–60.

69

An Unusual Cause of Cervical Dystonia: Porencephalic Cyst, Putaminal, Pallidal, and Cerebellar Atrophy, Aqueductal Stenosis, and Obstructive Hydrocephalus

MICHELLE FERREIRA AND NÉSTOR GÁLVEZ-JIMÉNEZ

THE CASE

JM was a 41-year-old woman who presented to us on January 23, 1997, with a chief complaint of neck pain and head spasms. She first noticed the pain in 1977, after lifting some heavy boxes, which brought about acute neck pain followed by stiffness. At first, the neck symptoms were not associated with neck muscle spasms. However, they progressed and were associated with contractions that were characterized by a sense of pulling, preferentially toward the back and side of her neck. She began using a soft neck collar, but the pain continued, becoming constant and affecting her ability to initiate sleep. Before coming to our center, she received the diagnosis of torticollis and was treated with diazepam, which provided mild relief to some of her painful symptoms. At the time of first diagnosis, no further neurologic, laboratory, or imaging assessments were made, despite the presence of some atypical features on history and examination.

She was born with congenital aqueductal stenosis, which was undiagnosed until later in life when its course was complicated by hydrocephalus needing a ventriculoperitoneal shunt at 18 years of age, requiring a revision 2 years later. Her neurologic history was further complicated by childhood seizures and behavioral difficulties. Although she required psychological intervention, formal psychiatric care and exposure to mood stabilizers and antipsychotics were not given. At the time of our consultation, she was not taking medications and was on permanent disability.

On examination, she was a woman of average build, quite animated when speaking, but behaving at a level expected for a 10- to 12-year-old child. It was clear she had diminished intelligence with the tendency to use colorful and expletive language. In addition, during mental status and psychiatric testing, she would use childhood metaphors when asked questions about similarities and differences among objects. She would also get easily frustrated with mental tasks.

On neurologic examination, retrocollis was present accompanied by slight rightward chin deviation while sitting in neutral position. The abnormal head and neck movements were most evident when walking, with a slight dystonic tremor superimposed on retrocollis and a mild right shoulder elevation. With synkinetic maneuvers, the torticollis/retrocollis and dystonic tremor worsened. There were areas of muscle tenderness to palpation most notably in the paraspinal muscles bilaterally. However, there was no micrographia, writing, postural, kinetic, or rest tremor noted in the examination. She has a lordotic spastic gait and increased generalized deep tendon reflexes.

THE APPROACH

We were puzzled and concerned by her history of congenital stenosis, status post-ventriculoperitoneal shunt placement, seizures, and intellectual impairment and began a neurologic workup for secondary causes of dystonia. Secondary causes of dystonia, particularly cervical dystonia, should always be entertained, especially when a patient presents with atypical features or diverse historical neurologic background (1). A multitude of disorders of the grey and white matter, basal ganglia, posterior fossa, craniocervical junction defects, and upper cervical cord should be considered, particularly when the neurologic examination demonstrates focal or asymmetric features (see Table 69.1).

We tried the patient on high doses of trihexyphenidyl and clonazepam. However, there were no significant improvements in her movements. We obtained an MRI of her cervical spine, which showed anterior spondylolisthesis of C4 over C3 with resultant diffuse central disc bulge and posterior osteophytosis. We attributed these findings to her chronic cervical dystonia and neck deviation. A brain MRI showed bilateral dilated lateral ventricles with a large area of porencephalic cyst involving the left posterior-dorsal-frontal lobe, dorsolateral medial lobe, and ventral left parietal lobe. The majority of the left temporal lobe, and mesial left temporal lobe, appeared to be in communication with the lateral ventricle. The corpus callosum was stretched and thinned dorsally with a concave appearance. The medial ventral cerebellum was atrophic. The lateral ventricles were stretched, resulting in diminished white matter volume in the centrum semiovale on the right hemisphere, more posterior than anteriorly. A small rim of cortical tissue filled most of the posterior cranium, with ventricular ex-vacuo dilatation, left greater than right, consistent with hydrocephalus. Atrophic changes were present in the left cerebral cortex, most significant in the occipital and posterior-parietal lobes. The third ventricle was markedly

TABLE 69.1
Causes of the So-Called Symptomatic or Secondary Torticollis and Its Mimickers.

o Klippel-Feil syndrome

o Herniated cervical disk

o Atlantoaxial subluxation

o Posterior fossa and spinal cord tumors (glioma, astrocytoma, ependymoma, hemangioblastoma, meningioma, Schwannoma)

o Arnold-Chiari malformation

o Arachnoid cyst

o Multiple sclerosis

o Brainstem, striatal, or cerebellar stroke (hemorrhagic, infarction)

o Arteriovenous malformation and cavernomas

o Labyrinthine disease (particularly in the chronic phases of Meniere's disease and endolymphatic hydrops and/ or during an acute mild to severe attack of vertigo)

o Abscess in the posterior pharynx, soft tissues, and deep neck spaces

o Syringomyelia (in association with other tumors such as glioma and astrocytomas)

o *Drugs*

• Dopaminergic medications (levodopa in mid to late stage Parkinson's disease (drug-induced dystonia/ dyskinesia)

• Stimulants

• Dopamine-blocking agents (typical or atypical neuroleptics)

• Metoclopramide

• Selective serotonin reuptake inhibitors (fluoxetine)

o Cerebellar lesions

o Fourth nerve palsy (head deviation/tilting to correct vertical diplopia)

Modified from Wiener W, Lang AE. *Movement Disorders: A Comprehensive Survey.* Future Publisher, LeDouex, Galvez-Jimenez (unpublished observations) (4–10).

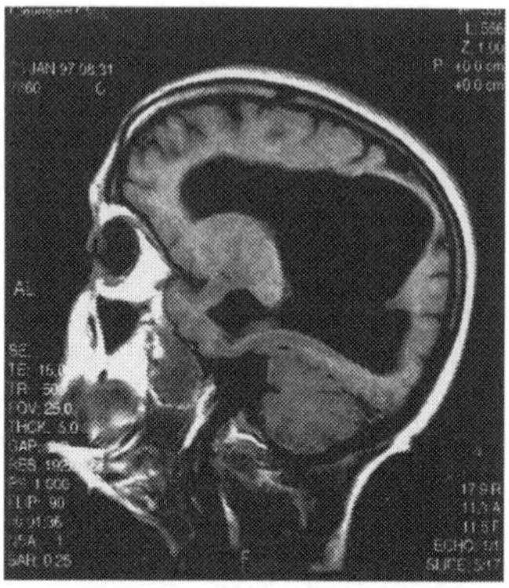

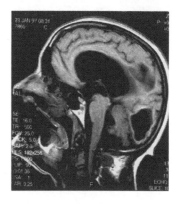

FIGURE 69.1
MRI scan showing dilated lateral ventricles with a large area of porencephalic cyst atrophy of medial cerebellum.

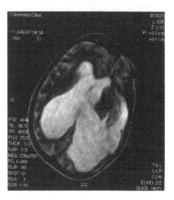

FIGURE 69.2
Thinned corpus callosum and cortical atrophy.

FIGURE 69.3
A large area of porencephalic cyst.

dilated, including the supraoptic, thinned lamina terminalis and infundibular recesses. The aqueduct showed minimal cerebrospinal fluid (CSF) signal, with an apparent normal size fourth ventricle. The posterior porencephalic cyst appeared to be compressing the lateral hemispheres of the cerebellum. As a consequence of the downward expansion of the occipital portion of the porencephalic cyst, the posterior fossa appeared small (see Figures 69.1–69.3).

Because of these findings, particularly with the history of aqueductal stenosis and two prior shunts, we obtained a cisternogram to understand her CSF dynamics. This showed persistent ventricular activity in keeping with communicating hydrocephalus. A revision of the shunt was performed in hopes of relieving some of the presumed increased pressures, particularly in the posterior fossa. Unfortunately, drainage of this cyst through a third ventriculoperitoneal shunt did not improve her symptoms and was associated with postoperative complications, including a subdural hematoma. However, she did get significant symptomatic relief with botulinum toxin therapy.

THE LESSON

Cervical dystonias are characterized by sustained, involuntary, active contractions of cervical muscles resulting in abnormal head movements or postures. The majority of cases are idiopathic or familial. Cervical dystonias as a symptom of other secondary causes are uncommon. Secondary cervical dystonias have been associated with vascular, traumatic, infectious, and toxic processes affecting the central or peripheral nervous systems (see Table 69.1). They have also been associated with heredodegenerative diseases such as Wilson's disease, progressive supranuclear palsy, neuroacanthocytosis, and corticobasal degeneration.

Structural lesions of the central nervous systems have been associated with the presence of cervical dystonias (1–3). A recent case review by LeDoux demonstrated that most lesions associated with cervical dystonia are localized to the brainstem and cerebellum. Nine of the 25 cases (36%) were secondary to cerebellar lesions (4). This patient's cervical dystonia was likely secondary to a combination of factors, including chronic cerebellar compression by a large porencephalic cyst, upstream basal ganglia dysfunction, and alterations in the cortical and white matter fiber tracts.

● Although most cases of cervical dystonia are "idiopathic," familial, or may represent a focal form (*form frustes*) of generalized dystonia, cervical dystonia may be a syndrome or a clinical finding suggesting a structural brain lesion, malformation, or drug exposure.
● Perhaps the most common form of secondary or so-called symptomatic cervical dystonia observed in a busy clinical practice is drug induced (neuroleptics, stimulants, or dopaminergic medications such as levodopa in Parkinson's disease), but as this case clearly demonstrates, a thorough neurologic assessment should be performed when there are atypical features on history, on examination, or when significant comorbidities exist, betraying the presence of an underlying structural lesion(s).
● In some patients, as our example and those of LeDoux and Brady demonstrate, the lesion(s) may be widespread, affecting the whole "motor system" including cortical, subcortical, diencephalic, brainstem, cerebellar, and cord structures. Therefore, the practicing neurologist should be particularly careful in first assuming the cause to be idiopathic when a secondary or structural lesion may be present.

REFERENCES

1. Cammarota A, Gershanik OS, Garcia S, et al. Cervical dystonia due to spinal cord ependymoma: involvement of cervical cord segments in the pathogenesis of dystonia. *Mov Disord*. 1995;10:500–503.
2. Krauss JK, Seeger W, Jankovic J. Cervical dystonia associated with tumors of the posterior fossa. *Mov Disord*. 1997;12:443–447.

3. Molho ES, Factor SA. Basal ganglia infarction as a possible cause of cervical dystonia. *Mov Disord.* 1993;8:213–216.
4. LeDoux MS, Brady KA. Secondary cervical dystonia associated with structural lesions of the central nervous system. *Mov Disord.* 2003;18:60–69.
5. Diler RS, Yolga AY, Avci A. Fluoxetine-induced extrapyramidal symptoms in an adolescent: a case report. *Swiss Med Wkly.* 2002;132:125–126.
6. Fahn S, Bressman SB, Marsden CD. Classification of dystonia. In: Fahn S, Marsden CD, DeLong M, eds. *Dystonia 3. Advances in Neurology,* Vol. 78. Philadelphia, PA: Lippincott-Raven Publishers; 1998:1–10.
7. Kasantikul D, Kanchanatawan B. Antipsychotic-induced tardive movement disorders: a series of twelve cases. *J Med Assoc Thai.* 2007;90:188–194.
8. Okumura K, Ujike H, Akiyama K, et al. BMY-14802 reversed the sigma receptor agonist-induced neck dystonia in rats. *J Neural Transm.* 1996;103:1153–1161.
9. William JW, Anthony EL. *Movement Disorders: A Comprehensive Survey.* Mt. Kisco, NY: Futura Publishing Company, Inc.; 1989:735.
10. Yumru M, Savas HA, Selek S, et al. Acute dystonia after initial doses of ziprasidone: a case report. *Prog Neuropsychopharmacol Biol Psychiatry.* 2006;30:745–747.

VI

Ataxia

70

The ABC of Ataxia Should Also Include the E

HASMET A. HANAGASI AND MURAT EMRE

THE CASE

The patient was a 28-year-old man who had progressive gait ataxia since the age of 16 years. Pregnancy and delivery were normal; his developmental milestones and motor function were normal until the age of 16 years. At this age, motor difficulties began, characterized by unsteadiness, head titubation, and tremor of the hands. Within a year, he developed dysarthria, followed by difficulties with fine finger movements.

He was born to nonconsanguineous parents, and none of the family members had similar complaints. His height and weight were normal; his systemic functions were normal; he had no gastrointestinal symptoms.

On examination, he had bilateral pes cavus and moderate scoliosis. Retinal and fundoscopic examinations were normal. On neurologic examination, he was alert and fully oriented. Speech was dysarthric. The cranial nerves and muscle strength were normal. He had gait and truncal ataxia with intention tremor, head tremor (titubation), dysmetria, dysdiadochokinesia, areflexia at lower limbs, bilateral Babinski sign, absent position and vibration senses in the feet, and positive Romberg's sign. Neuropsychological examination revealed signs of minimal executive dysfunction.

THE APPROACH

Hematologic and biochemical screening, erythrocyte sedimentation rate, protein electrophoresis, urine analysis, levels of organic acids, thyroid and parathyroid function tests, serum levels of vitamin B12, serum levels of vitamin A and vitamin D, serum copper and ceruloplasmin, total copper in 24-hour urine, pyruvate and lactate levels in serum, serum alpha-fetoprotein, analysis of feces, and serologic tests were all normal. Cerebrospinal fluid investigations including oligoclonal bands and serologic tests were unremarkable. Electromyography and nerve conduction velocity studies revealed moderate axonal sensory neuropathy, and the cortical responses of somatosensory-evoked potentials of the medial and tibial nerve stimulation were absent. MRI of the brain showed mild cerebellar atrophy. Spinal cord MRI was normal.

Serum vitamin E concentration was extremely low, <0.10 mg/dL (normal 0.5–1.8 mg/dL). Tests for cholestatic liver disease, fat malabsorption, and abetalipoproteinemia showed no pathologic findings. Vitamin E supplementation up to 900 mg/d resulted in serum vitamin E levels within normal ranges and a moderate improvement in the ataxia, postural tremor, and head tremor over a follow-up period of 3 years. Reflexes remained abolished and posterior column findings unchanged.

THE LESSON

Ataxia with vitamin E deficiency (AVED) is a rare autosomal recessive neurodegenerative disease caused by mutations in the α-tocopherol transfer protein (α-TTP) gene, which is located at chromosome 8q13 (1). Neurologic findings include spinocerebellar degeneration and mild to moderate axonal sensory neuropathy, with clinical features of ataxia, hyporeflexia, dysarthria, and impaired proprioception. Cardiac function (cardiac arrhythmias, cardiomyopathy) and cognition may be affected in later stages; rarely retinitis pigmentosa also occurs. The Friedreich ataxia-like phenotype is the most common clinical presentation.

Patients with AVED have normal gastrointestinal absorption of lipids. Mutations in the α-*TTP* gene lead to a failure of intrahepatocytic incorporation of α-tocopherol in very low-density lipoprotein, resulting in low vitamin E serum concentrations and a subsequent decrease in α-tocopherol transport to neuronal tissue. Neuropathologic studies show loss of Purkinje cells, degeneration of the posterior column, posterior root ganglia, and retina. Different mutations have been reported among various ethnic groups in the world. Most patients with AVED are reported from the Mediterranean region (2).

Supplementation with vitamin E in patients with AVED may improve neurologic symptoms and favorably influence prognosis. Therefore, screening for vitamin E deficiency is important in patients with ataxia of unknown etiology. Genetic analysis and early recognition of AVED may allow early introduction of effective treatment and appropriate genetic counseling.

REFERENCES

1. Mariotti C, Gellera C, Rsimoldi M. Ataxia with isolated vitamin E deficiency: neurological phenotype, clinical follow-up and novel mutations in TTPA gene in Italian families. *Neurol Sci.* 2004;25:130–137.
2. Marzouki N, Benomar A, Yahyaoui M. Vitamin E deficiency ataxia with (744 del A) mutation on alpha-TTP gene: genetic and clinical peculiarities in Moroccan patients. *Eur J Med Genet.* 2005;48:21–28.

71

Speech and Gait Problems in a Patient Being
Treated for Schizophrenia: A Lesson on Psychiatric
Comorbidity From an Afro-Caribbean Man

RUTH H. WALKER

THE CASE

A psychiatrist colleague asked for help with a patient who was currently on the psychiatry ward with psychotic symptoms. The patient was 31 years old at this time and was otherwise in good health with no history of alcohol or drug abuse.

The patient was of Afro-Caribbean ancestry and had developed paranoid, psychotic symptoms at the age of 21. There was no family history of neurologic or psychiatric disease. Although his father did not live nearby and he had not seen him in person for a while, the patient reported that he spoke to him regularly on the telephone and that he sounded well.

The patient had had paranoid symptoms that other people were "out to get him," but prominent delusions were somatic, that his brain was swollen and moved, and "had a sore on it," and that his left eye rolled back in his head. Over the next few years, he was treated with a variety of atypical antipsychotics, with partial control of his psychotic symptoms.

Our patient continued to report somatic symptoms of tightness around the eyes and stiffness in the head, neck, and knees. These complaints were interpreted as being an elaboration of side effects of his neuroleptics. However, despite decreasing doses and trying a variety of antipsychotic medications, the symptoms persisted. The addition of benztropine, to treat presumptively parkinsonian side effects, did not result in significant improvements.

At age 27, the patient reported that he had started to stutter, mainly when he was anxious, which was becoming more frequent. He also reported twitching of the lip and mouth. He felt off balance and clumsy, which interfered with his work in a technical position. His psychiatrist noted that he had oral dyskinesias and slurred speech at this time. His somatic complaints and speech difficulty progressed.

At age 31, he started to complain of dysphagia with solids, dizziness with position change, cramping of his hands and occasional spasms when holding objects, dry mouth, and blurred vision. The treating psychiatrist was concerned about the possibility of motor neuron disease because of involvement of speech and swallowing. When a neurologist colleague examined him, she found that he had mild dysarthria but that the remainder of the neurologic examination, including deep tendon reflexes and motor and sensory examination, was normal and not suggestive of the diagnosis of motor neuron disease. Otolaryngological evaluation at this time revealed a hyperfunctioning larynx, with scissoring of the left arytenoid cartilage.

I first saw him 5 months after this initial neurologic examination, during a psychiatric hospitalization, and noted dysarthric speech, normal eye movements, diminished deep tendon reflexes throughout, mild distal vibration loss, and mild gait ataxia. Limb movements showed somewhat mild but slightly more prominent ataxia.

When I examined the patient for the second time 6 months later, it was clear that there had been a progression of his neurologic disease. He had experienced a marked decline in cognitive function. He had now developed mild generalized chorea; his cerebellar findings still mild but more pronounced, with a more ataxic gait; inability to perform tandem gait; and clumsiness on repetitive movements. His voice was noted to be tight and choppy, suggestive of adductor spasmodic dysphonia. Eye movements were still normal. He had completely lost his deep tendon reflexes, and his sensory loss was more severe with diminished joint position and vibration sense in the toes and fingers bilaterally. Neuropsychological testing revealed significant impairments in some, but not all, domains and were interpreted as indicating subcortical rather than cortical dementia.

MRI showed minimal bilateral periventricular and subcortical high-signal white matter changes, most consistent with chronic microvascular ischemic changes, and moderate bilateral cerebellar atrophy; the pons seemed to be slightly symmetrically reduced in size.

Electromyography was normal except for absent H reflexes.

Modified barium swallow showed mild spasms at the distal esophagus, and laryngoscopy showed cricopharyngeal spasm and dystonia (spasmodic dysphonia).

THE APPROACH

The combination of longstanding psychiatric disease with a more recent development of neurologic signs and symptoms made it critical to exclude Wilson's disease as a treatable etiology. Normal liver enzymes made this diagnosis less likely, as did the absence of Kayser-Fleischer rings, but it was completely excluded by normal ceruloplasmin levels and normal 24-hour urinary copper excretion.

The patient's young age made a paraneoplastic syndrome less likely but was important to exclude as a potentially reversible cause of a cerebellar syndrome of subacute duration. Serum was sent for anti-Ri, anti-Hu, and antineuronal nuclear antibodies, which were all normal. A subacute cerebellar presentation may also be consistent with Creutzfeldt-Jakob disease; however, cerebrospinal fluid (CSF) was negative for 14-3-3 protein, and other CSF parameters were normal. Electroencephalography showed mild, diffuse slowing.

With the time course of slow progression over several years, we considered other neurodegenerative disorders. One direction was to evaluate for those affecting the cerebellum, as indicated by the brain MRI and clinical examination. However, if we considered his psychiatric symptoms to be part of the same disease process as his neurologic disease, this directed us more toward the basal ganglia as a cause of psychiatric disease and hyperkinetic movements.

Despite the absence of apparent family history, we considered autosomal dominant disorders, because anticipation might result in later onset in the parent. Testing for Huntington's disease was negative (14/19 CAG repeats). Huntington's disease–like 2 would also have been a consideration given his African ancestry.

Neuroacanthocytosis syndromes (autosomal recessive chorea-acanthocytosis and X-linked McLeod syndrome) can present in adulthood with psychiatric symptoms followed by hyperkinetic movements and peripheral neuropathy. Although we did not pursue definitive testing, both of these diagnoses were much less likely in the presence of a normal peripheral blood smear and normal liver enzymes and creatine kinase. Clear cerebellar findings were also inconsistent with these diagnoses.

Making the alternative assumption that psychiatric disease was not primarily related to our patient's neurologic complaints led us to focus on the inherited cerebellar disorders. In the absence of family history, autosomal recessive disorders were considered more likely. The most likely of these to have adult onset was Friedreich's ataxia (others might include ataxia telangiectasia and ataxia with oculomotor apraxia types I and II). Although onset is usually in childhood, Friedreich's ataxia may occasionally present in adulthood, when the GAA trinucleotide repeat expansion is at the lower end of the pathologic range. However, the results of genetic testing in our patient did not indicate this diagnosis.

Bassen-Kornzweig syndrome, in which acanthocytes can be seen, along with cerebellar findings and peripheral neuropathy, is an autosomal recessive disorder that usually presents in childhood. Steatorrhea is typical due to malabsorption of lipids from the gut and was not observed in our patient. Normal levels of apolipoprotein B excluded this diagnosis.

The clinical examination did not permit us to narrow down the differential diagnosis with respect to a possible autosomal dominantly inherited spinocerebellar ataxia (SCA), because our patient had truncal and limb ataxia, but normal eye movements, in addition to peripheral neuropathy. The presence of a movement disorder suggested SCA3 (Machado-Joseph disease; the most common etiology in North American populations) or SCA1; we also could not exclude SCA2 or SCA6.

We obtained a panel of genetic tests, including SCA1, 2, 3, and 6. SCA1 showed 26/30 repeats (normal <34); SCA6 showed 11/11 repeats (normal <18); SCA3 showed 23/29 repeats (normal 12–40). Finally, SCA2 testing showed 22 CAG repeats on one allele and 41 on the other (upper limit of normal = 31!).

The patient's chorea has remained mild and variable and has not been problematic for him. He underwent injections of botulinum toxin to the vocal cords with improvement in the choppiness of his speech. His ataxia is slowly progressing, but he remains ambulatory and independent in all activities of daily living. Fortunately, after much urging and several near misses, he decided to give up driving. His paranoid ideation remains predominantly resistant to treatment.

THE LESSON

The relationship between this young man's psychiatric disease and his neurodegenerative condition is unclear. Psychosis is not typical of the SCAs in general, although other psychiatric and cognitive problems are reported (1,2). It is tempting to hypothesize that the hyperkinetic movements observed in the form of chorea and dystonia were due to involvement of the caudate-putamen, and that the psychosis was an early manifestation of this; however, the time interval of 10 years to neurologic presentation may argue against this. However, it is more likely that this young man suffered from one common psychiatric disease and one rare neurodegenerative disorder.

The more important point brought out by this case is that neurologic symptoms were reported by the patient and were dismissed for many years as being side effects of medication. It remains unknown whether his early complaints, attributed to psychosis, were his interpretations of somatic symptoms caused by SCA2. Serial neurologic examinations clearly demonstrated progression of neurologic findings.

Schizophrenia is a common illness, and the medications used to treat it frequently have side effects. Although the newer atypical neuroleptics have less dopamine receptor-blocking actions, both parkinsonism and tardive hyperkinetic movement disorders can be seen. I suspect that our patient's reports of stiffness, clumsiness, and unsteadiness were all related to his cerebellar disease. Psychiatrists need to be particularly alert to the presence of atypical neurologic signs and symptoms and to unusual progression of any psychiatric illness.

REFERENCES

1. Brandt J, Leroi I, O'Hearn E, et al. Cognitive impairments in cerebellar degeneration: a comparison with Huntington's disease. *J Neuropsychiatry Clin Neurosci.* 2004;16:176–184.
2. Liszewski CM, O'Hearn E, Leroi I, et al. Cognitive impairment and psychiatric symptoms in 133 patients with diseases associated with cerebellar degeneration. *J Neuropsychiatry Clin Neurosci.* 2004;16:109–112.

Suggested Reading
Durr A. Autosomal dominant cerebellar ataxias: polyglutamine expansions and beyond. *Lancet Neurol.* 2010; 9:885–894.

72

How Wiggling Movements in a 13-Year-Old Girl Helped Diagnose a Longstanding Ataxia

DAVID SALAT AND OKSANA SUCHOWERSKY

A 13-year-old girl was referred to the movement disorders clinic for the assessment of long-standing ataxia.

The patient had been born at full term, after an uneventful pregnancy, through cesarean section performed for suspected fetal distress. She had required oxygen supplementation for several days, but initially, she did not seem to have sequelae. Her parents became concerned when she was not walking by the age of 18 months. Pediatric neurologic consultation at 22 months found truncal ataxia. Despite comprehensive evaluation, congenital and acquired causes were not found, and no definite diagnosis was reached.

Over the following years, additional mild neurologic features were found, including slight speech delay (although her overall cognitive development was believed to be appropriate), hypotonia, fidgetiness, and abnormal inward posturing of her feet when walking. On general examination, she was consistently found to be below the 10th percentile for height and weight. Significant delay of her gross motor development was noted, but all significant milestones were eventually met: she was able to walk independently at the age of 3 and run at 7, and she was able to participate in sports by the age of 11. Nevertheless, she was somewhat "clumsy" and continued to fall occasionally. Her only limitation in school was that she required a longer time than her peers to write. A trial of levodopa was recommended at the age of 11. The drug transiently improved the dystonic foot posturing but was discontinued because of loss of benefit.

Aside from recurrent urinary tract infections (which led to a diagnosis of spastic neurogenic bladder and transient treatment with oxybutinin), her medical history was unremarkable. On review of family history, her father had been diagnosed with essential tremor, but no other member had neurologic problems.

When seen in the movement disorders clinic, her height and weight were below the fifth percentile when adjusted for age and sex. No dysmorphic features, skin lesions, and abnormal findings in the cardiopulmonary and abdominal examinations were identified. She was alert, oriented, and cooperative throughout the neurologic examination. Cranial nerve, motor, and sensory examinations were normal. She was mildly hypotonic. No dysmetria or abnormalities on rapid alternating movements were noticed in her arms. Her reflexes were 2/4 throughout and plantar responses downgoing. When asked to hold her arms outstretched, continuous low-amplitude, involuntary, nonsuppressible, and nonaction-induced movements (believed to be most consistent with chorea) were noticed in her fingers. Motor impersistence was not apparent. While seated, her trunk constantly moved in a rather unpredictable manner, but when she stood, her posture was normal. Gait was unsteady and wide based, and she was unable to walk heel-to-toe. Slight inversion of both feet was noted during ambulation.

THE APPROACH

The patient's clinical picture is that of a nonprogressive childhood-onset movement disorder, including truncal ataxia, hypotonia, chorea, task-specific foot dystonia, no cognitive abnormalities or systemic symptoms, and a negative family history.

The earliest and most prominent symptoms in this case were related to gait and coordination. Investigations during her childhood included brain MRI, which had showed an empty sella turcica but no structural abnormalities, and blood tests (complete blood count and basic chemistry and thyroid function testing), which disclosed only a slightly increased thyroid-stimulating hormone (TSH) with T4 within the normal range (subclinical hypothyroidism). Neuroacanthocytosis, spinocerebellar ataxias (SCA) 1, 2, 3, 6, 7, and 8, Wilson's disease, Friedreich's ataxia, ataxia-telangiectasia, lysosomal and amino acid disorders, and accumulation of paramagnetic materials in the basal ganglia had all been ruled out. Both the empty sella turcica and the thyroid function abnormality were considered to be not significant, and we arrived at the working diagnosis of static encephalopathy causing truncal ataxia.

On careful examination in our clinic, however, we felt that her chorea was a significant part of her symptom complex. As a result, the differential diagnosis of the patient's condition was expanded (1,2).

On clinical grounds alone, the nonprogressive course and the lack of systemic involvement made the diagnosis of any of the secondary causes of chorea (including systemic lupus erythematosus, the antiphospholipid syndrome, Sydenham's chorea, encephalitis, and AIDS) unlikely. Finally, there was no history of exposure to any of the drugs known to potentially lead to the development of chorea.

With respect to primary diseases characterized by chorea, the nonprogressive course and the lack of cognitive impairment argued against both a diagnosis of Huntington's disease (HD) and dentatorubral-pallidoluysian atrophy (DRPLA). Childhood-onset HD is uncommon (<2% of cases) and manifests as a parkinsonian syndrome ("Westphal variant") with seizures; neuroimaging may disclose signal abnormalities in the putamen and caudate early in the disease course. DRPLA is most often found among patients of Asian descent, manifesting predominantly as a myoclonic epilepsy, and is accompanied by diffuse atrophy and white matter changes on neuroimaging. The symptoms were not episodic, and there was no evidence of consistent triggers; therefore, the paroxysmal dyskinesias (3) were also felt to be an unlikely diagnosis.

Given the gradual, albeit delayed, meeting of motor milestones over childhood, the clinical picture, despite the negative family history, was most suggestive of benign hereditary chorea (BHC) (4), an autosomal dominant disease with an estimated prevalence of around two cases per million.

Genetic testing of the patient disclosed a large deletion involving all three exons of the thyroid transcription factor 1 (*TITF-1*) gene on the long arm of chromosome 14 (14q13) (5). Genetic testing was also performed in the patient's parents, and they were shown not to harbor the mutation. Although the possibility of a falsely attributed fatherhood could not be completely excluded, the case was assumed to represent a "de novo" mutation. Although accurate data on the frequency of de novo mutations are unknown, Krude et al. (6) found it to be the case in two of their five (40%) study subjects.

The diagnosis of BHC was originally restricted to patients presenting with isolated nonprogressive chorea and a positive family history with autosomal dominant mode of inheritance. After genetic testing became widely available, this entity was placed within the spectrum of *TITF-1* mutations. In addition to the "classical BHC" phenotype, it is now recognized that patients can have a variety of other neurologic abnormalities, such as ataxia, hypotonia, intention tremor, sensorineural deafness, seizures, developmental delay (with eventual acquirement of the relevant milestones during childhood), and even mental retardation. Non-neurologic features, which are associated with larger deletions, include hypothyroidism and pulmonary abnormalities [the so-called brain-thyroid-lung syndrome (6)], hypospadias, psychosis, and short stature. In our case, the subclinical hypothyroidism and the fidgetiness (which had been described as tics, myoclonus, or chorea in different consultations) had been discarded as important diagnostic clues.

The short stature was finally attributed to growth hormone (GH) deficiency, possibly in relation with the empty sella turcica. A recent description of an Italian family with BHC (7) reported a higher than expected incidence of empty sella turcica, and the authors postulated the involvement of *TITF-1* in the proper development of the sellar diaphragm. Previous reports of short stature in the context of BHC had not ascribed it to GH deficiency, but given the possible relation of *TITF-1* mutations to development of empty sella turcica and the fact that this condition is frequently associated with GH deficiency, we considered the hormonal deficiency as a nonneurologic constituent of this patient's phenotype.

THE LESSON

Reaching a diagnosis of BHC allowed us to inform the patient and her parents about the expected clinical course, which has contributed markedly toward their emotional well-being. In addition, the identification of the mutation will enable genetic counselling, if requested, when the patient becomes pregnant.

Although the typical course of the disease includes little or no progression, and most patients have no impairment in activities of daily living by adulthood, worsening of symptoms up to the age of 20 years is occasionally seen. Information on appropriate pharmacologic management in the medical literature is limited to a report on the beneficial effect of levodopa on two patients who were safely treated with a dose of up to 20 mg/kg/d and experienced improvement in both their gait and choreic movements within 6 weeks (8).

BHC should be included in the differential diagnosis of nonprogressive movement disorders with onset in childhood, even if chorea is not prominent and family history is negative.

REFERENCES

1. Gilbert DL. Acute and chronic chorea in childhood. *Semin Pediatr Neurol.* 2009;16:71–76.
2. Mathews KD. Hereditary causes of chorea in childhood. *Semin Pediatr Neurol.* 2003;10:20–25.
3. van Rootselaar AF, van Westrum SS, Velis DN, et al. The paroxysmal dyskinesias. *Pract Neurol.* 2009; 9:102–109.
4. Kleiner-Fisman G, Lang AE. Benign hereditary chorea revisited: a journey to understanding. *Mov Disord.* 2007;22:2297–2305.
5. Breedveld GJ, van Dongen JW, Danesino C, et al. Mutations in TITF-1 are associated with benign hereditary chorea. *Hum Mol Genet.* 2002;11:971–979.
6. Krude H, Schütz B, Biebermann H, et al. Choreoathetosis, hypothyroidism, and pulmonary alterations due to human NKX2–1 haploinsufficiency. *J Clin Invest.* 2002;109:475–480.
7. Salvatore E, Di Maio L, Filla A, et al. Benign hereditary chorea: clinical and neuroimaging features in an Italian family. *Mov Disord.* 2010;25:1491–1496.
8. Asmus F, Horber V, Pohlenz J, et al. A novel TITF-1 mutation causes benign hereditary chorea with response to levodopa. *Neurology.* 2005;64:1952–1954.

Suggested Reading

Kleiner-Fisman G, Rogaeva E, Halliday W, et al. Benign hereditary chorea: clinical, genetic, and pathological findings. *Ann Neurol.* 2003;54:244–247.
Mahajnah M, Inbar D, Steinmetz A, et al. Benign hereditary chorea: clinical, neuroimaging, and genetic findings. *J Child Neurol.* 2007;22:1231–1234.
Asmus F, Devlin A, Munz M, et al. Clinical differentiation of genetically proven benign hereditary chorea and myoclonus-dystonia. *Mov Disord.* 2007;22:2104–2109.
Willemsen MA, Breedveld GJ, Wouda S, et al. Brain-thyroid-lung syndrome: a patient with a severe multisystem disorder due to a de novo mutation in the thyroid transcription factor 1 gene. *Eur J Pediatr.* 2005;164:28–30.

Moya CM, Perez de Nanclares G, Castaño L, et al. Functional study of a novel single deletion in the TITF1/NKX2.1 homeobox gene that produces congenital hypothyroidism and benign chorea but not pulmonary distress. *J Clin Endocrinol Metab.* 2006;91:1832–1841.

Devos D, Vuillaume I, de Becdelievre A, et al. New syndromic form of benign hereditary chorea is associated with a deletion of TITF-1 and PAX-9 contiguous genes. *Mov Disord.* 2006;21:2237–2240.

Provenzano C, Veneziano L, Appleton R, et al. Functional characterization of a novel mutation in TITF-1 in a patient with benign hereditary chorea. *J Neurol Sci.* 2008;264:56–62.

Glik A, Vuillaume I, Devos D, et al. Psychosis, short stature in benign hereditary chorea: a novel thyroid transcription factor-1 mutation. *Mov Disord.* 2008;23:1744–1747.

Ferrara AM, De Michele G, Salvatore E, et al. A novel NKX2.1 mutation in a family with hypothyroidism and benign hereditary chorea. *Thyroid.* 2008;18:1005–1009.

Kleiner-Fisman G, Calingasan NY, Putt M, et al. Alterations of striatal neurons in benign hereditary chorea. *Mov Disord.* 2005;20:1353–1357.

Maccabelli G, Pichiecchio A, Guala A, et al. Advanced magnetic resonance imaging in benign hereditary chorea: study of two familial cases. *Mov Disord.* 2010;25:2670–2674.

Acquired Cerebellar Ataxia Associated With Glutamic Acid Decarboxylase in a 52-Year-Old Brazilian Woman

HÉLIO A.G. TEIVE

THE CASE

A 52-year-old female patient, who presented initially with diplopia, had difficulty walking and had progressively worsening balance, with a marked deterioration over 20 days. The patient had an ophthalmologic assessment, which proved inconclusive, and was referred for neurologic assessment in her hometown. Neurologic examination revealed gait ataxia, difficulty with tandem gait, and the presence of horizontal gaze-evoked nystagmus. The patient was on thyroid hormone replacement therapy (100 mcg/d). Further investigation revealed normal routine blood tests except for an erythrocyte sedimentation rate (ESR) of 60. Brain neuroimaging (computed tomography [CT] and MRI) was normal. Cerebrospinal fluid (CSF) examination revealed the presence of 16 cells (100% lymphomononuclear) without other abnormalities. Over time, the patient complained of nausea and vomiting and used an antiemetic (metoclopramide), dimenhydrinate, and clonazepam. Viral cerebellitis was suspected. She later presented with a clinical picture of urinary infection, which subsequently improved with norfloxacin. The clinical picture of ataxia remained unchanged, and 30 days later, the patient presented with a generalized tonic-clonic seizure while asleep, which recurred the following day. The patient was hospitalized, and phenytoin was administered intravenously. Neurological examination demonstrated cerebellar ataxia with nystagmus and diplopia. The repeat brain MRI was normal. Phenytoin was replaced by lamotrigine at a daily dose of 200 mg, and methylprednisolone pulse therapy (1 g/d for 5 days) was started. At the end of the 5 days, this was substituted by prednisone (40 mg/d). New CSF tests were normal. A further detailed investigation, including tests for vasculitis, screening for an occult neoplasm, and screening for infections (serologic tests to detect antibodies against HIV, Epstein-Barr, varicella-zoster, and herpes simplex viruses) and Hu, Ri, and Yo antibodies, was normal. The electroencephalogram was also normal.

THE APPROACH

Because the patient's clinical picture deteriorated, she was referred for specialist assessment in Curitiba, Paraná, Brazil. At this time, she continued to complain of dizziness, imbalance, and diplopia, and the neurologic examination revealed marked gait ataxia (she could not perform tandem gait unsupported) with horizontal and vertical gaze-evoked nystagmus and slight dysarthria.

Because autoimmune cerebellar ataxia was suspected, further investigations were again performed, including routine blood chemistry, Venereal Disease Research Laboratory (VDRL), complete blood count, coagulogram, ESR, hepatic function, thyroid tests, anti-DNA tests, and a new MRI and CSF examination in addition to measurement of antigliadin, antithyroglobulin, and antiperoxidase antibodies, all of which were normal. Anti–glutamic acid decarboxylase (GAD) level was 39 IU/mL (normal value <1.0 IU/mL).

Given a diagnosis of cerebellar ataxia and epileptic seizures associated with anti-GAD antibodies, the patient underwent intravenous immunoglobulin treatment (4 g/kg) for 5 days followed by a single monthly intravenous dose (for 12 months) and subsequently used aza-thioprine orally (2 mg/kg/d). There was a gradual improvement in the clinical picture, and 1 year after the start of the specific treatment, neurologic examination showed only mild gait ataxia (more apparent in tandem gait) and the presence of mild horizontal nystagmus on both extreme gazes. Lamotrigine (200 mg/d) orally and clonazepam (1.0 mg/night) were continued; complete blood count and hepatic function were normal, and azathioprine was discontinued.

THE LESSON

Ataxia associated with GAD autoantibodies is a very rare condition and is considered to be a component of a polyglandular autoimmune syndrome in patients with circulating GAD antibod-ies. Most patients with ataxia and anti-GAD antibodies are women and have insulin-dependent diabetes mellitus. In general, there is a slowly progressive pancerebellar syndrome, and cerebel-lar atrophy is sometimes found in MRI examinations (1).

Anti-GAD syndrome includes stiff person syndrome (SPS), which is characterized by stiff-ness that is prominent in axial muscles together with sudden episodic spasms, and its variants, such as stiff trunk syndrome, stiff limb syndrome (stiff leg syndrome, stiff three-limb syndrome), progressive encephalomyelitis with rigidity, and SPS-plus, and epilepsy and ataxia with the pres-ence of anti-GAD antibodies (2–4). Anti-GAD syndrome is often found in association with other autoimmune disorders such as diabetes and those caused by antithyroid, antinuclear, and antiparietal cell autoantibodies (3,4). Anti-GAD antibodies are considered a serologic marker of the disease. Purkinje cells are very sensitive to and affected by anti-GAD antibodies, and this in turn may affect cerebellar GABAergic transmission (1–3).

Cerebellar ataxia with anti-GAD antibodies may respond to intravenous immunoglobu-lins or plasma exchanges. Other immunotherapies can be used, but the results are contro-versial (4,5).

REFERENCES

1. Klockgether T. Acquired cerebellar ataxias and differential diagnosis. In: Brice A, Pulst SM, eds. *Spinocerebellar Degenerations. The Ataxias and Spastic Paraplegias.* Philadelphia, PA: Butterworth Heinemann Elsevier; 2007:61–77.
2. Vasconcelos OM, Dalakas MC. Stiff-person syndrome. *Curr Treat Options Neurol.* 2003;5:79–90.
3. Barker RA, Revesz T, Thom M, et al. Review of 23 patients affected by the stiff man syndrome: clinical subdivision into stiff trunk (man) syndrome, stiff limb syndrome, and progressive encephalomyelitis with rigidity. *J Neurol Neurosurg Psychiatry.* 1998;65:633–640.
4. Vulliemoz S, Vanini G, Truffert A, et al. Epilepsy and cerebellar ataxia associated with anti-glutamic acid decarboxylase antibodies. *J Neurol Neurosurg Psychiatry.* 2007;78:187–189.
5. Dalakas MC. The role of IVIg in the treatment of patients with stiff person syndrome and other neurologi-cal diseases associated with anti-GAD antibodies. *J Neurol.* 2005;252(Suppl 1):19–25.

Suggested Reading
Manto MU. Immune diseases. In: Manto MU, ed. *Cerebellar Disorders. A Practical Approach to Diagnosis and Management.* Cambridge, UK: Cambridge University Press; 2010:102–112.
Pittock SJ, Yoshikawa H, Ahlskog E, et al. Glutamic acid decarboxylase autoimmunity with brainstem, extra-pyramidal, and spinal cord dysfunction. *Mayo Clin Proc.* 2006;81: 1207–1214.

74

Ataxia With Oculomotor Apraxia Type 2 in a 58-Year-Old Computer Programmer Without Oculomotor Apraxia

FRANCES M. VELEZ-LAGO AND S.H. SUBRAMONY

THE CASE

A 58-year-old, right-handed man presented with a history of ataxia "all of his life." He was born prematurely but attained his milestones in a normal fashion and seemed to be doing well for the first 10 years. During middle school and high school, he was able to play non-competitive sports such as baseball, basketball, and football. He was clumsy as a kid and as a teenager. Then, he gradually began having increasing walking difficulties, and by age 27, he was wheelchair bound and has been for the past 31 years. He also developed dysarthria. He has had a gradual decline in his functions and is to the point where he is barely able to transfer himself. He had significant wasting and sensory loss of his distal upper and lower extremities. His speech was dysarthric but intelligible, and he did not complain of any visual difficulties such as diplopia, oscillopsia, visual loss, or night blindness. There was no history of cognitive dysfunction or dysphagia. He had some urinary urgency but no other significant sphincter complaints.

He is a retired computer programmer. He had to quit his job when he could no longer use the keyboard. Recently, he was diagnosed with hypothyroidism for which he takes low doses of thyroxine. There is a history of glycosuria without hyperglycemia. He has no history of heart or lung disease. He also denied any history of gastrointestinal illnesses or liver disease. There was no history of cancer or prostate hypertrophy. He denied any alcohol or tobacco use.

Both of his parents are alive; both are in their early 100s. They have no ataxic difficulties. He has three sisters, none of whom have any ataxic difficulties. He had no children.

Our examination revealed an alert and oriented man. General examination was unremarkable, except for a mild curvature of his thoracic spine and few subcutaneous soft nodules in the back. There were no other neurocutaneous stigmata. Neurologic examination was remarkable for prominent saccadic intrusions in ocular pursuit. There was high-amplitude nystagmus, particularly on left lateral gaze. Saccades were normal with normal velocity, but accuracy was diminished. Hearing was mildly decreased to finger rub. Motor examination revealed severe atrophy in the intrinsic hand muscles and in the distal forearm. He had severe, symmetric atrophy in both legs below the knees and in distal thigh muscles. Occasional fasciculations over the thighs were observed on both legs. Wrist extensors and flexors were 4/5 bilaterally, and intrinsic hand muscles were 0 to 1/5; otherwise, strength in the proximal arms was normal. In the legs, iliopsoas and hamstrings were 3 to 4/5, and distal leg muscles, including the gastrocnemius, tibialis anterior, and intrinsic foot muscles, were 0/5. He was areflexic. Sensory examination revealed a profound loss of touch extending to above the knees in both legs and above the wrist in both hands. Vibration in legs was impaired all the way up to the knees and to the elbows in the arms; proprioception was affected in both arms and legs. No dystonia or extrapyramidal features were observed. He had evident finger-to-nose abnormalities with significant tremor and dysmetria. Rapid alternating movements were decomposed. Heel-shin testing was not performed. He was unable to stand up by himself.

THE APPROACH

He had seen numerous physicians in the past and had testing, including brain and cervical spine MRIs and electromyography (EMG) and nerve conduction studies (NCS), more than 5 years ago. His cervical spine MRI showed no spinal cord atrophy, but there seemed to be some atrophy of the cerebellum in the midline. He had genetic testing for Friedrich's ataxia and spinocerebellar ataxia type 1 (SCA1), both of which were negative. This man had a slowly progressive ataxia with sensorimotor neuropathy that seemed consistent with an autosomal recessive ataxia because of its age at onset. Initial differential diagnosis included ataxia with oculomotor apraxia (AOA), POLG gene mutation, or a mitochondrial mutation. Initial blood work requested included lactate and pyruvate levels, copper, ceruloplasmin, very long-chain fatty acids, and serum alpha-fetoprotein (AFP). On subsequent follow-up, the blood work showed normal copper and ceruloplasmin levels and normal long-chain fatty acids, pyruvate, and lactate in plasma. Phytanic acid and hexosaminidase A were also normal. He had increased levels of AFP in the serum at 33.1 ng/mL (normal 0.0–8.7 ng/mL). In view of this latter finding, genetic testing to look for mutations in the Senataxin (*SETX*) gene was requested. The genetic panel revealed that he possessed a mutation in the *SETX* gene, confirming a diagnosis of AOA type 2 (AOA2).

THE LESSON

Recessive ataxias with severe sensory-motor neuropathy include those related to AOA and mitochondrial mutation. A predominantly sensory neuropathy is seen in Friedreich ataxia and ataxia with vitamin E deficiency. Our patient with AOA2 shows some classic features of this disease such as slowly progressive ataxia with an early age of onset and a severe sensorimotor neuropathy with profound sensory loss and muscle weakness. However, he lacked significant oculomotor abnormalities such as oculomotor apraxia! This characteristic eye movement abnormality characterized by poor ability to initiate saccades has been associated with three different ataxic diseases: ataxia telangiectasia, AOA1, and AOA2 (1). All of these seem to involve genes involved in DNA break repair mechanisms (1). The clinical characteristics of AOA2 include young age of onset (usually between ages 3 and 30 years), cerebellar ataxia, slow progression, areflexia and a peripheral axonal sensorimotor neuropathy (>90%), and oculomotor apraxia (51%) and pyramidal features (20.5%), and less commonly dystonia, chorea, or strabismus (1,2). Oculomotor apraxia has been defined as dissociation of eye-head movement where the head reaches the lateral target before the eyes (2). In AOA2, there is a lack of cardiac involvement, predisposition to cancer or immunodeficiency, and rare or absent telangiectasia (2). Other common findings in AOA2 include cerebellar atrophy on MRI, increased levels of AFP, and, less commonly, increased levels of creatine kinase (CK). The combination of ataxia, neuropathy, and increased AFP makes AOA2 highly likely even in the absence of "oculomotor apraxia." The defective gene in AOA2 is Senataxin mapped at 9q34, by Moreira et al., and encodes a large protein, senataxin (SETX), which shows homology to the helicase domain suggestive that this protein is involved in nucleic acid processing (RNA transcription and regulation), DNA repair, and telomere stability (3). Managing a patient with AOA2 can be challenging, and a multidisciplinary approach is recommended. Many patients are wheelchair bound by age 30. As the disease progresses, they may need speech recognition computers and special keyboards to compensate for difficulties in reading (secondary to the oculomotor apraxia) and for typing (secondary to the ataxia) to communicate.

REFERENCES

1. Anheim M, Monga B, Fleury M, et al. Ataxia with oculomotor apraxia type 2: clinical, biological and genotype/phenotype correlation study of a cohort of 90 patients. *Brain.* 2009;132:2688–2698.

2. Moreira MC, Koenig M. Ataxia with oculomotor apraxia type 2. *GeneReviews* [Internet]. Seattle, WA: University of Washington; 1993–2004. Accessed March 24, 2009.
3. De Amicis A, Piane M, Ferrari F, et al. Role of senataxin in DNA damage and telomeric stability. *DNA Repair.* 2010: doi:10.1016/jdnarep.2010.10.012.

Suggested Reading

Aicardi J, Barbosa C, Andermann E, et al. Ataxia-ocular motor apraxia: a syndrome mimicking ataxia telangiectasia. *Ann Neurol.* 1988;24:497–502.
Gazulla J, Benavente I, Lopez-Fraile IP, et al. Sensory neuronopathy in ataxia with oculomotor apraxia type 2. *J Neurol Sci.* 2010;298:118–120.
Gazulla J, Benavente I, Lopez-Fraile IP, et al. Sensorimotor neuronopathy in ataxia with oculomotor apraxia type 2. *Muscle Nerve.* 2009;40:481–485.
Moreira MC, Klur S, Watanabe M, et al. Senataxin, the ortholog of a yeast RNA helicase, is mutant in ataxia-ocular apraxia 2. *Nat Genet.* 2004;36:225–227.

75

A Patient With a Progressive Ataxia and Brain Iron Accumulation

ELISABETH WOLF AND WERNER POEWE

THE CASE

This 47-year-old gentleman was referred to the neurology department of Innsbruck Medical University because of a history of unexplained progressive worsening of a pre-existing gait disorder. At age 23, he had sustained a severe head injury in a car accident, and after a long period of rehabilitation therapy, he was eventually left with a moderate residual left-sided spastic hemiparesis. He was able to walk unaided, and his left arm was held in a fixed flexed posture with some residual movements of the fingers. There was no ataxia or other movement disorder, and his cognition remained largely intact. The patient was able to re-enter his professional career as a carpenter, however, with some limitation to the scope of his activity and performance. At the time of hospital treatment for his head injury, diabetes mellitus (DM) had been first diagnosed, and he had been put on insulin treatment.

Twenty years later, at age 43, he began to notice new gait difficulties: he became unsteady and started to have regular falls. In addition, his speech became slurred, and he complained of clumsiness of his previously unaffected right hand. These symptoms progressed over the following 3 years, and he became eventually unable to continue working in his profession. He presented to our department at the age of 46. At the time of admission, there was slight to moderate hypomimia, his speech was slurred, and there was some abnormality of eye movements with saccadic hypometria in the horizontal and vertical plane. Further findings included left-sided spastic hemiparesis with fixed flexion dystonia of his arm at the elbow and dystonic finger flexion. He was unable to lift up the paretic arm but could actively open his hand. There was dysmetria and intention tremor when performing finger-to-nose testing with his right arm and alternating hand movements were slow and reduced in amplitude. His gait was severely impaired by a combination of left-sided spastic paresis and marked truncal ataxia; he was still able to walk unaided.

His medical history included reports of unexplained anemia, and his family history revealed that one of his sisters, aged 38, also suffered from DM since age 11 and a second sister, aged 36, developed chronic iron deficiency after the birth of her only child. His two other brothers aged 42 and 47 and his 75-year-old mother were reported to be well. His father had died of colon cancer at the age of 65 years.

THE APPROACH

This is a 46-year-old patient who experienced newly progressive gait problems against the background of a pre-existing post-traumatic left-sided spastic hemiparesis, which had been stable for approximately 20 years. He now presented with progressive ataxia gait with falling, right-hand dysmetria and incoordination, dysarthria, and oculomotor abnormalities consistent with a cerebellar syndrome. On the other hand, there was no indication that his previous focal deficit had deteriorated, suggesting a new-onset condition. To rule out structural pathology in the cerebellum, a brain MRI examination was included in his initial workup. This revealed cerebellar atrophy and on MRI T2 sequences images showed marked hypointensities bilaterally in the putamen, GPi, caudate nuclei, thalamus, and dentate nuclei, suggestive of brain iron deposition (1).

Given this patient's history of DM since age 23 and of unexplained anemia plus diabetes and anemia in his two sisters, there was a strong possibility for a diagnosis of aceruloplasminemia—one of the four main types of neurodegeneration with brain iron accumulation (NBIA). This was eventually substantiated by a number of laboratory abnormalities, including mild normocytic anemia with a hemoglobin of 121 g/L (normal 130–177 g/L), marked hyperferritinemia (1171 mcg/L; normal 30–400 mcg/L), low serum iron concentration (5.2 μmol/L; normal 11–28 μmol/L), and reduced transferrin saturation (10%; normal 16%–45%). Serum ceruloplasmin (CP) was not detectable, and serum copper was reduced (2.1 μM; normal 11–22 μM), establishing the diagnosis of aceruloplasminemia. MRI T2* imaging of the liver revealed signs of iron overload, and hepatic iron concentration in tissue obtained from a liver biopsy was increased (22915 μg iron/g liver; normal 300–1400 μg iron/g liver).

Sequencing the *CP* gene in this patient revealed a novel homozygous mutation (deletion) in intron 14 (2).

The two brothers and two sisters of our patient underwent a neurologic and genetic examination, where one of his sisters, aged 38, who also had DM, showed a postural tremor of both hands with mild bradykinesia when finger tapping on the right hand. His other sister, aged 36, was neurologically normal, but both sisters had the same laboratory findings of anemia, aceruloplasminemia, and iron deposition in the brain and liver on MRI studies. They were both homozygous for the *CP* gene mutation found in the index case. The two brothers were clinically unaffected and showed normal laboratory tests. One of them was heterozygous for the mutation as was the mother of the patient.

The patient was started on treatment with the iron-chelating agent deferasirox (15 mg/kg body weight). Serum ferritin concentration decreased within 3 months to nearly normal levels, and liver iron deposition as assessed by MRI showed a marked decrease. Unfortunately, there was no effect on his neurologic symptoms and brain MRI showed no sign of decreased iron accumulation. Despite alternative iron-chelating therapy with deferiprone and an oral zinc sulfate therapy, this patient's ataxia slowly worsened so that the patient now needs walking assistance. His sisters were also treated and so far have not shown signs of clinical progression.

THE LESSON

The combination of a progressive cerebellar syndrome and brain iron deposition in the basal ganglia and dentate nuclei in our patient placed him into the category of conditions subsumed under the label of NBIA. NBIAs consist of four main types, including pantothenate kinase-associated neurodegeneration (PKAN), neuroferritinopathy, infantile neuroaxonal dystrophy (INAD), and aceruloplasminemia. Patients with PKAN present either as early-onset, rapidly progressive classic disease patients with age of onset in the first decade or as having an atypical disease with later onset in the second or third decade and slower progression (3). Clinically, these patients typically present with dystonic or parkinsonian symptoms and almost all show typically the eye-of-the-tiger sign on MRI (1), which was not seen in our patient. The clinical presentation of our case was also not typical for neuroferritinopathy, which results from mutations in the gene encoding ferritin light chain on chromosome 19q13.3–q13.4 (4) and is clinically characterized by progressive dystonia usually with prominent orofacial dystonia. Patients with neuroferritinopathy may show cystic degeneration in the pallida and putamen in addition to iron deposition (1), again absent in this case. On the other hand, the combination of MRI signs of NBIA with a history of diabetes and anemia plus a positive family history for both abnormalities was suggestive for aceruloplasminemia (5).

Aceruloplasminemia is a rare autosomal recessive disorder of iron metabolism caused by mutations of the *CP* gene (5). Patients present with a typical triad of neurologic symptoms, DM, and retinal degeneration (5,6). DM and anemia usually precede neurologic manifestations. The latter typically include dysarthria, ataxia, and movement disorders such as rigidity, tremor, bradykinesia, or dystonic symptoms. Some patients also develop cognitive impairment. Onset of neurologic symptoms is usually in adulthood (5). The mutation of the *CP* gene results in absence of serum CP. CP functions as a multicopper ferroxidase, which is responsible for iron binding to transferrin and promotes iron export from glial cells, hepatocytes, and macrophages (7). As a result of reduced iron binding to transferrin, iron accumulates in the central nervous system, in the liver and pancreas, and in the retina. The typical laboratory signature found in patients with aceruloplasminemia is a combination of absent CP with mild anemia, low serum iron concentration, and hyperferritinemia and low serum copper (5). Iron deposition involves the cerebral cortex, globus pallidus, putamen, caudate, thalamus, substantia nigra, and the dentate nuclei (1) but, in contrast to other NBIAs, is not restricted to the brain and involves the liver, pancreas, and retina. A diagnosis of aceruloplasminemia is confirmed through sequencing the *CP* gene for mutations.

Iron-chelating agents have been recommended as a treatment (5) and can decrease serum ferritin concentrations and liver iron deposition. The response of neurologic symptoms and the brain iron overload to this form of therapy is inconsistent, and some patients may progress despite treatment (2,5,6).

REFERENCES

1. McNeill A, Birchall D, Hayflick SJ, et al. T2* and FSE MRI distinguishes four subtypes of neurodegeneration with brain iron accumulation. *Neurology*. 2008;70:1614–1619.
2. Finkenstedt A, Wolf E, Hoefner E, et al. Hepatic but not brain iron is rapidly chelated by deferasirox in aceruloplasminemia due to a novel gene mutation. *J Hepatol*. 2010;53:1101–1107.
3. Hayflick S, Westaway SK, Levinson B, et al. Genetic, clinical, and radiographic delineation of Hallervorden-Spatz syndrome. *N Engl J Med*. 2003;348:33–40.
4. Curtis AR, Morris CM, Bindoff LA, et al. Mutation in the gene encoding ferritin light polypeptide causes dominant adult-onset basal ganglia disease. *Nat Genet*. 2001;28:350–354.
5. Miyajima H. Aceruloplasminemia. In: Pagon RA, Bird TD, Dolan CR, Stephens K, eds. *GeneReviews* [Internet]. Seattle, WA: University of Washington; August 1993–2003. Accessed May 15, 2008.
6. McNeill A, Pandolfo M, Kuhn J, et al. The neurological presentation of ceruloplasmin gene mutations. *Eur Neurol*. 2008;60:200–205.
7. Vassiliev V, Harris ZL, Zatta P. Ceruloplasmin in neurodegenerative diseases. *Brain Res Rev*. 2005; 49:633–640.

76

Evaluating Ataxia: The Eyes Have It—Or Do They?

Robert L. Rodnitzky

THE CASE

A 24-year-old man was referred to me for evaluation of unsteady gait and progressively slurred speech since age 11. He denied any cognitive, visual, or sensory symptoms and was not aware of any weakness. His mother confirmed that he had not been subjected to severe or frequent infections in the past. There was no history of neurologic impairment in his parents or in his one sibling. He was married but had no children.

On examination, there was significant scanning dysarthria but normal language functions. His gait was wide based and ataxic. He broke stance after two steps when attempting tandem gait. Finger-nose and heel-knee-shin testing revealed marked dyssynergy bilaterally. Finger tapping was slow and arrhythmic bilaterally. His stretch reflexes were normally active and symmetric. Sensory examination was normal, including pin prick, touch, position sense, and vibration. Plantar responses were flexor bilaterally. Examination of his eyes revealed subtle conjunctival telangiectasia, mildly slowed saccades in both the horizontal and vertical plane, and equivocal oculomotor apraxia. I did not appreciate any skeletal abnormalities.

THE APPROACH

My patient has significant cerebellar dysfunction with no first-degree family members who are similarly affected. A variety of toxic, metabolic, demyelinating, nutritional, or genetic conditions could result in a syndrome like this. Diagnostic tests were obtained, including an MRI scan, which revealed moderate pancerebellar atrophy with no abnormality of supratentorial structures. Additional diagnostic tests that were normal included antigliadin and anti–glutamic acid decarboxylase (GAD) antibodies, vitamin E levels, thyroid-stimulating hormone (TSH) and T4, serum copper and ceruloplasmin, and very long-chain fatty acids. Genetic testing for Friedreich's ataxia was negative. Serum alpha-fetoprotein level was obtained and was found to be markedly increased. Serum immunoglobulins, including IGA, IGM, and IGG, were normal. The finding of a markedly increased alpha-fetoprotein plus ocular telangiectasia in an ataxic patient suggested the diagnosis of ataxia telangiectasia (AT) (1). Further testing included a colony survival test. In this procedure, the patient's lymphocytes are subjected to ionizing radiation, and the percentage of surviving cells is calculated. Because AT is a disorder of DNA repair, cells from patients with AT are very sensitive to damage caused by radiation. In this case, there was abnormal survival of lymphocytes, compatible with AT. On the basis of this finding and the previously noted increased alpha-fetoprotein, a presumptive diagnosis of AT was made. My patient continued to slowly worsen over the next few years. As additional genetic tests became more widely available, a mutation analysis of the *ATM* gene, the known cause of AT, was performed, and a chromosomal breakage study was obtained, another measure of defective DNA repair. The chromosomal breakage study was normal, a point against AT, and sequencing of the *ATM* gene revealed mutation in only one allele in this autosomal recessive condition. Thus, there were conflicting messages from the variety of laboratory and genetic test results. The increased alpha-fetoprotein and abnormal colony survival test suggest AT, but the normal chromosomal breakage study speaks against it. The finding of a mutation in only a single *ATM* allele suggests that the patient does not have AT or that the patient does have AT but is a compound heterozygote with the abnormality in the opposite allele having not yet been discovered. Because of the apparently negative evaluation for homozygous mutations of the *ATM* gene, further genetic testing was performed for a clinically similar condition, ataxia with ocular motor apraxia type 2 (AOA2), a condition caused by mutations in the *SETX* gene (2). In this case, the genetic analysis revealed an unusual, but definite, mutation of different identity in each of the two *SETX* alleles, strongly suggesting the diagnosis of AOA2.

THE LESSON

AT and ataxia with AOA1 and AOA2 are all autosomal recessive conditions; therefore, unless there is an affected sibling, family history is usually not very helpful in raising the suspicion of either of these conditions. But there are clinical and laboratory features of each sydrome that can be very suggestive of the correct diagnosis and can lead to targeted genetic testing, thereby reducing the often substantial expense of widespread genetic testing for a great number of different conditions. In this case, the colony survival test strongly suggested AT; however, one additional test, the chromosomal breakage study spoke against that diagnosis—therefore, clinical and laboratory findings gave mixed diagnostic signals. Ultimately, formal evaluation of the *ATM* gene revealed an abnormality in only one allele, casting further doubt on the diagnosis of AT. Without genetic testing, distinguishing between AOA1, AOA2, and AT in this case would have been difficult if not impossible, because there is considerable clinical and diagnostic testing overlap between these three conditions. AOA1 is not associated with either increased alpha-fetoprotein or an abnormal colony survival assay as is the case in AT, and ataxia with AOA2, although sharing the characteristic of increased alpha-fetoprotein with AT, does not typically exhibit an abnormal colony survival study as was seen in this case (3). All three conditions can manifest varying degrees of oculomotor apraxia.

The lesson here is that phenotypes of clinically similar conditions can overlap so much as to render a diagnosis made solely on either clinical or laboratory grounds very unreliable. In cases such as this with potentially misleading clinical or laboratory findings, a formal genetic analysis is necessary to arrive at the correct diagnosis. This is a lesson that has already been learned in other aspects of clinical movement disorders practice such as diagnosing the various parkinsonisms. Although distinct clinical syndromes are classically associated with each of the forms of parkinsonism, it is not uncommon for significant clinical overlap to exist among them and for the final diagnosis to depend on the ultimate definitive test—in this case, an autopsy examination of the brain. The clinician should not feel diminished by the specter of a genetic analysis or an autopsy examination of the brain reversing his or her diagnosis but rather should view this experience as an opportunity to further hone one's understanding of the potential variability of these clinical syndromes and always reserve final judgment on a diagnosis until the most definitive diagnostic study has been done.

REFERENCES

1. Lavin MF. Ataxia-telangiectasia: from a rare disorder to a paradigm for cell signaling and cancer. *Nat Rev Mol Cell Biol*. 2008;9:759–769.
2. Liu W, Narayanan V. Ataxia with oculomotor apraxia. *Semin Pediatr Neurol*. 2008;15:216–220.
3. Nahas SA, Duquette A, Roddier K, et al. Ataxia-oculomotor apraxia 2 patients show no increased sensitivity to ionizing radiation. *Neuromuscul Disord*. 2007;17:968–969.

77

A Zebra Can Change Its Stripes: A Case of Inherited Ataxia

LIANA S. ROSENTHAL, SHAWN F. SMYTH, AND JOSEPH M. SAVITT

THE CASE

Our patient is a 61-year-old woman who came to our clinic seeking to improve her quality of life. For the past 17 years, she has suffered from increasingly poor balance, frequent muscle jerking, and bulbar dysfunction. While walking, her feet frequently catch on rugs or other objects, often leading to falls and significant trauma, including bilateral ankle fractures. There is difficulty walking on uneven ground, and she now requires a walker most of the time for ambulation. The rapid and brief muscle jerking developed a few years after the onset of imbalance, and she found these jerks even more bothersome. When we saw her in clinic, the jerking was only partially treated through the use of lamotrigine and zonisamide. Her speech was understandable, although she had developed dysarthria and dysphagia. Previous medical history included arthritis and bilateral sensorineural hearing loss since childhood. Similar hearing loss was present in her nephew, maternal grandmother, and mother, but no dysarthria or imbalance. Her mother suffered from seizures. Our patient's older sister and daughter had recently developed frequent falling. She has a niece with developmental delay. No one in the family had muscle jerks. Our patient denies heavy alcohol use, drug exposure, and occupational exposures.

On examination, she was cognitively intact. There are dysmetric saccades, occasional facial myokymia, mild dysarthria, and an impaired vestibulo-ocular reflex. There is dysmetria on finger-to-nose testing and a wide-based gait. Both of her hands display dystonic posturing, and we noted occasional, low-amplitude myoclonic jerks.

THE APPROACH

When this patient came to clinic, we sought to find a unifying diagnosis and to offer improved symptomatic treatment. In regard to her diagnosis, she had been tested for treatable causes of ataxia and for genetic etiologies given her positive family history. Treatable causes of ataxia include paraneoplastic syndromes, toxins, Wilson's disease, and numerous immune-mediated syndromes, including anti-GAD and antigliadin antibodies. Given this patient's protracted and progressive course, paraneoplastic disease was considered highly unlikely. Tests for Wilson's disease and autoimmune disorders were unremarkable. She was previously tested for spinocerebellar ataxia (SCA) types 1, 2, 3, 6, and 7. We expanded genetic testing to include DYT1 mutations given her dystonia, mitochondrial disorders, and maternal family history. Her clinical picture was consistent with mitochondrial epilepsy with ragged red fibers (MERRF), and subsequent testing revealed the A8344G mutation of the mitochondrial DNA consistent with MERRF.

In regard to symptomatic treatment, the patient's biggest concern was the myoclonic jerking. We initiated clonazepam 0.25 mg nightly and as needed, which provided some relief. Switching from zonisamide and lamotrigine to levetiracetam monotherapy at 1000 mg twice a day resulted in a significant reduction in the frequency and severity of her myoclonic jerking. Physical and speech therapy have shown some success in maintaining her function.

THE LESSON

This case exemplifies much of what I find fascinating and rewarding about treating patients with ataxia. The genetic syndromes that lead to ataxia are a complex group associated with many different, frequently overlapping phenotypes. However, this particular patient, like many of the other patients with ataxia we see in clinic, had specific components of her history and examination that typified a particular ataxia syndrome. Her myoclonus, sensorineural hearing loss, and family history of hearing loss all directed us toward testing for mitochondrial disorders, specifically MERRF.

Patients with MERRF typically present with myoclonus and subsequently develop ataxia, myopathy, and generalized seizures (1). Like many mitochondrial diseases, patients with MERRF may also develop sensorineural hearing loss, poor vision, and cognitive dysfunction (2). The diagnosis is based on detection of the A8344G mutation in mitochondrial DNA that was found in our patient, although other rare mutations have been noted in this clinical syndrome. The A8344G mutation of the mitochondrial tRNA lysine is believed to eliminate the "wobble" uridine, resulting in a deficiency of protein synthesis because the codons of the mutant mitochondrial tRNA cannot be decoded (3). Family members with the same mutation may have different manifestations due to heteroplasmy, thus explaining why our patient's family members had only hearing loss or epilepsy.

This case highlights a number of important insights regarding the care of patients with ataxia:

1. The medical and family history should be extensively probed for clues regarding diagnosis.
2. Mitochondrial dysfunction is the cause of numerous neurodegenerative syndromes, including those with ataxia (4).
3. Physical therapy is an effective form of managing ataxic symptoms (5).

REFERENCES

1. Fukuhara N, Tokiguchi S, Shirakawa K, et al. Myoclonus epilepsy associated with ragged-red fibres (mitochondrial abnormalities): disease entity or a syndrome? Light- and electron-microscope studies of two cases and review of the literature. *J Neurol Sci.* 1980;47:117–133.
2. Ilg W, Synofzik M, Brotz D, et al. Intensive coordinative training improves motor performance in degenerative cerebellar disease. *Neurology.* 2009;73:1823–1830.
3. Morava E, van den Heuvel L, Hol F, et al. Mitochondrial disease criteria: diagnostic applications in children. *Neurology.* 2006;67:1823–1826.
4. Schapira AHV. Mitochondrial dysfunction in neurodegenerative diseases. *Neurochem Res.* 2008;33:2502–2509.
5. Suzuki T, Nagao A, Suzuki T. Human mitochondrial diseases caused by lack of taurine modification in mitochondrial tRNAs. *Wiley Interdiscip Rev RNA.* 2011;2:376–386.

78

Abrupt Onset "On Stage Ballerina-Like" Stair Descent in an Art Student

MARCELO MERELLO

THE CASE

I first saw this 19-year-old fine arts college student who was also a very good athlete back in the year 2000 when her psychiatrist had sent her to me. She excelled in volleyball in an amateur club and was also a very good student, and when I saw her, she showed no significant personal antecedents. Her problem seemed to have started while walking down the stairs at her university, while on her way to the cafeteria. From the top of the stairs, while on her way down, she saw an old friend whom she had been emotionally involved with years ago, at the bottom of the staircase looking up at her. She became petrified and could not detach her feet from the floor. After some time (as she referred to as being a few minutes) with great effort, she reached down with her left leg to the first step and to her surprise noticed that it behaved in a very funny manner. Lifting upward as if it were performing a martial maneuver, it then come down swaying, and her foot twisted inward as it landed on the step below. It only occurred with her left foot, and it happened repeatedly throughout the day. It was so evident that it amused those around her who laughed openly, making her feel extremely embarrassed and causing her to burst into tears. Ever since then, it has affected her so much that she has not been able to go down a stairway without having difficulties. The very thought of this experience made her cry. She would try to overcome her fear by going down the stairs when no one was looking, but it never worked. She could walk and go upstairs and play volleyball without any difficulties, but when it came to going down a stairway, her difficulties persisted. She saw a clinician who recommended that she see a psychiatrist, who then diagnosed her with a psychogenic gait and prescribed clonazepam and later seritonine reuptake inhibitors (IRSS), but no improvements were noted. Therefore, after 1 year of treatment, the patient decided to visit a second psychiatrist. At that time, she presented with dysthymia according to the *DSM-III*, and the movement disorder persisted unmodified. She underwent intravenous placebo therapy, but it never worked, and a year after she began with the difficulty in walking downstairs, her new psychiatrist sent her to our clinic.

With a sport biotype, fit as a result of her intensive training, without antecedents of alcohol or drugs, smoking 10 cigarettes daily, and taking oral contraceptives, the office checkup was completely normal. Her eye movements were normal as were the cranial pairs, strength, and muscle tone, deep tendon reflexes, and the sensitivity. Extrapyramidal and cerebellar signs were not found, and her postural reflexes were normal. We took the patient to a corridor we currently use to see the way patients walk, and it was normal; however, when we led her to the stairs, we noticed this particular movement difficulty. Bending her knee 90 degrees over her thigh, the patient extends her thigh over her hip almost 90 degrees, performing an abduction of 30 degrees. Then, with a circular movement of the foot, it falls on the step, as would a ballerina when performing on stage. Her right leg was normal, and she can walk upstairs with both legs without any difficulty.

An electromyography (EMG) was performed that did not reveal any cocontraction; however, the examination was performed on the examination bed and not on the stairs. Sensitivity and motor conduction were normal. An MEP showed a slight delay in central conduction time to the inferior limb on the left side. MRI scans of the brain and spine were normal. Copper in blood and urine, thyroid function, peripheral blood search of acanthocytes, ASTO, and ASLO, just like the VSG, were normal.

She went on to mention that her 65-year-old mother was currently bedridden, and at the age of 40 years, she had had difficulties in speaking and loss of balance. Her sister who was 35 years old had a few months earlier noticed some changes in the way she spoke, and finally, the characteristics that they both held were those that her maternal grandmother also had had 30 years before she passed away.

The patient's mother and sister came to the clinic and evident clinical ataxia was confirmed in both individuals with severe dysarthria and difficulties in walking without aid. There were no other neurologic symptoms or extra neurologic signs other than mild increase in deep tendon reflexes. A dosage of B12 folic and vitamin E and VDRL were requested, as well as Ac ultrasensitive antiperoxidase and Ac antiglobulin. The mother has undergone studies with Ac anti–Hu Yo Ri and a genetic study for spinocerebellar ataxia (SCA) 1, 2, 3, 6, 7, and 8 and later on FA, FRAX, and Ac anti-GAD—all the results proved negative. Other mutations have not been explored because the studies are not available locally.

The patient continued under observation with the same symptom evident until 2005; however, a significant attenuation has been seen since then. Response to 10 mg of trihexyphenidyl was good, but medication was suspended because it interfered significantly with her studies and she had difficulty concentrating. Eye movement began to reveal certain abnormalities in pursuit movements and nystagmus was detected in far-sighted vision in both directions; saccades were abnormal. An increase of the deep tendon reflexes was detected; however, the rest of the examination was normal.

Years later, she developed an increase in basal sustentation and alterations in her postural reflexes, therefore developing difficulties with walking as the disease progressed. She has almost completely recovered from the movement interpreted as "task-specific dystonia" because it has been predominantly replaced by pancerebellar ataxia with few extracerebellar signs. A new MRI scan showed cerebellar atrophy.

Currently, at age 32, 12 years after the initial difficulty of walking down the stairs, the patient walks with difficulty and needs help. The dysarthria is very evident and distressing, and she has difficulties with reading because of diplopia and severe nystagmus.

THE APPROACH

The description of the involuntary movement this patient presents corresponds to a sporadic movement related to a specific task that compromises only one limb in a stereotype manner. It is slow and continuous, therefore generating an abnormal stance. It disappears when the patient is resting, and there is no other cause that triggers it. Even though the movement disorder could be described as choreic, the clear connection with a specific movement together with the twitching (twisting) characteristic and being both slow and not compatible with ballistic movements describes most probably a movement within the category of dystonia. Dystonia triggered by a specific task is a manner of task-specific dystonia. Bearing in mind the strong hereditary antecedent the patient holds and the clinical characteristics she presented, the case was interpreted as task-specific dystonia as an early and unusual symptom of hereditary ataxia.

THE LESSON

This is a fascinating case of which unfortunately we do not have a confirmed genetic result, but it does hold a series of important messages for the reader. It points out and emphasizes once again the importance of questioning the patient and the information we get of the antecedents, even years before the disease unfolds. Another interesting issue to draw out is that involuntary movements that take place in a specific setting must be investigated by the doctor within the same scenario (in this case, the stairway). And finally, the diagnosis of psychogenic movements must always be the last option to bear in mind once the organic causes have been ruled out.

Psychogenic gait disorders may occur either isolated or as part of a more complex generalized disorder.

The term psychogenic is used for those disorders that are not caused by known structural or neurochemical diseases. The fourth edition of the *Diagnostic and Statistical Manual of Mental Disorders* identifies three pertinent categories: somatoform disorders, factitious disorders, or malingering. Abnormal gait can be an isolated phenomenon in patients with psychogenic movement disorders or mixed with other clinical manifestations. Psychogenic pictures are not uncommon, accounting for 1.5% to 26% of all patients admitted to a neurologic service (1–3). Although the psychogenic nature of the gait is in general quickly apparent to an experienced observer, these are often difficult patients, and optimal diagnostic and management requires extra time. Imaging studies are easily justified and are sometimes informative even if the suspicion of organic disease is low. Diagnosis relies mainly on the observation of bizarre motor behavior, discrepancy between obvious dysfunction and normal diagnostic evaluation, and evidence of psychiatric abnormalities; nevertheless, many cases without bizarre features remain obscure despite careful investigations and are clarified only on follow-up.

This patient met almost all the criteria proposed by Fahn and Williams, despite the patient not having a psychogenic movement disorder.

Focal and generalized forms of dystonia have been documented in SCA 1, 2, 3, 6, 7, 12, 14, 17, and 20; however, they are mainly associated with SCA17, SCA3, and SCA2 with frequency estimates of around 53%, 24%, and 14%, respectively.

In some SCA17 families, individuals may have focal dystonia as the first symptom, which may be the case in our patient. An initial presentation with cervical dystonia has also been documented in SCA 1, 2, and 14 and writer cramps in SCA6. Limb dystonia, which has been described in association with SCA3, and retraction of the eyelids causing bulging eyes, has been regarded as a clinical hallmark of Machado-Joseph disease (MJD) in patients of Portuguese background. In addition, cervical or facial dystonia has been described in other families (5,6).

Chorea is a particularly common feature of SCA17, with a reported prevalence between 20% and 66%. Because cognitive decline and behavioral disturbances are other potential features within the SCA17 profile, the clinical presentation might mimic Huntington's disease (HD). Therefore, SCA17 is also referred to as HD-like syndrome. Chorea can also be encountered in SCA 1, 2, 3, 14, and 27.

Shoulder girdle and upper limb dystonia have been recently reported as SCA6 presentation (7). In addition, Muzaimi et al. (8) described a case of SCA6 with a focal dystonia preceding the onset of gait or limb ataxia within a period of at least 5 years as one of the most similar cases that has been presented in reported literature.

Movement disorders like parkinsonism, tremor, myoclonus, chorea, or even dystonia are among the most common noncerebellar features in SCAs. The observed movement disorder, when present in combination with cerebellar ataxia, could provide clues to the underlying genotype. When cerebellar ataxia is mild or even absent, an SCA might not at first seem to be the cause. Useful clues to raise suspicion might be cerebellar atrophy on brain imaging or a family history suggesting an autosomal dominant disorder.

REFERENCES

1. Bhatia KP. Psychogenic gait disorders. *Adv Neurol.* 2001;87:251–254.
2. Keane JR. Hysterical gait disorders: 60 cases. *Neurology.* 1989;39:586–589.
3. Lempert T, Brandt T, Dieterich M, et al. How to identify psychogenic disorders of stance and gait: a video study in 37 patients developed for diagnostic purposes. *J Neurol.* 1991;238:140–146.

4. Fahn S, Williams PJ. Psychogenic dystonia. *Adv Neurol.* 1988;50:431–455.
5. Sudarsky L, Coutinho P. Machado-Joseph disease. *Clin Neurosci.* 1995;3:17–22.
6. Cardoso F, de Oliveira JT, Puccioni-Sohler M, et al. Eyelid dystonia in Machado-Joseph disease. *Mov Disord.* 2000;15:1028–1030.
7. Sethi KD, Jankovic J. Dystonia in spinocerebellar ataxia type 6. *Mov Disord.* 2002;17:150–153.
8. Muzaimi MB, Wiles CM, Robertson NP, et al. Task specific focal dystonia: a presentation of spinocerebellar ataxia type 6. *J Neurol Neurosurg Psychiatry.* 2003;74:1444–1445.

VII

Tics and Stereotypies

79

Hereditary Syndrome With Multiple Tics: A Lesson on the Phenotypic Variability of Huntington's Disease

CARLO COLOSIMO, GIOVANNI FABBRINI, AND ALFREDO BERARDELLI

THE CASE

A 30-year-old man came to our clinic with multiple abrupt, stereotypic, and jerky movements. The involuntary movements had begun insidiously about 10 years earlier, initially only affecting his limbs and later involving his trunk, neck, and face. The involuntary movements were occasionally accompanied by sounds of throat clearing. Examination revealed normal mental status, oculomotor function, strength, coordination, and deep tendon reflexes. There was generalized anxiety and depressive symptoms with initial social withdrawal. As the early symptomatology was generally mild, the patient was able to go on working as a state clerk.

THE APPROACH

No family history of neurologic disorders was reported, and the brain MRI scan was unremarkable. However, during a second consultation, we noticed that his 65-year-old father, who had accompanied him on this occasion, also had very subtle involuntary movements, such as eye blinking, facial twitching, and shoulder elevation. He was healthy otherwise and was unaware of those movements. Given the multiple tic-like movements, mood disorder, probable positive family history, normal investigations, and relatively mild neurologic picture, a diagnosis of atypical Gilles de la Tourette syndrome was made on the basis of the late age of symptom onset, stable symptomatology, and lack of voluntary suppressibility of the involuntary movements (1). The neurologic and psychiatric symptoms of the patient rapidly progressed over the following 2 years, resulting in increasingly severe involuntary movements and profound mood disorder that required high-dose antidepressant therapy. After this worsening, the patient was referred to our senior psychiatrist for further advice. This psychiatrist was not convinced by our clinical diagnosis and suggested further diagnostic tests. Among others, a genetic screening for Huntington's disease (HD) showed 45 repeats of the CAG trinucleotide.

THE LESSON

HD is a hereditary neurologic disorder characterized by the typical triad of dominant inheritance, choreoathetosis, and dementia. However, the presence of other involuntary movements, such as tics, dystonia, and tremor, may in some cases render the clinical diagnosis of this disease more difficult, as the case presented in this report shows. The mean age at onset of HD is around 40 years, and once symptoms first appear, the disease progresses relentlessly and usually results in death within 10 to 20 years. The diagnosis is straightforward in families with fully developed HD, although genetic screening helps to confirm the diagnosis in atypical cases and in patients with an earlier onset of symptoms. If the gene encoding the huntingtin protein located on the

TABLE 79.1

Huntington's Disease: Diagnostic Categories According to the Number of CAG Repeats
(American College of Medical Genetics Huntington's Disease Working Group)

CATEGORY	CAG NUMBER	PHENOTYPE
Normal allele	<26	Normal
Normal allele but susceptible to mutation	27–35	Normal
Pathologic allele with reduced penetrance	36–39	Normal/HD
Pathologic allele	>40	HD

short arm of chromosome 4 has more than 36 repeats of the CAG trinucleotide, the disease is confirmed, as it was in this patient (2,3). We may hypothesize that the patient's father had a HD premutation (i.e., borderline number of CAG), resulting in minor manifestations of the disease (late-onset mild involuntary movements), whereas his son developed the full-blown form of HD because of the well-known anticipation phenomenon (see Table 79.1) (4). For ethical reasons, we decided not to disclose our hypothesis to the family and not to ask for genetic testing of the patient's father.

The symptoms in this patient, who continues to be seen regularly by us, have worsened rapidly. He is now wheelchair bound and has a severe cognitive dysfunction, apathy, anarthria, and severe dysphagia, for which he has received a percutaneous gastrostomy.

REFERENCES

1. Jankovic J. Tourette's syndrome. *N Engl J Med.* 2001;345:1184–1192.
2. Gusella JF, Wexler NS, Conneally PM, et al. A polymorphic DNA marker genetically linked to Huntington's disease. *Nature.* 1983;306:234–238.
3. Huntington's Disease Collaborative Research Group. A novel gene containing a trinucleotide repeat that is expanded and unstable in Huntington's disease chromosomes. *Cell.* 1993;72:971–983.
4. Trottier Y, Biancalana V, Mandel JL. Instability of CAG repeats in Huntington's disease: relation to parental transmission and age of onset. *J Med Genet.* 1994;31:377–382.

80

Affective Changes and Involuntary Movements in a
29-Year-Old Man: Do Not Forget to Review
the Medication List!

KATHLEEN M. SHANNON

THE CASE

A 29-year-old man with a history of bipolar affective disorder (type II) presented with involuntary movements. He had been treated for his psychiatric illness for many years with a variety of dopamine receptor blocking agents, including haloperidol, risperidone, and aripiprazole.
Extrapyramidal symptoms and signs had never been noted. Eventually, he stabilized on a combination of mirtazepine 45 mg daily and lithium 900 mg daily and then remained stable until
5 months before presentation. At that time, he became acutely manic. Bupropion 150 mg daily,
lamotrigine (LTG) 200 mg daily, clonazepam 2 mg thrice a day, and zolpidem controlled release
12.5 mg daily were added to his regimen. Within a few weeks, he began to have involuntary
movements of his face and shoulders. The movements were frequent and stereotyped. He had
repeated eyelid closure, lower facial grimacing movements, and shoulder shrugging. The movements were associated with a premonitory urge and were partially suppressible by voluntary effort.
Suppressing the movements produced an unpleasant sensation that was relieved by letting the
movements happen. There were no vocalizations. There was no history of involuntary movements, behavior, or attention disorder in childhood, and this was confirmed by his mother. There
was no family history of Gilles de la Tourette syndrome or tics. His psychiatrist thought the movement disorder might represent Huntington's disease and referred him for diagnostic testing.

General examination and vital signs were normal. Bedside cognitive testing was normal.
Cranial nerve, sensory, and cerebellar examination were normal. Motor strength and tone and
deep tendon reflexes were normal, and there were no pathologic reflexes. He had stereotyped
repetitive movements of the face, neck, and shoulder. These were voluntarily suppressible. There
were no other involuntary movements or extrapyramidal signs.

THE APPROACH

Stereotyped and suppressible movements associated with a premonitory urge are most likely tics.
Onset of tics in adulthood is rare, and in many cases, a detailed history unveils a childhood history of tics. Chouinard and Ford (1) reviewed 22 patients with tic disorders presenting after age
21 from a database that included 411 patients with tic. Mean age of onset in these 13 cases was
40 years (range 24–63 years). Nine of the patients had a childhood history compatible with
Gilles de la Tourette syndrome, but 13 first had onset in adulthood. Nearly half of these with first
onset in adulthood cases developed symptoms in association with an external trigger (infection,
trauma, cocaine use, and neuroleptic exposure).

The patient did not have a history of childhood tics, attention deficit disorder, obsessive-
compulsive disorder, or other behaviors suggestive of Gilles de la Tourette syndrome. A detailed
history of the movements in relation to medication changes suggested that LTG may have been
the causative agent, and the tics resolved after LTG was discontinued.

THE LESSON

LTG (3,5-diamino-6-(2,3-dichlorophenyl)-1,2,4-triazine) is a newer anticonvulsant used in the treatment of partial and generalized epilepsy in all age groups. LTG is believed to exert its anticonvulsant effect through inhibition of transmitter release (primarily glutamate) through its action at voltage-sensitive sodium channels (2). LTG treatment has been associated with a number of movement disorder side effects, including dystonia, chorea, tremor, myoclonus, and tics (3–5). There are now several reports of tics in adults and children treated with LTG. Sotero de Menezes et al. (6) reported five children between 2.5 and 12 years old who developed new onset of tics within 10 months of onset of LTG. Tics were mostly simple motor tics, but one person had vocal tics. Tics resolved within 1 to 4 months of discontinuation of the LTG, and two patients had recurrence on rechallenge with LTG. Seemüller et al. reported a 55-year-old woman with bipolar affective disorder who developed multifocal motor and vocal and phonic tics 3 months after starting LTG. She had a remote history of tics in childhood and rare tics in the 2 months before initiating LTG. Tics resolved after stopping LTG (7). A 49-year-old woman developed motor tics, blepharospasm, repetitive touching, echopraxis, and phonic and vocal tics associated with obsessive thoughts during titration of LTG for the treatment of depression. Symptoms improved when LTG was decreased, although it did not resolve until risperidone was added (8).

Other drugs that have been associated with the development of tics include dopaminergic drugs, stimulants, neuroleptics, cocaine, and carbamazepine (1,9–11).

When a movement disorder begins in a child or adult who is being treated with LTG, an LTG-induced movement disorder should be considered in the differential diagnosis.

REFERENCES

1. Chouinard S, Ford B. Adult onset tic disorders. *J Neurol Neurosurg Psychiatry*. 2000;68:738–743.
2. Leach MJ, Marden CM, Miller AA. Pharmacological studies on lamotrigine, a novel potential antiepileptic drug: II. Neurochemical studies on the mechanism of action. *Epilepsia*. 1986;27:490–497.
3. Das KB, Harris C, Smyth DP. Unusual side effects of lamotrigine therapy. *J Child Neurol*. 2003;18:479–480.
4. Fernandez Corcuera P, Pomarol E, Amann B, et al. Myoclonus provoked by lamotrigine in a bipolar patient. *J Clin Psychopharmacol*. 2008;28:248–249.
5. Rosenhagen MC, Schmidt U, Weber F, et al. Combination therapy of lamotrigine and escitalopram may cause myoclonus. *J Clin Psychopharmacol*. 2006;26:346–347.
6. Sotero de Menezes MA, Rho JM, Murphy P, et al. Lamotrigine-induced tic disorder: report of five pediatric cases. *Epilepsia*. 2000;41:862–867.
7. Seemüller F, Dehning S, Grunze H, et al. Tourette's symptoms provoked by lamotrigine in a bipolar patient. *Am J Psychiatry*. 2006;163:159.
8. Alkin T, Onur E, Ozerdem A. Co-occurence of blepharospasm, tourettism and obsessive-compulsive symptoms during lamotrigine treatment. *Prog Neuropsychopharmacol Biol Psychiatry*. 2007;31:1339–1340.
9. Dafotakis M, Fink GR, Nowak DA. Dopaminergic drug-induced tics in PARK2-positive Parkinson's disease. *Mov Disord*. 2008;23:628.
10. Kurlan R, Kersun J, Behr J, et al. Carbamazepine-induced tics. *Clin Neuropharmacol*. 1989;12:298–302.
11. Lal S, Al Ansari E. Tourette-like syndrome following low dose short-term neuroleptic treatment. *Can J Neurol Sci*. 1986;13:125–128.

Suggested Reading

Detweiler MB, Kalafat N, Kim KY. Drug-induced movement disorders in older adults: an overview for clinical practitioners. *Consult Pharm*. 2007;22:149–165.
Gilbert DL. Drug-induced movement disorders in children. *Ann N Y Acad Sci*. 2008;1142:72–84.
Jimenez-Jimenez FJ, Garcia-Ruiz PJ, Molina JA. Drug-induced movement disorders. *Drug Saf*. 1997; 16:180–204.
Rodnitzky RL. Drug-induced movement disorders. *Clin Neuropharmacol*. 2002;25:142–152.

81

Hereditary Stereotypies From a Family in Canada

JUSTYNA R. SARNA AND OKSANA SUCHOWERSKY

THE CASE

An 8-year-old boy was seen at the movement disorders clinic accompanied by his mother for an assessment of abnormal movements. The referral was precipitated by a history of similar move-ments in the patient's 4-year-old brother who was developmentally delayed and eventually diag-nosed with fragile X syndrome. The mother described the movements as paroxysmal, repetitive, and highly stereotyped consisting of hand flapping, dystonic posturing of hands and feet, facial grimacing, and occasional associated pacing. The boy was not fully aware of the movements and could not suppress them. The episodes were as frequent as 10 times daily, lasting from 10 seconds to 30 minutes. Typical triggers included fatigue, stress, or excitement. There was no associated loss of awareness. He was otherwise healthy and exceled in school. Neurologic exam-ination was normal.

Detailed family history inquiry revealed similar paroxysmal movements in other family mem-bers. Available family members were assessed at a subsequent visit. The patient's 4-year-old brother had developmental delay consistent with fragile X phenotype and was later confirmed to have fragile X syndrome. There were no other known members of the family with fragile X syndrome. The boy's sister was healthy and had no abnormal movements. The boy's 43-year-old father had similar repetitive and patterned movements since childhood. The movements would occur on average 10 times daily and last from 10 seconds and up to 75 minutes. There was no preceding warning. He described the episodes starting out as a "trance" or daydream and then progress to involuntary symmetric dystonic posturing involving his hands and occasionally his feet and frequent pacing. He could suppress the movements for minutes to hours and conscious-ness was preserved throughout the episode. He was otherwise healthy and had a normal neu-rologic examination. MRI of the brain and electroencephalography (EEG) were normal. The father's brother and sister who were otherwise healthy also reported similar movements.

Finally, the patient's grandfather, aged 67 years, experienced similar movements since child-hood that resolved during his 40s. He described it as a semi-fugue state with involuntary tens-ing of his muscles lasting for 15 seconds. He could suppress these, and there was no associated buildup or an urge. His neurologic examination was unremarkable.

THE APPROACH

The family is characterized by repetitive, paroxysmal, and highly stereotyped movements that start in infancy or early childhood. The movements are not preceded by a premonitory urge and have not waxed and waned over time. There were no associated tics or obsessive-compulsive symptoms. On the basis of the description and nature of the movements, complex motor stereo-typy was diagnosed in this family.

Stereotypies are most commonly defined as involuntary, purposeless, and highly patterned movements that are performed in a monotonous manner during times of boredom, anxiety, or excitement. The differential diagnosis of stereotypy is extensive (see Table 81.1), and the diagnosis can often be challenging.

Complex motor tics in developmentally normal children can be particularly difficult to distinguish from complex motor stereotypies. The approach in differentiating these two movements includes (1) age of onset (stereotypy present by approximately age 2, whereas tic onset typically around 6 years of age); (2) pattern (fixed and stereotyped in stereotypies, whereas ever evolving and waxing and waning for tics); (3) rhythm (generally rhythmical movements in stereotypies and more random movements in tics); (4) duration (longer and continuous in stereotypies); (5) lack of premonitory urge in stereotypies; and (6) distraction (stereotypies can cease with distraction, whereas tics have to be intentionally suppressed), among others (1,2).

Obsessive-compulsive behaviors also need to be considered in the differential diagnosis of stereotypies. Compulsions are repetitive motor or mental rituals aimed at reducing anxiety in response to obsessions (intrusive, recurrent, and unwanted thoughts that increase anxiety) (2,3). Motor stereotypies do not share these features, but their repetitive nature may blur the distinction. Similarly, epileptic automatisms are highly stereotyped and can be especially difficult to identify in developmentally delayed and noncommunicative children in whom impaired consciousness may not be immediately obvious. Correlation of the repetitive movement with concurrent changes on EEG is required to confirm the diagnosis in these cases.

Mannerisms are also motor acts performed in a distinctive pattern and have been defined as an unusual and peculiar way of completing a purposeful act (4), distinguishing it from the purposeless aspect of stereotypy. Drug-induced dyskinesias can also appear highly stereotyped; a careful drug history (past and/or present) will typically unveil this diagnostic entity. Paroxysmal dyskinesias represent episodic movements or postures lasting from minutes to hours that are triggered by movement (kinesogenic) or exertion starting in early childhood. The movements are distinguished from stereotypies by the episodic occurrence and preserved mentation (3). Inner restlessness typifies both akathisia and restless leg syndrome (when confined to limbs) and with appropriate history can usually be clearly discerned from stereotypy.

The family in this case is characterized by early onset of repetitive, highly stereotyped hand movements, and dystonic posturing most often triggered by excitement or stress. The distinctive, static, and nonevolving nature of the movements with no preceding premonitory urge distinguishes it from complex motor tics. According to history from the older members of the family, the motor acts are not voluntarily performed rituals aimed at suppressing an unwanted intrusive thought (obsession), distinguishing them from compulsions. Paroxysmal dyskinesia is also unlikely, because these movements are not characterized by episodic chorea or dystonia, although this diagnostic entity on the differential diagnosis cannot be definitively ruled out.

TABLE 81.1
Differential Diagnosis of Complex Motor Stereotypy.

Complex motor tic

Obsessive-compulsive behaviors

Epileptic automatisms

Mannerisms

Drug-induced dyskinesias

Paroxysmal dyskinesias

Restless legs syndrome

Akathisia

Adapted from Ref. 3.

TABLE 81.2
Secondary Causes of Stereotypy.

Autism/autistic spectrum disorder

Rett syndrome and other etiologies of mental retardation

Inborn errors of metabolism

Sensory deprivation

Drug-induced

Infection

Tumor

Psychiatric

Adapted from Ref. 2.

THE LESSON

Our case highlights the importance of diligent and detailed history taking, including family history. The presenting complaint of repetitive hand flapping and intermittent posturing in the hands was initially raised by the family in their developmentally delayed son who had autistic-like features and was later diagnosed with fragile X syndrome. Stereotypies are most commonly seen in the context of autistic spectrum disorder or other disorders that affect normal development, including inborn errors of metabolism (e.g., Lesch-Nyhan, neuroacanthocytosis), Rett syndrome, and sensory deprivation (congenital blindness, deafness) among others (2,5; Table 81.2). Therefore, the stereotypy observed in this patient may have been easily attributed to the coexisting developmental delay, and only meticulous family history inquiry revealed similar movements in other developmentally normal family members.

There is a paucity of research evaluating stereotypies in developmentally normal individuals. These nonpathologic or physiologic stereotypies have been classified in the literature into three subtypes: (1) common (thumb sucking, body rocking, nail biting, and hair twisting); (2) head nodding; and (3) complex motor (hand shaking, posturing, flapping, or posturing) (2,5). Complex motor stereotypies, as described in this case, have been associated with high rates of comorbid conditions, including attention deficit hyperactivity disorder (ADHD), tics, and obsessive-compulsive behaviors (1). The movements tend to have a chronic, fixed course contrary to the previously believed transient nature of stereotypies in normally developing children.

There are few studies specifically examining familial association of complex motor stereotypies, although high rates of positive family history have been reported in studies (one third of patients in Ref. 6; 25% in first- or second-degree relatives in Ref. 1; 17% in first-degree relatives and 25% in any relative in Ref. 7). Most of these have implicated an autosomal dominant mode of inheritance, as described in this family, although no gene has thus far been identified.

REFERENCES

1. Mahone EM, Bridges D, Prahme C, et al. Repetitive arm and hand movements (complex motor stereotypies) in children. *J Pediatr.* 2004;145:391–395.
2. Muthugovindan D, Singer H. Motor stereotypy disorders. *Curr Opin Neurol.* 2009;22:131–136.
3. Friedman JH. Stereotypy and catatonia. In: Jankovic J, Tolosa E, eds. *Parkinson's Disease and Movement Disorders.* Lippincott Williams and Wilkins, Philadelphia, PA; 2007:468–474.

4. Lees AJ. Facial mannerisms and tics. *Adv Neurol.* 1988;49:255–261.
5. Singer HS. Motor stereotypies. *Semin Pediatr Neurol.* 2009;16:77–81.
6. Castellanos FX, Ritchie GF, Marsh WF, et al. DSM-IV stereotypic movement disorder: persistence of stereotypies of infancy in intellectually normal adolescents and adults. *J Clin Psychiatry.* 1996;57:116–122.
7. Harris KM, Mahone EM, Singer HS. Nonautistic motor stereotypies: clinical features and longitudinal follow-up. *Pediatr Neurol.* 2008;38:267–272.

Suggested Reading

Muthugovindan D, Singer H. Motor stereotypy disorders. *Curr Opin Neurol.* 2009;22:131–136.
Singer HS. Motor stereotypies. *Semin Pediatr Neurol.* 2009;16:77–81.

82

Tics From a Church Choir: A Unique Case Illustrating the Challenge of Distinguishing Organic From Psychogenic Tics

NELSON HWYNN, GENKO OYAMA, AND MICHAEL S. OKUN

THE CASE

A 50-year-old man came to us for an evaluation of a tic disorder. He unfortunately was the restrained driver of a vehicle traveling at a speed of approximately 65 mph before becoming involved in a head-on collision with another moving car that resulted in two fatalities. He was extracted from the vehicle. The medical records cited loss of consciousness, although the duration was uncertain. He underwent a computed tomography (CT) scan of the head on the day of injury, which was reported as normal. He also sustained various orthopedic injuries, including fractures to the ribs and sternum, along with lacerations to the liver and spleen. He had open fractures to the right upper extremity requiring surgical intervention and ultimately these left him with a chronic right ulnar nerve palsy. Two days after the accident, he developed intractable hiccups, which were treated with intravenous chlorpromazine for 1 day. This medication was discontinued later that same day at the request of his wife, and it is unclear how many total doses he was given.

Approximately 3 months after the accident, he experienced an abrupt onset of vocal and motor tics consisting of stuttering and grunting, as well as tics involving the arms and legs. The episodes were more likely to occur in the presence of strangers or when he was emotionally aroused, particularly when having nonscripted conversations in public. He had a time before he saw us when the stuttering was beginning to subside, but it fully reappeared after he spent time with a friend who stuttered. His stuttering also disappeared when he sang, as he often did in the church choir. He did not have any premonitory sensations before the tics occurred and believed that deep breathing lessened the duration and intensity of the tics, although he was ultimately unable to completely suppress the movements. He also did not feel any relief with carrying out the tics.

His previous medical history was significant for hypertension. There was no history of psychiatric problems or treatment predating the motor vehicle accident that was suggestive of a previous depressive episode, manic episode, obsessive-compulsive traits, or attention deficit hyperactivity disorder (ADHD). His family history was not significant for psychiatric disorder or any obvious tic disorders or subtle tics such as throat clearing or sniffing.

He was the product of a normal pregnancy and birth, and he reached developmental milestones at appropriate ages. Early history of physical, verbal, or emotional abuse was denied. He attended regular classes throughout school without any academic problems or learning difficulties. He was gainfully employed, had been happily married for 28 years, and had two adult children.

On examination, he was a gregarious man with prominent vocal and motor tics that waxed and waned over time. His conversational speech was sometimes dysfluent because of vocal tics that included grunting and, less frequently, stuttering. Occasionally, he abruptly reiterated single words or short phrases repetitively, before suddenly initiating a fluent stream of speech to complete his sentence. The patient also exhibited prominent motor tics consisting of jerking of his trunk and proximal upper extremities, jerking of his legs, blinking, and, rarely, jerking of his neck. His constellation of symptoms sometimes escalated to marked episodes involving stuttering, grunting, labored breathing, and repetitive jerks lasting up to 10 or 15 minutes. Cognitively, he was a good historian with logical and linear thinking. His affect appeared normal without demonstrating any evidence of depressed affect or anxiety. Aside from the aforementioned abnormalities, the remainder of his neurologic examination was unremarkable.

THE APPROACH

Before he presented to us, he was treated by his primary physician with alprazolam (0.5 mg three times a day) and escitalopram (20 mg daily), both of which failed to improve his motor and vocal symptoms.

His previous diagnostic workup at an outside institution included a normal electroencephalogram (EEG) and MRI of the brain without gadolinium without significant findings.

Because of the diagnostic uncertainty of whether his abrupt- and late-onset tics were organic, psychogenic, or mixed, we started him on risperidone and titrated up to a dose of 0.5 mg twice a day, which he stated led to the complete resolution of his tics 5 months later. He then slowly tapered off the risperidone. He is no longer taking risperidone and has remained asymptomatic to date.

THE LESSON

Our case illustrates the complexity of differentiating organic from psychogenic tic disorders. The details of this case are suggestive of the diagnosis of a psychogenic post-traumatic tic disorder that was characterized by the abrupt onset and marked resolution of his vocal and motor tics after a very brief treatment and did not reappear after treatment discontinuation. In addition, his age of onset and lack of family history were also contributory to a psychogenic diagnosis. He did not feel the inner tension building to perform the movement, nor did he have suppressibility or release of his tics, which are the common features often accompanying organic tic disorders. The inconsistency of stuttering was also a suspicious feature. He did not have any obvious psychiatric premorbid conditions. The case illustrates the importance of a careful and thoughtful workup in differentiating organic from psychogenic tic disorder.

Another consideration for adult-onset tic disorder would be tardive tics from neuroleptic exposure. Our patient had neuroleptic exposure for at most 1 day, and he developed the tics approximately 3 to 4 months after exposure. Previously reported cases of tardive tics included exposure to chronic dopamine receptor blocking agents for several years (1,2). Secondary tics from vascular causes have been described (3), but the MRI findings in our case did not reveal extensive white matter changes. Finally, our case was not likely a transient tic disorder, which usually occurs before adulthood and persists less than a year (4).

Separating organic tic disorders from psychogenic tics can be extremely challenging and difficult because at this time there are no definitive tests or imaging to prove or disprove the presence of an organic syndrome. There are no stringent criteria for distinguishing between organic tic disorders versus psychogenic tics. Complicating matters, psychogenic tics can coexist with organic tic disorders (5) in the way that pseudoseizures can coexist with true epileptic seizures. Thomas and Jankovic (6) list the presence of an abrupt onset, response to placebo, selective disability, marked resolution, an increase with attention, and cessation of movements with distraction as possible ways to differentiate general psychogenic movement disorders from organic movement disorders. Although helpful, these criteria are not definitive. Moreover, as noted by Sampaio and Hounie (5), these criteria were not specifically devised for differentiating psychogenic and organic tic disorders, and patients with tic disorders have been known to demonstrate abrupt onset, waxing and waning course, and exacerbation with attention.

It has been argued that psychogenic disorders should be diagnosed early in their course to obtain the best possible treatment. In a recent review by Gupta and Lang, it was noted that making the diagnosis within 6 to 12 months after symptom onset seemed to be optimal. This early identification reduced the risk of multiple referrals, unnecessary tests, perpetuation of the belief of organic illness, and unecessary medications (7). Random controlled trials in treating and managing psychogenic movement disorders are currently not available. In light of diagnostic uncertainty of an organic, psychogenic, or mixed etiology at the initial visit, we treated this patient as if he had an organic tic disorder. His marked resolution after a short course of medication therapy, which was maintained after discontinuation, helped solidify the diagnosis of a psychogenic etiology. The clinical neurologic and neuropsychological examination paired with close clinical follow-up all contributed to obtaining the correct diagnosis in this challenging case.

REFERENCES

1. Yamauchi K, Ohmori T. Two cases of tardive Tourette syndrome. *Seishin Shinkeigaku Zasshi.* 2006; 108:459–465.
2. Reid SD. Neuroleptic-induced tardive Tourette treated with clonazepam: a case report and literature review. *Clin Neuropharmacol.* 2004;27:101–104.
3. Gomis M, Puente V, Pont-Sunyer C, et al. Adult onset simple phonic tic after caudate stroke. *Mov Disord.* 2008;23:765–766.
4. Kenney C, Kuo S, Jiminez-Shahed J. Tourette's syndrome. *Am Fam Physician.* 2008;77:651–658.
5. Sampaio A, Hounie AG. Organic vs. psychogenic tics. *Rev Bras Psiquiat.* 2005;27:163.
6. Thomas M, Jankovic J. Psychogenic movement disorders: diagnosis and management. *CNS Drugs.* 2004;18:437–452.
7. Gupta A, Lang AE. Psychogenic movement disorders. *Curr Opin Neurol.* 2009;22:430–436.

VIII
Myoclonus and Startle Syndromes

83

The Challenging Case of a Man With Paroxysmal Irregular Jerking of the Right Arm

A. ZANGERLE, J. WILLEIT, AND W. POEWE

THE CASE

When first seen at our department in January 2008, a 54-year-old man had a 4-month history of brief attacks of involuntary repetitive movements of the right arm. Typical attacks lasted for less than 10 seconds and were especially likely to occur after rising from sitting or lying positions, whereas limb position or exertion was not a provocative factor. Frequency of attacks was up to five times a day.

The patient was admitted to the neurology department of Innsbruck Medical University for further workup, and his neurologic examination at admission was unremarkable. His previous medical history included hyperlipidemia and arterial hypertension. His family history was negative for movement disorders (MDs), mental illness, or epilepsy. A videotape recorded by his wife demonstrated a typical episode showing abrupt onset of irregular jerks restricted to his right arm and involving both proximal and distal muscles lasting for approximately 10 seconds. There was no sign of abnormal consciousness during the attack, and there was no paresis immediately afterward.

THE APPROACH

This patient presented with a 4-month history of a paroxysmal MD involving his right arm. Paroxysmal kinesigenic choreoathetosis (PKC) was not a likely differential diagnosis because there was no consistent provocation by sudden movement, although attacks tended to occur when rising from a sitting or lying position. Restriction of attacks to the right arm also would be unusual for PKC and attack frequency was low, as opposed to up to 100 per day in classical PKC. Lower attack frequencies are typical for other paroxysmal dyskinesias such as paroxysmal dystonic choreoathetosis (PDC) or exertional paroxysmal dystonia, but the respective provoking factors typical for these disorders (sudden movement, caffeine, alcohol, or prolonged exertion) were not reported here. The phenomenology caught on video by his wife showing brief irregular jerking for less than 10 seconds raised a serious consideration of focal epilepsy. The patient's interictal electroencephalogram (EEG) was free of epileptic discharges, and he was transferred to our EEG monitoring unit for continuous video EEG monitoring over 72 hours. During monitoring, a single attack with irregular cloni of the right hand was captured, and there was no accompanying epileptic activity, strongly arguing against an epileptic origin of his attacks.

MRI was performed to rule out focal basal ganglia pathology and revealed multiple clinically silent borderzone infarctions on the left middle cerebral artery (MCA) territory. High-resolution ultrasound and contrast-enhanced magnetic resonance angiography revealed occlusion of the left internal carotid artery (ICA) leading to a diagnosis of "limb shaking" transient ischemic attacks (TIAs) with carotid artery occlusive disease. Transcranial duplex sonography (TCD) detected a significantly impaired blood flow in the left MCA with a loss of autoregulation during hypercapnia. There was no evidence of cross-flow via the anterior or posterior communicating arteries. Collateral blood flow was demonstrated via the ophthalmic artery and leptomeningeal pathways. A Tc-99m single photon emission computed tomography (SPECT) with an acetacolamide challenge showed reversible hypoperfusion in frontal and parietal cortical areas on the left side.

Antithrombotic treatment with aspirin or warfarin and modifications of the antihypertensive regimen (mildly hypertensive blood pressure) did not affect the frequency of attacks. Because symptoms persisted and neither endarteriectomy nor carotid artery stenting of the ICA occlusion was possible, a superficial temporal artery–MCA (STA-MCA) anastomosis was successfully performed in October 2008. Afterward, focal blood flow and vasoreactivity improved, and the patient has since remained asymptomatic (last visit in July 2010).

THE LESSON

Limb shaking TIA is a symptom of carotid occlusive disease first described by Fisher in 1962 (1,2). Limb shaking attacks (LSAs) occur in 10% to more than 20% of patients with ICA occlusion, according to recent series (3,4). LSAs more often involve the arm than the leg, almost always last for less than 5 minutes, typically for less than a minute and have a mixed phenomenology of brief jerking with elements of myoclonus and chorea. Provoking factors of rising from a sitting or lying position as seen in this case are found in about 40% and may also include other activity, giving rise to potential confusion with other paroxysmal MDs such as PKC. Transient weakness of the involved limb after an attack was reported in about 80% of cases in a recent survey and has been taken as an argument for a possible epileptic origin of LSAs (4).

Different from focal seizures, TIAs with limb shaking are usually arrhythmic and have never been reported to spread along the limbs in a jacksonian march fashion, and several series failed to detect epileptic EEG activity during or between the attacks. In addition, anticonvulsant medication has not been successful in controlling LSAs (5).

On the other hand, limb shaking is often precipitated by standing or walking and is promptly alleviated by assuming a supine position, arguing for a hemodynamic ischemic mechanism (1).

A variety of techniques has been applied to measure a compromised cerebral blood flow (CBF) in patients with LSAs and carotid occlusion—including positron emission tomography (PET), 123 I SPECT, stable xenon computed tomography (CT), and TCD with and without vasodilatory stimuli. Measurement of CO_2 reactivity by TCD is the least invasive and least expensive method and does not involve the use of radioactive tracers (6,7). Vasomotor reactivity seems to be compromised over the entire cerebral hemispheres opposite to the involuntary movements (1). In our patient, perfusion was reduced focally in the frontal and parietal cortical areas in the symptomatic hemisphere. Specific and consistent areas of regional cerebral ischemia in patients with limb shaking have not been found thus far, although basal ganglia hypoperfusion may well play a role in producing these involuntary movements, which often contain elements of chorea or, rarely, may resemble focal ballism.

Consistent with ischemia as the main mechanism, a decreased frequency or complete cessation of limb shaking TIAs after extracranial/intracranial (EC/IC) bypass or carotid endarteriectomy has been described (1,8–10), and our patient has had no further attacks after this procedure. In addition, there are reports that limb shaking TIAs disappeared after reduction of the antihypertensive regimen (5), as an option for patients who are not candidates for surgical revascularization treatments.

Limb shaking TIAs caused by carotid artery occlusive disease are an important differential diagnosis in patients presenting with a history of brief focal episodes of jerky involuntary movements affecting one limb and should be seriously considered in subjects with vascular risk factors.

REFERENCES

1. Baumgartner RW. Vasomotor reactivity is exhausted in transient ischaemic attacks with limb shaking. *J Neurol Neurosurg Psychiatry*. 1998;65:561–564.
2. Fisher CM. Concerning recurrent transient cerebral ischemic attacks. *Can Med Assoc J*. 1962;86:1091–1099.
3. Knoflach M, Matosevic B, Meinhart M, et al. Prognostic relevance of limb shaking in symptomatic carotid artery occlusion. *Cerebrovasc Dis*. 2011;32:35–40.
4. Persoon S, Kappelle LJ, Klijn CJ. Limb-shaking transient ischaemic attacks in patients with internal carotid artery occlusion: a case-control study. *Brain*. 2010;133:915–922.
5. Leira EC, Ajax T, Adams HP, Jr. Limb-shaking carotid transient ischemic attacks successfully treated with modification of the antihypertensive regimen. *Arch Neurol*. 1997;54:904–905.
6. Ogasawara K, Ogawa A, Yoshimoto T. Cerebrovascular reactivity to acetazolamide and outcome in patients with symptomatic internal carotid or middle cerebral artery occlusion: a xenon-133 single-photon emission computed tomography study. *Stroke*. 2002;33:1857–1862.
7. Klijn CJ, Kappelle LJ, van Huffelen AC, et al. Recurrent ischemia in symptomatic carotid occlusion: prognostic value of hemodynamic factors. *Neurology*. 2000;55:1806–1812.
8. Baquis GD, Pessin MS, Scott RM. Limb shaking—a carotid TIA. *Stroke*. 1985;16:444–448.
9. Tatemichi TK, Young WL, Prohovnik I, et al. Perfusion insufficiency in limb-shaking transient ischemic attacks. *Stroke*. 1990;21:341–347.
10. Yanagihara T, Piepgras DG, Klass DW. Repetitive involuntary movement associated with episodic cerebral ischemia. *Ann Neurol*. 1985;18:244–250.

84

A Stiff and Jerky Person: How Useful Is a DAT Scan in the Differential Diagnosis?

NICOLA MODUGNO, GIOVANNI FABBRINI,
CARLO COLOSIMO, AND ALFREDO BERARDELLI

THE CASE

A 55-year-old general practitioner was seen in our department because of severe generalized stiffness and involuntary movements in the left lower limb. Symptoms had begun 6 years earlier with clumsiness in the left leg when walking. In the subsequent years, his gait difficulties progressively increased, with jerks in the left lower limb and falls. In the year before coming to our attention, he was unable to walk and had started displaying speech problems and urinary incontinence. An initial neurologic evaluation suggested a diagnosis of "upper motor neuron syndrome or stiff person syndrome." He underwent numerous diagnostic tests, including spine and brain MRI; serologic tests for Borrelia, EBV, VZV, HTLV 1, HSV, CMV, HIV, and VDRL; research for anticerebellar, antigliadin, antiglutamic acid decarboxylase, and anti-TP b2 glycoprotein antibodies; and genetic testing for SPG4 and SPG7 mutations, although all were negative. Cerebral 18-fluorodeoxyglucose positron emission tomography (18FDG-PET) disclosed hypometabolism in the right medial and superior motor cortex, particularly in the leg and foot area.

THE APPROACH

When we first saw the patient, the neurologic examination disclosed stiffness in the lower extremities (very severe in the left lower limb). He also had dystonia in the left upper limb and jerks in the left lower and upper limbs. The patient was unable to stand or walk unassisted. Tendon reflexes were bilaterally brisk but Babinski's sign was absent. Apraxia was observed in the left arm. He had severe dysarthria and displayed delayed initiation of the horizontal saccadic eye movements. Neuropsychological testing yielded a normal Mini-Mental State Examination (MMSE) score of 30, although deficits in attention, constructive praxis, and visuospatial memory were detected. A brain MRI (3T) revealed mild atrophy of the rolandic and postrolandic cortical regions, with paramagnetic deposition in the cortical layers. Surface electromyography (EMG) investigation of the muscles in the lower limbs unveiled the presence of noncontinuous, arrhythmic, short bursts in the left arm and leg at rest, during voluntary activity, and after acoustic and exteroceptive stimuli, which were compatible with a diagnosis of myoclonic jerks. Somatosensory evoked potentials showed slight asymmetry in the P33-N40 amplitude (left > right). The electroencephalography (EEG) recording was normal. Because the presence of rigidity and jerks pointed to a possible parkinsonism, we investigated the presynaptic dopaminergic terminals by assessing the striatal dopamine transporter (DAT) with single photon emission tomography (SPECT). This examination revealed an asymmetric (right > left) and severely reduced distribution of radiotracer in the caudate and putamen. Attempts to find an effective therapy using levodopa, diazepam, baclofen, amantadine, and anticholinergics did not yield any improvement in the motor symptoms.

THE LESSON

Several possible diagnoses, including motor neuron disease, stiff person syndrome, and atypical parkinsonism, were considered for this patient. A progressive asymmetric pyramidal syndrome was suspected by the neurologist who first saw this patient. Although primary lateral sclerosis can start in the lower limb asymmetrically, the absence of clear pyramidal signs and the presence of jerks, dystonia, and apraxia would be unusual in a pure disorder of the pyramidal system (1). Stiff person syndrome is usually characterized by progressive muscular rigidity affecting the axial muscles in the back, abdomen, hips, and shoulders and stiffness of the legs when walking. Stiff person syndrome may present with initial or major involvement of a lower limb. The diagnosis of stiff person syndrome was, however, unlikely given the lack of painful spasms, the presence of dystonia and apraxia, and EMG-documented continuous voluntary contraction activity of the agonist and antagonist muscles (2); finally, serum high-titer anti-GAD antibodies, which are present in the majority of patients with stiff person syndrome (3), were absent in this patient. Bearing in mind the asymmetrical motor involvement observed in this patient, yet another possibility was corticobasal degeneration (CBD). The diagnosis of CBD may prove difficult, as suggested by a recent report indicating that movement disorders specialists correctly identify only 45% of patients with this disease (4). The presence of myoclonic jerks and limb apraxia supported the hypothesis of CBD in the patient we describe here. A recent clinicopathologic study of corticobasal syndrome suggested that the main clinical features in patients with pathologically proven CBD are a varying combination of clumsy useless limb, apraxia, action myoclonus, focal limb dystonia, cortical sensory loss, alien limb, stimulus-sensitive myoclonus, and delayed initiation of horizontal saccades (4). Some of these symptoms were present in our patient, although the onset in the lower limb as opposed to the upper limb (5) and the early inability to walk cannot be considered classic features of CBD. The striatal DAT assessment with SPECT proved to be extremely useful in this patient by revealing reduced dopaminergic presynaptic terminals. Indeed, although the DAT scan does have diagnostic limitations, including possible false-positive and false-negative results (and it has never been studied in stiff person syndrome), in this case, it played a crucial role by demonstrating dopaminergic degeneration, suggesting a possible diagnosis of CBD.

REFERENCES

1. Gordon PH, Cheng B, Katz IB, et al. The natural history of primary lateral sclerosis. *Neurology*. 2006;66, 647–653.
2. Lockman J, Burns TM. Stiff-person syndrome. *Curr Treat Options Neurol*. 2007;9:234–240.
3. Alexopoulos H, Dalakas MC. A critical update on the immunopathogenesis of Stiff Person Syndrome. *Eur J Clin Invest*. 2010;40:1018–1025.
4. Ling H, O'Sullivan SS, Holton JL, et al. Does corticobasal degeneration exist? A clinicopathological re-evaluation. *Brain*. 2010;133:2045–2057.
5. Lalive PH, Personeni O, Slosman DO, et al. Lower limb corticobasal degeneration. *Eur Neurol*. 2000;44:248–249.

85

The Torture of Tortuosity: Lessons From a 45-Year-Old Woman With Myoclonus, Dystonia, Chorea, and Ataxia

BART P.C. VAN DE WARRENBURG AND BASTIAAN R. BLOEM

THE CASE

A 45-year-old woman was referred to us because of severe right arm weakness during chemotherapy that she received as part of treatment for her right-sided breast cancer. She had already undergone a radical mastectomy and radiotherapy over the ipsilateral chest wall and supraclavicular and axillary lymph node regions (total dose of 45 Gy in 20 daily fractions). In summary, a diagnosis of radiation-induced brachial plexopathy was made, but the radiotherapist felt that this complication was unexpected given the relatively low (45 Gy) dose. Noticeable also was a desquamation involving more than half of the irradiated area, which developed about 3 weeks after radiotherapy.

Her previous medical history revealed longstanding, unexplained choreoathetosis. Involuntary movements were already apparent in her first year of life, evident as twisting movements of the neck and arms, with additional jerks of the head and shoulders. She underwent extensive investigations in the pediatric department, of which we have no records. The involuntary movements did not show much progression, and the jerks turned out to respond to alcohol. At the age of 40 years, she was investigated in another hospital, and a diagnosis of myoclonus dystonia was made. However, mutation analysis of the epsilon-sarcoglycan gene (*DYT11*) was negative. When we first saw her, she mentioned that gait and balance difficulties had evolved over the past few years, and more recently, she had also noticed speech difficulties. Family history revealed breast carcinoma in the mother but no neurologic diseases.

On examination, we noted skin fibrosis over the right chest wall; tortuous and dilated vessels in the medial corner of the left eye; a severe disturbance of voluntary gaze in all directions, compatible with oculomotor apraxia; cerebellar dysarthria; dystonia of the neck and left arm; lightning jerks of the head and neck; generalized but mild chorea; some upper limb ataxia; an ataxic gait; complete right-arm paralysis; absence of tendon reflexes; and downgoing plantars. Investigations were requested (see below).

During the following years, our patient was increasingly suffering from radiation-induced complications, including a mediastinal shift due to progressive chest fibrosis. Three years after radiotherapy, a Philadelphia translocation–positive chronic myeloid leukemia was diagnosed, which was successfully treated. She was then admitted repeatedly because of herpes simplex I infection, pneumonia, and gastroenteritis. Her neurologic condition worsened, and 4 years after her initial diagnosis of breast cancer, the patient died.

THE APPROACH

When confronted with a patient with a mixed, complex movement disorder, we advocate the approach as shown in Figure 85.1A (1). How this approach works for the case presented here is illustrated in Figure 85.1B.

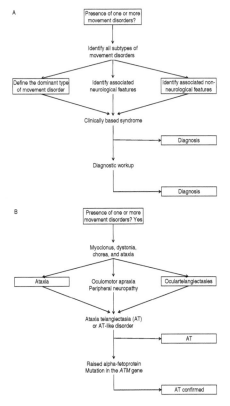

FIGURE 85.1

(A) Systematic approach to the diagnosis in patients presenting with movement disorders. (B) The approach applied to the case presented here. Adapted from Ref. 1.

Central to this approach is the identification of all different types of movement disorders that are present within a given patient. This is then followed by labeling one of these movement disorders as the dominant one. The term "dominant" here applies to the movement disorder that offers the best leads with respect to the differential diagnosis and the subsequent diagnostic workup. The dominant movement disorder is thus not necessarily the clinically dominant feature, but rather the diagnostically most informative one. This is particularly relevant for cerebellar ataxia, the presence of which—even when subtle—has great clinical value because it narrows the differential diagnosis significantly. For example, in a patient with marked action tremor of the hands, the presence of mild cerebellar ataxia should put us on the "ataxia path" rather than the "tremor path."

In our patient, the clinical picture was dominated by myoclonus dystonia, but mild chorea and cerebellar ataxia were also present. As pointed out earlier, we often select ataxia as the dominant feature when this is present. The next step in our diagnostic approach (Figure 85.1A) is to identify additional neurologic symptoms or signs, which in the present case were a gross abnormality in making any voluntary saccades (which is termed oculomotor apraxia) and perhaps a peripheral neuropathy (as suggested by the complete absence of deep tendon reflexes). Finally, one must then identify potentially relevant non-neurologic features, which in our patient was the presence of ocular telangiectasias, multiple forms of cancer, and the excessive skin response to radiation.

These combined, integrated elements lead to a clinically based syndrome. Our patient's clinical syndrome was that of ataxia telangiectasia (AT) or an AT-like disorder, such as ataxia with oculomotor apraxia types 1 and 2. Given the recent history of breast cancer at a young age, the second cancer type shortly thereafter (chronic myeloid leukemia), and the severe adverse events of low-dose radiotherapy, we had a strong suspicion that this was AT.

The initial confirmatory investigation that we requested was the alpha-fetoprotein level, which was 146.4 mcg/L (normal <3.0 mcg/L), followed by mutation analysis of the *ATM* gene. This showed a single mutation c.8147T>C (p.Val2716Ala) in exon 57 in the *ATM* gene. Although AT is a recessive disorder, a single heterozygote may also display symptoms. The course of the resulting disease is generally milder than in those with homozygous or compound heterozygous mutations, presumably because affected subjects still have some residual ATM kinase activity (2). The disease course in the case presented here testifies this.

THE LESSON

This case history teaches us at least three important lessons. The first is to adopt a systematic approach when a patient presents with a mixed movement disorder (Figure 85.1A) and, particularly, to invest in deciding which of the observed movement disorders is the dominant one, in terms of leading the diagnostic path. The individual weight that can be attributed to the various types of movement disorders differs. For example, it is low for tremor, whereas it is high for cerebellar ataxia. If physical examination shows cerebellar ataxia, even when mild, it is often rewarding to classify this as the dominant movement disorder.

Second, AT can present with atypical phenotypes. Classic AT, usually related to homozygous or compound heterozygous *ATM* mutations, is characterized by early-onset progressive cerebellar ataxia, oculomotor apraxia, oculocutaneous telangiectasias, immunodeficiency, diabetes, a predisposition to malignancies, and an increased sensitivity to radiation and alkylating drugs. Median age at death is approximately 20 years. Milder phenotypes occur not only in patients with only one mutation but also in those carrying two mutations and are often characterized by a childhood-onset extrapyramidal movement disorder (mostly chorea, dystonia, or both), with cerebellar ataxia manifesting much later, often in adulthood. The importance of making the correct diagnosis is the fact that patients with these milder phenotypes still have an increased risk of malignancies (3).

Third, there is also a lesson for oncologists and radiotherapists. When they see a patient with a malignancy who has a history of unexplained ataxia or other movement disorders, AT should be suspected and investigated for before installing treatment. Increased levels of alpha-fetoprotein almost prove the diagnosis in this setting, and thus offer an easy screening tool. If the malignancy does require radiation treatment or chemotherapy with alkylating agents, one should be very cautious about—and possibly refrain from—radiotherapy. This particular message motivated us to also write up this case for oncologists and radiotherapists (4).

REFERENCES

1. Abdo WF, van de Warrenburg BP, Burn DJ, et al. The clinical approach to movement disorders. *Nat Rev Neurol.* 2010;6:29–37.
2. Taylor AM, Byrd PJ. Molecular pathology of ataxia telangiectasia. *J Clin Pathol.* 2005;58:1009–1015.
3. Verhagen MM, Abdo WF, Willemsen MA, et al. Clinical spectrum of ataxia-telangiectasia in adulthood. *Neurology.* 2009;73:430–437.
4. Mandigers CM, van de Warrenburg BP, Strobbe LJ, et al. Ataxia telangiectasia: the consequences of a delayed diagnosis. *Radiother Oncol.* 2011;99:97–98.

86

On the Priority of Clinical Diagnosis:
A Complex Case With Myoclonus

FRANZISKA HOPFNER AND GÜNTHER DEUSCHL

THE CASE

An 18-year-old woman was referred by another neurologic hospital to clarify the etiology of her symptoms leading to intensive care treatment. When she was transferred to our department, she was sedated, ventilated through a tracheostoma, and feeded with a percutaneous endoscopic gastrostomy (PEG). She was positive for methicillin-resistant *Staphylococcus aureus* (MRSA), was anemic with a need for erythrocyte concentrates, and showed latent thyroid hypofunction.

Two months before admission, she suffered from back pain and symptoms of fatigue, anosmia, and optical and acoustical hallucinations. Initially, drug intoxication was assumed, and she was admitted to a psychiatric hospital, but this diagnosis could not be confirmed. During hospitalization, she presented with a generalized seizure and myoclonus, which prompted referral to a neurologic hospital. In the course of days, she became progressively somnolent and was therefore admitted to an intensive care ward. In addition, she suffered from a movement disorder with progressive generalized myoclonus, choreatic movements, and intermittent severe rigidity. Pneumonia led to intubation, and because all attempts failed to terminate ventilation, the patient needed a tracheostoma. Despite sedation with propofol and midazolam, the patient developed episodes of progressive tachycardia, tachypnea, sweating, agitation, and severe myoclonus. Rigidity was slightly improved with L-Dopa. The patient reacted to optical, acoustical, and tactile stimuli by opening her eyes, but there was no way to get in contact with her. She was not able to follow requests.

The medical history of the patient was normal for seizures, intellectual impairment, abnormal reaction to vaccination, and meningitis or other infectious disease. In her family, no neurologic disorder was reported.

THE APPROACH

At admission in our department, the patient was ventilated and sedated. She had no reaction to painful stimuli. Brainstem reflexes were preserved. She had spontaneous myoclonic movements and a slight rigidity. Reflexes were brisk, no Babinski sign. She had intermittent episodes of tachycardia, sweating, and myoclonic storms.

Cerebrospinal fluid (CSF) was normal on visual inspection; the cell count (130 cells/μL) and cell differentiation of the CSF and chemical analyses of the blood revealed nonspecific inflammation. We could not detect any pathology with electrophysiologic tests (FAEPs and SEPs, electroencephalography) and computed tomography of thorax and abdomen, a full-body positron emission tomography (PET)–MRI, and MRI of the brain.

Gynecologic examination, including an ultrasound scan of the ovaries and the abdomen, showed a tumor of 2.05 inches at the left adnexal space. However, MRI tomography of the abdomen did not confirm this but showed a nonspecific contrast enhancement in the musculi glutei mediales, the musculus obturatorius on the right side, and the musculus abductor on the left side.

The medical history, including the information about sex and age, the symptoms seizure, hyperkinesia with myoclonic movements, and rigidity combined with the psychiatric features of hallucination, led to the working diagnosis of an anti–*N*-methyl D-aspartate (NMDA) receptor encephalitis. In 2007, the condition was still labeled ovarian teratoma-associated encephalitis.

Tumor markers were negative. Antibodies against NMDA receptors, amphiphysin, glutamic acid decarboxylase (GAD), islet cell IA2, and ganglioside GM1 IgM and IgG; antibodies against Yo, Hu, Ri, and Recurerin; antibodies against ganglioside GD1b IgM and IgG; antibodies against myelin-associated glycoprotein (MAG); and antibodies against basal ganglia tissue were tested.

To our surprise, all antibodies tested turned out to be in the normal range. Particularly, NMDA receptor antibodies were negative in a certified German central laboratory. Anyhow, we assumed an autoimmunologic etiology and started a therapy with steroids, which has shown no effect on the clinical picture. After 3 weeks, we initiated a plasma separation of whole blood using a Shaldon catheter for 5 days. She regained consciousness and started to communicate nonverbally because of tracheostoma. Myoclonus was ongoing but improving. Nevertheless, the patient developed a further pneumonia as a result of *Candida* infection, a septic condition with *Acinetobacter baumanii* and *Staphylococcus hominis* and a subileus, which was treated conservatively. Overall, the general condition of the patient had worsened once again. In the meantime, a further test for antibodies against NMDA receptors was again negative, but given the clinical improvement of the first series, we decided to initiate a further daily plasma separation for 5 days.

After the second plasma separation, the patient further improved and was awake for long periods. She was able to communicate meaningfully despite tracheal cannula and indicated having had optical hallucinations.

The patient left the neurologic clinic with a significantly improved general condition to a rehabilitation hospital. After more than 8 weeks of intensive care treatment, with more than 2 weeks of artificial ventilation, a third analysis for antibodies performed in the British reference laboratory (Angela Vincent) revealed a positive result for antibodies against NMDA receptors already from the first CSF sample.

THE LESSON

We conclude that the patient was affected by an acute form of encephalitis, the anti-NMDA receptor encephalitis. It is caused by autoimmune reaction against NR1 and NR2 subunits of the glutamate NMDA receptor (1,2). Different descriptions and syndromal designations for this disease were available in the medical literature before 2007, when the cause was established and it finally received its current name (3). According to a review of 100 cases, 91 of the 100 patients were women, and mean age of all patients was 23 years (range 5–76 years) (4). The disease is associated with an initial phase of illness, psychiatric symptoms or memory problems, seizures, extrapyramidal symptoms, and tumors, mostly teratomas of the ovaries (5). Thus, it is considered a paraneoplastic syndrome. However, there are a substantial number of cases with no detectable cancer.

1. Medical history and symptom analysis are key to the diagnosis.
2. If you do not trust the laboratory results, continue to find better laboratories.
3. Remain critical with your clinical diagnosis and be prepared to change. However, if laboratory findings are conflicting with your clinical diagnosis, it is often the better strategy to stay with the clinical diagnosis and to adapt the treatment strategies accordingly.

REFERENCES

1. Vitaliani R, Mason W, Ances B, et al. Paraneoplastic encephalitis, psychiatric symptoms, and hypoventilation in ovarian teratoma. *J Ann Neurol. 2005*;58:594–604.
2. Iizuka T, Sakai F, Ide T, et al. Anti-NMDA receptor encephalitis in Japan: long-term outcome without tumor removal. *Neurology. 2008*;70:504–511.
3. Dalmau J, Tüzün E, Wu HY, et al. Paraneoplastic anti-N-methyl-D-aspartate receptor encephalitis associated with ovarian teratoma. *Ann Neurol. 2007*;61:25–36.
4. Dalmau J, Gleichman AJ, Hughes EG, et al. Anti-NMDA-receptor encephalitis: case series and analysis of the effects of antibodies. *Lancet Neurol. 2008*;7:1091–1098.
5. Dalmau J, Lancaster E, Martinez-Hernandez E, et al. Clinical experience and laboratory investigations in patients with anti-NMDAR encephalitis. *Lancet Neurol. 2011*;10:63–74.

IX

Psychogenic Movement Disorder Presentations

87

Walking Out of the Psychogenic "Bizarre-Gait" Pigeonhole: A Lesson From the Psychiatry Ward

Alberto J. Espay

THE CASE

Given my interest in psychogenic disorders, the consultation team at our hospital requested an outpatient evaluation for a 33-year-old woman who was to be discharged after an admission to the psychiatry ward for new-onset psychosis and psychogenic gait. The resident indicated that in addition to inappropriate behaviors, she was not making much sense, had developed "a little girl" speech, and had no memory of recent events. The evaluation was specifically meant for me to confirm that her bizarre gait was psychogenic because every other aspect of her function was deemed as such.

I evaluated her in my clinic 3 weeks after her discharge from the hospital. As I interviewed her, it emerged that she had spent approximately 3 weeks with intractable vomiting, reportedly triggered after a remorseful confession to her husband of an extramarital affair. Although she had no memories of other events leading to the hospitalization, the notes from her admission indicated convulsive-type movements in the arms and head, screaming episodes, and a bizarre gait. She also complained of feeling that "the ground is moving." She described it as the perception of objects around her moving up and down.

Her cognitive assessment revealed 0 out of 5 words recalled at 5 minutes. There were no other overt cognitive deficits. The oculomotor examination showed upbeat nystagmus, worse on primary gaze. Her gait was wide based, short stepped, and unsteady, but its severity and her need for a walker for most of her ambulation were in no way deserving of the "bizarre" epithet. There was no knee buckling or excessive swaying.

THE APPROACH

Elements of the history elicited doubts about the psychogenic nature of her problems. Her 3-week long intractable vomiting had caused an amnestic picture with retention of her identity (loss of identity would certainly increase the odds for a truly psychogenic presentation). The "ground is moving" complaint suggested oscillopsia and begged for a careful examination of her oculomotor function, which had not been previously done. She was confirmed to have upbeat nystagmus, much rarer in a movement disorders clinic than the downbeat variant. This finding in the setting of ataxia and amnesia, preceded by a history of protracted vomiting, should have brought to mind a nutritional disorder, particularly thiamine (B_1) deficiency. The brain MRI from her admission to the psychiatry ward was retrieved and reviewed in light of a revised assessment of her deficits. In fact, mild symmetric signal increase in the medial thalamic nuclei had been missed. Thiamine replacement was initiated intravenously (500 mg) for a week, followed by daily oral supplementation. Within a month, the oscillopsia disappeared and the abnormal signal intensity on MRI normalized. Her gait, however, improved only modestly, possibly due to a delay in initiation of therapy.

THE LESSONS

The statements regarding a "little girl" speech and "bizarre" gait wrongly seeded the mind of those assessing this patient in the psychiatry ward. She had been pigeonholed as psychogenic, and I bought the story and complied with the request of an outpatient evaluation without the urgency that her condition truly warranted. My complacency with the telephone summary of her case prevented an unbiased assessment of this patient and timely initiation of treatment. If a careful evaluation had taken place at the outset, the rapid development of ataxia and nystagmus in the setting of anterograde amnesia (with or without "bizarre" psychiatric elements) should have suggested the diagnosis of Wernicke's encephalopathy. Upbeat nystagmus is uncommon and has a relatively short differential list, which includes Wernicke's encephalopathy and paramedian lesions in the medulla and, less commonly, pons and midbrain (1). The upbeat nystagmus of Wernicke's encephalopathy should be present in primary gaze (not just evoked exclusively on upgaze) and may be suppressed or converted to downbeat nystagmus on convergence. In addition, there may be atypical symptoms such as optic neuropathy, papilledema, deafness, seizures, asterixis, weakness, or sensory and motor neuropathy developing as late as 18 months after bariatric surgery complicated with thiamine deficiency (2). The full triad of eye signs (nystagmus with or without ophthalmoplegia and ptosis), global confusion and ataxia of gait, is seen only in a minority of patients.

REFERENCES

1. Kim JS, Yoon B, Choi KD, et al. Upbeat nystagmus: clinicoanatomical correlations in 15 patients. *J Clin Neurol.* 2006;2:58–65.
2. Singh S, Kumar A. Wernicke encephalopathy after obesity surgery: a systematic review. *Neurology.* 2007;68: 807–811.

88

My Unforgettable Parkinson Patient With Psychogenic Tremors

KELVIN L. CHOU

THE CASE

I will never forget this patient. He was a 62-year-old right-handed man who presented to the movement disorders clinic with incoordination of his right hand and micrographia. He had also noticed dragging of the right leg but did not have a tremor. My examination demonstrated a mildly masked facial expression, soft speech, bradykinesia, and mild rigidity confined to the right side, but no rest or action tremor. He had no other significant medical or psychiatric history. I initiated pramipexole therapy at a dose of 1.5 mg daily. He had improved function in his right hand and was happy with the treatment.

About 1 year after starting pramipexole, he came back to the clinic urgently with the sudden onset of right-hand tremor. It had started over a weekend and was present "constantly." On examination, it was moderate in severity and present both at rest and with maintenance of posture. The tremor improved with finger-nose-finger testing but did not go away. The tremor did not diminish when going from resting state to a postural state; therefore, it was not a "re-emergent" rest tremor. There was a pill-rolling component to the tremor at rest, but it seemed faster than the typical 3 to 6 Hz seen in Parkinson's disease. It was not distractible, nor was there obvious variability. He had cogwheeling in the right hand but not the left. He had diminished amplitude with fine finger movements on the right but not the left. He did not have any other neurologic signs such as weakness, numbness, and speech or vision problems. His other parkinsonian symptoms did not seem to be worse at the time, although he was having difficulty using that right hand to write and type. If that was the only limitation, he stated that he could work around those problems because he owned his own insurance company. However, he felt that he was losing clients because of the visibility of the tremor.

THE APPROACH

Because of the rather sudden onset of his tremor, MRI brain imaging was obtained, which was unremarkable. Complete blood counts, a comprehensive metabolic panel, thyroid-stimulating hormone, and urinalysis were within normal limits. The rest of his neurologic examination, including mental status, cranial nerves, strength, sensation, and coordination, was unremarkable. Although the onset of tremor was unusual, because it was unilateral and he had a diagnosis of Parkinson's disease with response to dopaminergic medications, his pramipexole was increased over the next few weeks to 4.5 mg daily. Despite the increase in dosage, the severity of his tremor worsened. Over the next 3 months, trihexyphenidyl was added and titrated up to 6 mg daily without effect on the tremor. Levodopa was then started and titrated to 600 mg daily, also without effect on the tremor.

After being on these medications for about a month, his wife started calling, saying that her husband was having strange behaviors. For example, in the middle of the night, he would get up to go to the bathroom, but instead of urinating in the toilet, he would urinate in the garbage can in the kitchen. He was also having visual hallucinations, and he was not able to complete tasks at work.

He was brought back to the clinic for a re-evaluation. He performed well on bedside mental status testing and stated that he could not recall any of the events his wife had related. He had continued severe tremor present at rest and with maintenance of posture in the right hand only without significant impairment in bradykinesia or gait. Again, this tremor was not clearly distractible, nor was it inconsistent. At this visit, I specifically asked him about stress in his life, and he denied any. There were no problems with work that occurred before the onset of his tremor, and he denied marital or family problems. There was no personal history of physical or sexual abuse. Blood work and urinalysis were repeated but were again unremarkable. Routine electroencephalography (EEG) was read as normal. I recommended that he wean off his trihexyphenidyl and pramipexole because of the hallucinations but instructed him to stay on his levodopa.

He then was lost to follow-up, but about a year after this visit, he showed up in clinic again. He was taking only 600 mg of levodopa, and he had no tremor. The rest of his examination was virtually unchanged from a year before. He told me that his wife had divorced him 3 months ago, and the day after the papers were signed, his tremors disappeared. His business was starting to improve, and he stated that he had a new and improved outlook on life. I saw him once more before I accepted a position at another institution, but he continued to have no evidence of tremor.

THE LESSON

Psychogenic movement disorders are movement disorders believed to be the result of underlying psychological factors and unrelated to a primary neurologic or medical cause (1). They comprise 3% to 4% of all patients seen in movement disorders clinics (2,3), with psychogenic tremor being the most common form (4,5).

Although tremor is common in Parkinson's disease, there were a few features of the tremor in this case that were inconsistent with a typical Parkinsonian tremor. First, the tremor seemed to be equally severe at rest and with maintenance of posture without a short period of improvement that would suggest a re-emergent rest tremor. This would be an unusual combination for parkinsonian tremor. The tremor was also faster than the typical parkinsonian frequency of 3 to 6 Hz. By themselves, these features would not necessarily suggest a psychogenic tremor, but this patient had a fairly sudden onset of tremor, appearing over the course of a weekend, which would be consistent with a psychogenic tremor (6). Unfortunately, I could not convince myself that the tremors were variable in amplitude, direction, or frequency. They also were not entrainable or distractible, other features commonly seen with psychogenic tremor (4). The patient denied stress or other psychological causes for his tremor. It was not until the tremor disappeared and the stressful cause of it was identified that the diagnosis of a psychogenic tremor became clear. In hindsight, the patient admitted that he and his wife had arguments fairly frequently, but he thought that "all married couples did that." Because I was not convinced that this was purely psychogenic, I still had to rule out other metabolic or infectious etiologies, and I ended up treating it as if it were a worsening of Parkinson's disease.

For me, this case was a great example of how stress can result in abnormal movements. It was even more difficult in this instance to diagnose because it occurred in a patient with a reason to have tremors (Parkinson's disease). I always use this case whenever I try to counsel someone whom I think has a psychogenic movement disorder because it demonstrates the connection between mental stress and physical manifestations of stress. It also demonstrates the fact that many patients may not be able to identify the source of the stress, even though it is clearly present.

REFERENCES

1. Kranick S, Ekanayake V, Martinez V, et al. Psychopathology and psychogenic movement disorders. *Mov Disord*. 2011;26:1844–1850.
2. Factor SA, Podskalny GD, Molho ES. Psychogenic movement disorders: frequency, clinical profile, and characteristics. *J Neurol Neurosurg Psychiatry*. 1995;59:406–412.
3. Portera-Cailliau C, Victor D, Frucht S, et al. Movement disorders fellowship training program at Columbia University Medical Center in 2001–2002. *Mov Disord*. 2006;21:479–485.
4. Bhatia KP, Schneider SA. Psychogenic tremor and related disorders. *J Neurol*. 2007;254:569–574.
5. Jankovic J, Vuong KD, Thomas M. Psychogenic tremor: long-term outcome. *CNS Spectr*. 2006; 11:501–508.
6. Kenney C, Diamond A, Mejia N, et al. Distinguishing psychogenic and essential tremor. *J Neurol Sci*. 2007;263:94–99.

89

Bizarre "Exorcist-Like" Movements and Behavioral Change in an Adolescent Filipino: A Mystery Case

LILLIAN V. LEE, MA. LOURDES EBERO,
NELMA MAGPUSAO, AND JOSE ROBLES

THE CASE

A previously healthy, third-year high-school, 14-year-old girl was brought to the emergency department (ED) because of "seizures." Two days earlier, she complained of right frontal throbbing headache followed a few minutes later by unresponsiveness, rolling of the eyeballs, chewing movements, and squeezing motions of both hands. The event lasted less than a minute. She had no recall of the event. The event recurred two more times, but on the day of admission, there was associated drooling noted. At the ED, she was afebrile with stable vital signs. Physical and neurologic examinations were normal. Routine blood works were also normal. In the wards, she had repeated unprovoked stiffening of all extremities for a few seconds with associated upward gaze. Electroencephalography (EEG) showed a single event with EEG correlate of slowing, but no epileptiform discharges were recorded. She was placed on an antiepileptic drug (AED) valproic acid and discharged for outpatient follow-up.

THE APPROACH

A day after discharge, jerking of all extremities recurred, prompting readmission. The dose of her valproic acid was increased. On her first hospital day, she was oriented with no neurologic deficits noted. However, she would look intermittently around the room as if searching for something. She started talking to herself and had episodes of blank staring. She could however follow commands and answered appropriately to questions in between the episodes. On the second hospital day, she developed intermittent low- to moderate-grade fever. She began to exhibit restlessness and agitation. She would often pace back and forth in her room. She had poor recall of recent events. Her valproic acid assay level at this time was increased to 173 mcg/mL; therefore, the dose of valproate was reduced. On the fifth day of hospital stay, there was resolution of fever. However, she started to have labile mood with inappropriate affect. She would "hum" to herself and would beat to a rhythm. She was extremely agitated and restless in the evening with shouting episodes. During such attacks, she appeared frightened of the people around her and would fling her arms in the air as if to ward off attackers. This occurred intermittently while awake. Cerebrospinal fluid (CSF) analysis was normal. MRI of the brain was unremarkable. The possibility of viral encephalitis was entertained, and she was started on intravenous acyclovir. During the succeeding days, she became disoriented, incoherent, and unable to follow commands. On her 10th hospital day, she became abulic and anorexic with persistent episodes of combativeness. She was started on low-dose risperidone and clonazepam. CSF studies for herpes simplex virus (HSV) and Japanese B. enzyme-linked immunosorbent assay (ELISA) were negative. For the remainder of the 5 days of her hospital stay, she exhibited a terrified look in her eyes, with episodes of opening her mouth wide and throwing her head back. She would draw her knees to her chest and thrust her head forward and would

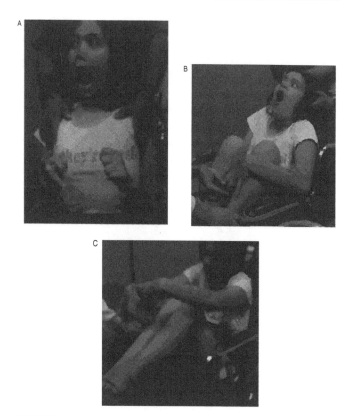

FIGURE 89.1
(A–C) Focus taken in sequence from a video clip showing the "possessed exorcist-like movements" as described in the text.

moan in pain. She uttered guttural sounds. She would extend her legs and raise her arms as if something was pulling them forward—her fingers twisted in a knot and her mouth wide open to let out a soundless scream. This recurred several times in an hour (see Figure 89.1). She was referred to a psychiatrist because of the "possessed exorcist-like" picture of her movements. An antipsychotic drug was prescribed (risperidone).

There was no significant improvement in her behavior. Therefore, her parents decided to bring her out of the hospital. She was brought to a faith healer with the parents thinking her symptoms were due to demonic possession. Her parents decided to discontinue all her medications. A week after leaving the hospital, she refused to eat and became withdrawn. Three days before she was brought to the hospital, she had episodes of jerking of all extremities. On the night of her death, she had generalized stiffening, which lasted for an hour. On the way to the hospital, she became cyanotic and apneic. An hour later, she was pronounced dead on arrival at the ED.

THE LESSON

This 14-year-old adolescent girl presented with seizures followed by psychotic-like behavior and bizarre movements. The possibility of a psychogenic movement disorder was initially entertained.

However, she deteriorated, clinically manifesting with more bizarre dyskinesias and more frequent "seizure-like episodes." When she was brought out of the hospital against medical advice, the medications, which included anticonvulsants, were abruptly withdrawn. It is very possible that the abrupt withdrawal of the AED precipitated status epilepticus and caused her death.

The possible considerations based on the triad of behavioral change, seizures, and dyskinesias are:

1. Viral encephalitis (however, no viral etiology was demonstrated by culture).
2. Immune-mediated limbic encephalitis.
3. Anti–*N*-methyl-D-aspartate encephalitis.
4. Paraneoplastic autoimmune encephalitis.
5. Subacute sclerosing panencephalitis (SSPE) (she however did not manifest the usual myoclonic movements seen in SSPE and no measles antibodies were demonstrated).

The paucity of imaging findings and the negative viral studies should have alerted the service to other causes such as paraneoplastic and nonparaneoplastic encephalitis and immune-mediated limbic encephalitis, including *N*–methyl-D-aspartate receptor encephalitis. A high index of suspicion is necessary for prompt institution of immunosuppressive treatment that might have modified the disease process and might have prevented a fatal outcome.

Suggested Reading

Kataoka H, Dalmau J, Ueno S. Paraneoplastic encephalitis associated with ovarian teratoma and *N*-methyl-D-aspartate receptor antibodies. *Eur J Neurol.* 2008;15:e5–e6.

Erdem T. Limbic encephalitis associated with antibodies to cell membrane antigens. *Arch Neuropsychiatry.* 2007;44:101–107.

Dalmau J, Gleichman AJ, Hughes EG, et al. Anti-NMDA-receptor encephalitis: case series and analysis of the effects of antibodies. *Lancet Neurol.* 2008;7:1091–1098.

Dale RC, Church AJ, Surtees RAH, et al. Encephalitis lethargica syndrome: 20 new cases and evidence of basal ganglia autoimmunity. *Brain.* 2004;127:21–33.

90

Intermittent Tunnel Vision in a Patient With Multiple Drug Abuse History

KATRIN BÜRK, ADAM STRELCZYK, AND WOLFGANG H. OERTEL

THE CASE

This 29-year-old male patient reported sudden attacks of intermittent neurologic deficits starting at the age of 18 years. During these episodes, his ability to see was impaired by some sort of tunnel vision, although he did not experience any problems in moving his eyes voluntarily. Furthermore, he was not able to speak properly, and he was not capable of properly moving his arms and legs. His limbs felt flabby and adynamic. He also reported mild dizziness. One attack would last 1 to 2 hours, and in rare cases, up to 4 hours. The frequency was two to three attacks per week with free intervals of up to 3 weeks. Episodes could be provoked by stress, heat, or excitement. During the attacks, there was no memory impairment or loss of consciousness. Attacks never occurred during sleep.

The patient had a history of multiple drug abuse (cannabis, heroine, amphetamines). He described relief of neurologic symptoms after amphetamine consumption. In other respects, the medical chart was unremarkable (normal pregnancy, birth, and motor milestones; no history of febrile seizures or generalized tonic-clonic seizures; no head trauma; no infections). The patient had been seen by many neurologists and psychiatrists before. So far, imaging and electroencephalographic investigations had always been considered normal. The patient was currently treated for depression with psychosomatic symptoms but had never received anticonvulsants.

The patient had two brothers and one sister. The latter has been followed up for behavioral problems. Both parents were still alive and denied any history of neurologic or psychiatric disorders.

The parents had divorced when the patient was 15 years old. After his certificate of secondary education, he had started vocational training as a gardener and painter but did not complete both. When working as a painter, he had dropped from the scaffold several times during attacks. Currently, he had not held down a job for about 8 years.

THE APPROACH

Because of the intermittent character of neurologic symptoms, epileptic seizures or transitory ischemic attacks could not be ruled out, and the patient was referred to the Department of Neurology.

Between attacks, the general physical and neurologic examination was normal except for impaired smooth pursuit to the left. A series of studies were then performed. Electrocardiogram (ECG) and echocardiography were normal. Caloric testing showed symmetrical vestibular excitability. Routine laboratory testing revealed a slight increase of creatine kinase, creatinine, and liver enzymes. Video-electroencephalographic monitoring (4 days and nights) revealed symmetrical occipital activity of 8/s with no focal dysfunction or epileptic discharges. Activity during sleep was unremarkable. During the monitoring, a 2-hour attack could be registered that was not accompanied by any EEG correlate. The patient complained of dizziness and tunnel vision. Clinically, he presented with marked dysarthria and moderate ataxia of stance and gait requiring assistance. Limb ataxia was more pronounced on the left side. Routine MRI excluded structural peculiarities. MRI spectroscopy yielded normal cerebellar pH values. During attacks, diffusion-weighted imaging did not show any abnormalities.

Recurrent episodes of intermittent cerebellar dysfunction with dysarthria and ataxia of gait, stance, and limbs suggested episodic ataxia (EA). The disease duration of several hours was compatible with EA type 2 (EA2). Indeed, direct sequencing established a molecular genetic diagnosis of EA2 with heterozygosity for exon 32 c.4984C>T, p.R1662X-mutation in the *CACNA1A* gene (1). The patient received acetazolamide up to a daily dose of 375 mg. To avoid low potassium levels, the patient was asked to follow a potassium-rich diet (bananas, apricots, etc.). After 4 weeks of treatment, the patient reported one single attack lasting 1 hour with dysarthric speech and tunnel vision, but no dizziness or unsteadiness. The attack had been provoked by a longer walk. During the attack, the patient remained ambulatory and was able to return home without support. ECG and laboratory tests were normal. Unfortunately, the patient did not show up during the following 15 months and increased his daily dose of acetazolamide to 750 mg. Single attacks lasted only 15 to 20 minutes, but the patient developed recurrent nephrolithiasis (calcium phosphate and calcium oxalate). Under concomitant EEG and ECG monitoring, treatment was shifted to 15 mg of 4-aminopyridine per day resulting in an increased frequency and severity of attacks and continuous dizziness that had not been present before. Symptoms did not improve after increasing the daily dose to 30 mg. The patient therefore insisted on receiving acetazolamide. To prevent further development of nephrolithiasis, alkaline treatment was introduced.

THE LESSON

The patient's history of multiple drug abuse had thrown multiple investigators off the scent. Psychiatric diagnosis seemed more obvious regarding the atypical description of intermittent symptoms, with speech problems and tunnel vision being most prominent. We were fortunate to document such an attack during EEG monitoring. Symptoms could be registered and objectified. To our surprise, limb ataxia seemed more pronounced on the left body half during attacks. Between attacks, the patient presented with saccadic pursuit only to the left. This asymmetry is rather astonishing because the voltage-gated calcium channel CACNA1A is expressed throughout the central nervous system (CNS). Similarly, the patient's statement of improvement after amphetamine consumption seemed rather implausible but could be confirmed from the literature. Another noted item is the negative family history: EA2 is an autosomal dominantly inherited disorder, but in contrast to spinocerebellar ataxias, EA2 is characterized by a highly variable penetrance (2). The fact that some mutations in this gene may even present with epilepsy does not really alleviate the diagnostic situation (3).

Taken together, the present case illustrates our challenge to keep an open-minded approach to each new patient even if the complaints do not seem to be compatible with what we normally see in our daily routine.

REFERENCES

1. Jodice C, Mantuano E, Veneziano L, et al. Episodic ataxia type 2 (EA2) and spinocerebellar ataxia type 6 (SCA6) due to CAG repeat expansion in the CACNA1A gene on chromosome 19p. *Hum Mol Genet.* 1997;6:1973–1978.
2. Denier C, Ducros A, Vahedi K, et al. High prevalence of CACNA1A truncations and broader clinical spectrum in episodic ataxia type 2. *Neurology.* 1999;52:1816–1821.
3. Rajakulendran S, Graves TD, Labrum RW, et al. Genetic and functional characterisation of the P/Q calcium channel in episodic ataxia with epilepsy. *J Physiol.* 2010;588:1905–1913.

91

"Psychogenic Tremor" in a 32-Year-Old Factory Worker: The Eyes Do Not Lie!

RICHARD M. ZWEIG

THE CASE

A 32-year-old man was referred for a fourth neurologic opinion, the second by a movement disorder specialist, for tremor and gait disorder. He reported the insidious onset of unsteady gait about 15 years earlier. This was at first very slight, worsening gradually over the years. He retired from construction work at age 26 because of unsteadiness. Nevertheless, his first neurologist noted an entirely normal examination (presumably including gait) at age 28. Within the year before my evaluation, the second neurologist described his gait as "somewhat spastic but unsteady and variable." The other movement disorder specialist noted a history of staggering and impaired balance and, on examination, described his gait as "wide-based and he had shuddering in his trunk. He walked up and down the hall; the best way to describe it would be like movie characterizations of Frankenstein's monster: stiff-kneed wide-based lunging steps with simian arm posture. He did not fall but did misstep on the turn so reached for the wall. Could not tandem."

I also obtained a 6- to 7-year history of clumsiness using his upper extremities for activities of daily living such as brushing teeth and cutting food, with some assistance accepted for the latter over the previous 3 to 4 years. His voice had also become somewhat slurred in recent years. Over the previous year, the second neurologist noted "hesitant speech" on one examination, but then normal at a second, later visit. Coordination was believed to be normal. The other movement disorder specialist thought that his speech was "accented but otherwise not impaired, not ataxic." He also noted that finger-to-nose movements were "not too accurate, but he tended to not look at the target consistently, so is hard to see how he could be accurate. He avoided eye contact with me. Affect was dysphoric. Heel shin coordination was jerky but not dysmetric. On testing alternating motion rates, his leg movements looked apraxic. Hand alternating movements were close to normal."

However, despite possible abnormalities of gait and coordination, all three neurologists focused their examination, and ultimately diagnosis, on the patient's tremor. He reported to me a 6- to 7-year history of a variable tremor of his head and to a lesser degree of his upper extremities and trunk. He acknowledged that the tremor would apparently start abruptly and persist for up to days to as long as about 2 weeks before stopping, often after a "hard sleep." And then, he could go for as long as a few months with little if any tremor. He acknowledged the possibility of some relationship between tremor and stress. He specifically noted that the gait disorder, speech difficulty, and clumsiness persisted with or without the tremor. Tremor was not noted on examinations provided by the first two neurologists. The other movement disorder specialist noted a "large amplitude shuddering, no-no motion of his head, about 4 Hz. but did fluctuate." His head tremor seemed to entrain with repetitive hand movements. He had no resting, postural, or action tremor of his extremities.

Other history of note: the patient had obstructive sleep apnea and was benefiting from continuous positive airway pressure (CPAP). He acknowledged a history of depression. He denied orthostatic lightheadedness or syncope, and he had no urinary or bowel complaints. He also had no cognitive difficulties and denied smoking, heavy alcohol use, or illegal drug usage. Family history was negative for movement disorder; however, the patient did not know his father and neither the patient nor his mother had any information concerning the father's family history.

Previous workup had included a brain MRI 2 years earlier, which was reportedly normal except that the medulla appeared "slightly small." No intraparenchymal signal changes were reported. Previous laboratory studies included normal copper and ceruloplasmin levels. Medications at the time of my examination included gabapentin 300 mg twice daily with unclear benefit, alprazolam 1 mg up to three times daily as needed for tremor (with apparent benefit), and escitalopram 20 mg daily.

The first three neurologists diagnosed the patient as having psychogenic tremor.

On my examination, the patient was euthymic and cognitive testing was normal. Extraocular movements were full without nystagmus, but he had very slow horizontal and, to a lesser degree, vertical saccades. He also had absent optokinetic nystagmus. His speech was dysarthric. Cranial nerve examination was otherwise normal. On motor examination, he had normal tone and strength throughout. He had occasional titubation while seated on the examination table and an intermittent, irregular head tremor when excited or stressed. There was no resting or postural upper extremity tremor. Finger-to-nose movements were moderately dysmetric, and he had an ataxic tremor with heel–shin movements. He had difficulty with rhythmic tapping, although repetitive finger movements were fairly normal. His gait seemed to be ataxic: moderately wide based and with decreased tandem. Sensory exam, Romberg, and reflexes were normal except for absent ankle reflexes.

THE APPROACH

This patient seemed to me to be ataxic, yet imbalance and dysmetria can be mimicked or psychogenic, which was the apparent impression of two neurologists (one a movement disorder specialist) who had examined the patient within the previous year of my examination. Similarly, what I heard as dysarthria struck the other movement disorder specialist as "accented," which in a native English speaker may be psychogenic. And all three of the other neurologists were obviously impressed by the variability and inconsistency of the patient's tremor, and to the other movement disorder specialist, by its entrainment with repetitive hand movements—all suggestive of a psychogenic etiology (1). And the head tremor and reported body "shuddering" may have been psychogenic or an embellished titubation. These movements did not appear on my examination (or my report) to be choreiform, dystonic, or myoclonic.

But what impressed me most were the slow saccadic eye movements. The other neurologists had not reported this, although the movement disorder specialist noted that there was no internuclear ophthalmoplegia, so presumably checked saccadic eye movements. Although benzodiazepines, even at low dosage, can slow some saccades (2), this was not a subtle slowing, and most definitely was not psychogenic. Thus, the differential diagnosis is of a slowly progressive (i.e., degenerative) ataxia, dysarthria, and slow saccadic eye movements in an otherwise healthy young adult.

In my experience, the most common degenerative causes of slow saccades are Huntington's disease and progressive supranuclear palsy. Although Huntington's patients can be ataxic, this patient had no chorea or bradykinesia/rigidity as may be seen in the Westphal variant. He did not have other features of progressive supranuclear palsy (where slow horizontal saccades should be accompanied by absent or at least more severely affected vertical saccades). He had no ophthalmoplegia, as might be seen with a mitochondrial disturbance. A disturbance of saccadic eye movements can be a "red flag" suggesting multiple system atrophy (MSA) in ataxic or parkinsonian patients, and MSA cerebellar type was in my original differential diagnosis. However, hypometric saccades are more typical of MSA than slow saccades as seen in this patient (3). This leaves the large family of inherited spinocerebellar ataxias (SCAs). Recall that this patient had no knowledge of his paternal medical history. Of the more common of these rather rare diseases, the one most associated with slow saccades is SCA-2, which can also be associated with reduced reflexes—this patient had no ankle reflexes—and tremor (4,5). At my first office visit with this patient, a screening SCA panel was obtained, which revealed 42 CAG repeats on the affected gene, confirming a diagnosis of SCA-2.

THE LESSON

Sometimes psychogenic, or apparent psychogenic, symptoms can be a "red herring," particularly in the setting of other symptoms or signs on examination that exclude a psychogenic diagnosis. The combination of slowly progressive ataxia and very slow horizontal saccadic eye movements pointed toward a diagnosis of SCA, possibly type 2, irrespective of an inconsistent tremor, that may or may not have been psychogenic.

REFERENCES

1. Bhatia KP, Schneider SA. Psychogenic tremor and related disorders. *J Neurol.* 2007;254:569–574.
2. Masson GS, Mestre DR, Martineau F, et al. Lorazepam-induced modifications of saccadic and smooth-pursuit eye movements in humans: attentional and motor factors. *Behav Brain Res.* 2000;108:169–180.
3. Anderson T, Luxon L, Quinn N, et al. Oculomotor function in multiple system atrophy: clinical and laboratory features in 30 patients. *Mov Disord.* 2008;23:977–984.
4. Rivaud-Pechoux S, Durr A, Gaymard B, et al. Eye movement abnormalities correlate with genotype in autosomal dominant cerebellar ataxia type 1. *Ann Neurol.* 1998;43:297–302.
5. Lastres-Becker I, Rub U, Auburger G. Spinocerebellar ataxia 2 (SCA2). *Cerebellum.* 2008;7:115–124.

About the Editors

Hubert H. Fernandez, MD
Professor of Medicine (Neurology)
Cleveland Clinic Lerner College of Medicine
and
Head of Movement Disorders
Center for Neurological Restoration, Cleveland Clinic
Cleveland, Ohio

Dr Fernandez received both his BS in Biology and MD degree in the Philippines at the University of Santo Tomas and Virgen Milagrosa Institute of Medicine. He completed his internship in internal medicine at University of Pennsylvania/Pennsylvania Hospital in Philadelphia, Pennsylvania; his residency in neurology at Boston University Medical Center in Boston, Massachusetts; and his fellowship in movement disorders at Brown University in Rhode Island.

Dr Fernandez is an internationally recognized expert in movement disorders who has been voted one of the best doctors in America by his peers. After completing his medical training, he joined the faculty of Brown University School of Medicine as assistant professor of the Department of Clinical Neurosciences and served as Associate Director of the Movement Disorders Unit and Neurological Director of its Functional Neurosurgical Program. In 2003, Dr Fernandez relocated to the University of Florida, where he eventually became director of the Clinical Research Unit for Neurological and Psychiatric Disorders, vice chair of Academic Affairs, and Professor of Neurology prior to joining Cleveland Clinic. Currently, he is professor of Medicine (Neurology) at the Cleveland Clinic Lerner College of Medicine, Case Western Reserve University and the head of Movement Disorders under the Center for Neurological Restoration at Cleveland Clinic in Cleveland, Ohio. An active and productive researcher, he has initiated or participated in more than 50 clinical trials and has published his findings in well over 300 articles and abstracts on Parkinson's disease and other movement disorders. He has nearly 40 published book chapters and books to his credit, and has served on the editorial board of *Movement Disorders* and is currently an editorial board member of the *American Journal of Clinical Neurology*, *European Neurological Journal*, and *Clinical Neuropharmacology*.

Dr Fernandez is a fellow of the American Academy of Neurology, and a member of the American Neurological Association. He is currently elected as the the Co-Chair of the Parkinson Study Group and a member of the executive committee of the Dystonia Study Group; he is also an executive board member of the World Neurology Foundation. He has served as President of the Florida Society of Neurology and is the current co-medical editor of the Movement Disorders Society Web site. He is married to Dr Maria Cecilia Lansang, an endocrinologist and director of the Cleveland Clinic Diabetes In-Patient Program. They have one daughter, Annella Marie Fernandez, who is currently in 7th grade.

Marcelo Merello, MD, PhD
Professor of Neurology and Director of Neuroscience Department
Raul Carrea Institute for Neurological Research (FLENI)
and
Clinical Researcher
Consejo Nacional de Investigaciones Científicas y Técnicas (CONICET)
Buenos Aires, Argentina

Born in Argentina in 1961, Marcelo Merello graduated from Buenos Aires University School of Medicine in 1987, where he later took his PhD degree. He completed an internal medicine residency at Centro de Educación Médica e Investigaciones Clínicas (CEMIC) and then neurology residency at the Raul Carrea Institute for Neurological Research (FLENI), both in Buenos Aires. He was a research fellow in neurology at the National Hospital for Nervous Diseases Queen Square and research registrar in neurology at the Middlesex Hospital, both in London. Currently, he is the head of the Movement Disorders Section and the director of Neuroscience at FLENI. He is also currently teaching at the University of Buenos Aires and is a Professor of Neurology at the Universidad de Ciencias Empresariales y Sociales (UCES), Pontificia Universidad Católica Argentina (UCA) and the Instituto Tecnológico Buenos Aires (ITBA). He was recently appointed clinical researcher of the Consejo Nacional de Investigaciones Científicas y Técnicas (CONICET) in Buenos Aires, Argentina.

He has coauthored over 100 papers in leading peer-reviewed journals in the field, with more than 200 abstracts presentations on Parkinson's disease, dystonia, and other movement disorders in International Congresses. He has written more than 20 book chapters on movement disorders, co-edited "New Trends in Parkinson's Disease Treatment" with Andrew J. Lees, and is the author of *Psychiatric Complications of Parkinson's Disease* for Cambridge University Press, among others. He was a member of the editorial board of *Disorders*, and is currently editor-in-chief of *Archives of Neurology, Neurosurgery and Psychiatry (ARG)*; he was a member of the International Executive Committee of the Movement Disorders Society and is currently serving as the co-medical editor of the society's web page. He is married and has three children.

Acanthocytosis, 156
ACE. *See* Angiotensin converting enzyme
Activities of daily living (ADLs), 179
Adenosine A$_{2A}$ receptor antagonist, 16
Adenosine triphosphate (ATP), 179
ADHD. *See* Attention deficit hyperactivity
    disorder
ADLs. *See* Activities of daily living
AED. *See* Antiepileptic drug
AFP. *See* Alpha fetoprotein
Akinetic-rigid syndrome. *See* Parkinsonism
Alpha-fetoprotein (AFP), 194, 250
α-tocopherol transfer protein (α-*TTP*), 238–239
Amantadine, 16
Angiotensin-converting enzyme (ACE), 145
Antiepileptic drug (AED), 295
Anti-GAD syndrome, 247–248
Anti-*N*-methyl D-aspartate (NMDA), 286
Antiphospholipid syndrome (APS), 153
Antistreptolysin (ASO), 168
AOA. *See* Ataxia with oculomotor apraxia
APS. *See* Antiphospholipid syndrome
Archimedean spiral test, 123, 140
ASO. *See* Antistreptolysin
AT. *See* Ataxia telangiectasia
Ataxia. *See also* Ataxia telangiectasia (AT);
    Episodic ataxia (EA); Friedreich's ataxia;
    Spinocerebellar ataxia (SCA)
    AOA2, 249–251
    AVED, 238–239
    BHC, 243–245
    PKAN, 252–254
    psychogenic gait disorders, 259–261
    schizophrenia, 240–242
Ataxia telangiectasia (AT), 194–195, 255–256,
    281–283. *See also* Ataxia
Ataxia telangiectasia mutated gene (ATM gene), 194
Ataxia with oculomotor apraxia (AOA), 250
    type 2 (AOA2), 249–251, 256
Ataxia with vitamin E deficiency (AVED),
    238–239
ATM gene. *See* Ataxia telangiectasia mutated gene

ATP. *See* Adenosine triphosphate
Attention deficit hyperactivity disorder
    (ADHD), 178, 270
Autosomal recessive juvenile onset Parkinson's
    disease (PARK 2), 66
AVED. *See* Ataxia with vitamin E deficiency

Basal ganglia calcifications, 115–117
Bassen-Kornzweig syndrome, 241–242
Benign hereditary chorea (BHC), 243–245
Bilateral posterior-ventral pallidal
    hyperintensities, 115
Bilateral striopallidodentate calcinosis
    (BSPDC), 162–164
Bizarre exorcist-like movements, 295–297
Blood pressure (BP), 225
Blood urea nitrogen (BUN), 168
Body mass index (BMI), 217
BSPDC. *See* Bilateral striopallidodentate calcinosis

CABG. *See* Coronary artery bypass grafting
Carbonic anhydrase II (CAII), 117
Catatonia, 50–52. *See also* Schizophrenia
Catatonic schizophrenia, 51
CBC. *See* Complete blood count
CBD. *See* Corticobasal degeneration
CBF. *See* Cerebral blood flow
CBGD. *See* Corticobasal ganglionic degeneration
Central nervous system (CNS), 68, 299
Central pontine myelinolysis (CPM), 105
Central pontine myelinolysis/extrapontine
    myelinolysis (CPM/EPM), 104–106
Cerebellar ataxia, 194, 195, 247–248, 282, 285.
    See also Ataxia
Cerebral blood flow (CBF), 277
Cerebral palsy, 211–214
Cerebrospinal fluid (CSF), 57
Ceruloplasmin (CP), 253
Cervical dystonia, 232–235. *See also* Dopa-responsive
    dystonia (DRD); DYT6 dystonia; Multifocal
    dystonia; Spasmodic dysphonia (SD); Task-
    specific action dystonia; Wilson's disease (WD)

Chorea. *See also* Huntington's disease (HD);
    Parkinsonism; Sydenham's chorea (SC)
    APS, 152–154
    BSPDC, 162–164
    defiant and rebellious behavior, 172–174
    HDL syndrome, 165–167
    HDL2, 158–159
    McLeod syndrome, 155–156
    movement disorder evolution, 168–170
    nvCJD, 175–177
CJD. *See* Creutzfeldt Jakob disease
Clinical Laboratory Improvement Amendments
    (CLIA), 212
CNS. *See* Central nervous system
Complete blood count (CBC), 7, 169
Complex motor stereotypy diagnosis, 269
Compulsive behaviors, 21. *See also* Impulsive
    behaviors
Computed tomography (CT), 81, 117
Continuous positive airway pressure (CPAP), 300
Coronary artery bypass grafting (CABG), 18
Corticobasal degeneration (CBD), 80, 81, 279–280
Corticobasal-ganglionic degeneration
    (CBGD), 71, 72
CP. *See* Ceruloplasmin
CPAP. *See* Continuous positive airway pressure
CPK. *See* Creatine phosphokinase test
CPM. *See* Central pontine myelinolysis
CPM/EPM. *See* Central pontine myelinolysis/
    extrapontine myelinolysis
C-reactive protein (CRP), 98, 168
Creatine kinase (CK), 24, 250
Creatine phosphokinase test (CPK), 192
Creutzfeldt-Jakob disease (CJD), 108
CRP. *See* C-reactive protein
CSF. *See* Cerebrospinal fluid (CSF);
    Minimal cerebrospinal fluid
CT. *See* Computed tomography

DAT. *See* Dopamine transporter
DAT SPECT. *See* Dopamine transporter
    single-photon emission computed
    tomography
DBS. *See* Deep brain stimulation
DDS. *See* Dopamine dysregulation syndrome
Deep brain stimulation (DBS), 27, 122, 169,
    198–200
Defiant and rebellious behavior, 172–174
Dementia, 109. *See also* Dementia with
    Lewy bodies (DLB)
    sCJD as, 78
    subcortical, 78
    VSGP with, 77
Dementia with Lewy bodies (DLB), 80, 107–109
De novo parkinsonism, 33–34. *See also*
    Parkinsonism
Dentatorubralpallidoluysian atrophy (DRPLA),
    187–190, 244

Depakote, 180. *See also* Movement disorder (MD)
Depression, 11, 33–34
Diabetes mellitus (DM), 252
DID. *See* Dystonia improvement dystonia
Diffusion-weighted imaging (DWI), 107
DIP. *See* Drug induced parkinsonism
Disabling postural and resting tremor, 140–143
DLB. *See* Dementia with Lewy bodies
DM. *See* Diabetes mellitus
Dopamine depletion, 142
Dopamine dysregulation syndrome
    (DDS), 10–12, 31, 32
Dopamine receptor blocking drugs (DRBD), 112
Dopamine replacement therapy (DRT), 11, 12
Dopaminergic blockade, 25
Dopamine transporter (DAT), 113, 279
Dopamine transporter single-photon emission
    computed tomography
    (DAT SPECT), 107, 109
Dopaminergic choreiform, 4
Dopa-responsive dystonia (DRD), 66–69,
    224–228. *See also* Cervical dystonia;
    Dystonia-improvement-dystonia (DID);
    DYT6 dystonia; Improvement-dystonia-
    improvement (IDI); Multifocal dystonia;
    Task-specific action dystonia
DRBD. *See* Dopamine receptor blocking drugs
DRPLA. *See* Dentatorubralpallidoluysian atrophy
DRT. *See* Dopamine replacement therapy
Drug-induced parkinsonism (DIP), 111–114
DWI. *See* Diffusion weighted imaging
Dyskinesia, 95–96
    amantadine dosage, 16
    dopaminergic choreiform, 4
Dystonia, 2–6
    AT, 194–195
    cerebral palsy, 211–214
    cervical dystonia, 232–235
    DBS, 198–200
    DRD, 224–226, 228–229
    DRPLA, 187–190
    embouchure, 202
    Friedreich's ataxia, 191–193
    GM1 gangliosidosis secondary, 196–197
    multifocal dystonia, 215–216
    PKAN, 184–186
    Satoyoshi syndrome, 217–221
    SCA, 207–209
    SD, 201–202
    task-specific action dystonia, 222–223
    WD, 204–205
    zolpidem effect on movement disorders,
        229–231
Dystonia-improvement-dystonia (DID), 2. *See also*
    Cervical dystonia; Dopa-responsive dystonia
    (DRD); DYT6 dystonia; Improvement-
    dystonia-improvement (IDI); Multifocal
    dystonia; Task specific action dystonia

DYT6 dystonia, 134–136. *See also* Cervical
    dystonia; Dopa-responsive dystonia (DRD);
    Dystonia-improvement-dystonia (DID);
    Improvement-dystonia-improvement (IDI);
    Multifocal dystonia; Task-specific action
    dystonia

EA. *See* Episodic ataxia
Ear, nose, and throat (ENT), 202
EC/IC bypass. *See* Extracranial/intracranial
    bypass
EDTA. *See* Ethylenediaminetetraacetic acid
ELD. *See* External lumbar drainage
Electroencephalogram (EEG), 51, 60
Electromyography (EMG), 199, 218
ELISA. *See* Enzyme linked immune sorbent assay
Embouchure dystonia, 202
Emergency department (ED), 5, 295
EMG. *See* Electromyography
ENT. *See* Ear, nose, and throat
Enzyme-linked immune-sorbent assay
    (ELISA), 160, 295
Episodic ataxia (EA), 299. *See also* Ataxia
    type 2 (EA2), 298–299
EPM. *See* Extrapontine myelinolysis
EPS. *See* Extrapyramidal side effects
Erythrocyte sedimentation rate (ESR), 98, 153
Essential tremor (ET), 122, 123, 140
ET. *See* Essential tremor
Ethylenediaminetetraacetic acid (EDTA), 41
Excessive daytime sleepiness (EDS), 81
Excessive diurnal sleepiness (EDS), 35
External lumbar drainage (ELD), 63
Extracranial/intracranial bypass
    (EC/IC bypass), 277
Extrapontine myelinolysis (EPM), 104, 105
Extrapyramidal side effects (EPS), 112

Fahr's disease, 163
FDG. *See* Fluorodeoxyglucose
6-[^{18}F]fluoro-l-DOPA (^{18}FDOPA-PET), 140, 142
Fluid-attenuated inversion recovery
    (FLAIR), 107
    multiple MS plaques, 147
    periventricular white matter plaques, 145
    white matter MS plaque, 146
    white matter T2 hyperintensity signal, 124
Fluorodeoxyglucose (FDG), 81, 115
FMR1. *See* Fragile X mental retardation 1
FOG. *See* Freezing of gait
Fragile X mental retardation 1 (FMR1), 124
    FXTAS, 129
    molecular genetic analysis, 125
    mutations in, 124
Fragile X syndrome, 124
Fragile X tremor ataxia syndrome (FXTAS),
    122–129
Freezing of gait (FOG), 80

Friedreich's ataxia, 123, 191–193, 241.
    See also Ataxia
Frontotemporal dementia (FTD), 71
Frontotemporal dementia and parkinsonism
    (FTDP), 80, 81
FXTAS. *See* Fragile X tremor ataxia syndrome

GABA-A receptor, 180
GAD. *See* Glutamic acid decarboxylase
Gamma-aminobutyric acid (GABA), 179, 230
Gaucher's disease, 67
General practitioner (GP), 60
GH. *See* Growth hormone
Gilles de la Tourette syndrome,
    264, 266. *See also* Tics
Globus pallidus interna (GPi), 199
Glutamic acid decarboxylase (GAD), 218, 247
GM1 gangliosidosis secondary dystonia, 196–197
GP. *See* General practitioner
GPi. *See* Globus pallidus interna
Growth hormone (GH), 245
GTP Cyclohydrolase I. *See* Guanosine
    triphosphate cyclohydrolase I
Guanosine triphosphate (GTP), 179, 228
Guanosine triphosphate cyclohydrolase I
    (GTP Cyclohydrolase I), 211
    autosomal dominant, 213
    deletion analysis, 212
    DRD, 228
    mutation effect, 211, 213

Hallervorden-Spatz disease. *See* Pantothenate
    kinase–associated neurodegeneration
    (PKAN)
Hallucinations, 7, 8, 13–15
HD. *See* Huntington's disease
HD-like 2 (HDL2), 158–159
HDL syndrome. *See* Huntington's
    disease-like syndrome
Heart rate (HR), 225
Herpes simplex virus (HSV), 295
HPRT. *See* Hypoxanthine-guanine
    phosphoribosyltransferase
HR. *See* Heart rate
HSV. *See* Herpes simplex virus
Huntington's disease (HD), 60–61, 158, 264–265.
    See also Chorea; Parkinsonism; Sydenham's
    chorea (SC)
Huntington's disease-like syndrome
    (HDL syndrome), 165–167
Hypomania, 21, 22
Hypophonia, 40–42
Hypoxanthine-guanine
    phosphoribosyltransferase (HPRT), 178

ICA. *See* Internal carotid artery
ICU. *See* Intensive care unit
IDI. *See* Improvement-dystonia-improvement

IFET. *See* Ischemic forearm exercise test
IM lorazepam. *See* Intramuscular lorazepam
Implantable pulse generator (IPG), 27, 199–200
Improvement-dystonia-improvement (IDI), 2.
    See also Cervical dystonia; Dopa-responsive
    dystonia (DRD); Dystonia-improvement-
    dystonia (DID); DYT6 dystonia; Multifocal
    dystonia; Task-specific action dystonia
Impulse control disorder (ICD), 7–8, 20–22
Impulsive behaviors, 21, 22. *See also*
    Compulsive behaviors
Infantile neuroaxonal dystrophy (INAD), 45, 253
Intensive care unit (ICU), 4
Internal carotid artery (ICA), 276
Intramuscular lorazepam (IM lorazepam), 52
Intravenous gamma globulin (IVIgG), 219
Iodine-121-metaiodobenzylguanidine
    single-photon emission computed
    tomography (MIBG SPECT), 107
IPG. *See* Implantable pulse generator
Ischemic forearm exercise test (IFET), 218
IVIgG. *See* Intravenous gamma globulin

Kayser-Fleischer ring, 204, 205
Kufor-Rakeb syndrome (KRD), 80, 81

Lamotrigine (LTG), 266, 267
Laterocollis, 232
LE. *See* Limbic encephalitis
Lesch-Nyhan syndrome (LNS), 178–180
Levodopa dosage, 16
Levodopa-responsive parkinsonism, 67, 75
Lewy body dementia. *See* Dementia with
    Lewy bodies (DLB)
Limbic encephalitis (LE), 139
Limb shaking attack (LSA), 277
Limb shaking TIA, 276–277
LNS. *See* Lesch-Nyhan syndrome
LP. *See* Lumbar puncture
LSA. *See* Limb shaking attack
LTG. *See* Lamotrigine
Lumbar puncture (LP), 50
Lysosomal storage disease, 44

Machado-Joseph disease.
    See Spinocerebellar ataxia: type 3
Magnetic resonance imaging (MRI), 102
    brain MRI in, 142
    cerebellar atrophy on, 45
    edema in midbrain periaqueductal area, 58
    ependymitis signs, 58
    eye of the tiger sign, 185
    hydrocephalus, 58
    hypointensity of globus pallidus, 44, 45
    inhomogeneous area in left thalamus, 96
    intraventricular cysts, 58
    marked hyperdense bilateral lesions, 104
MCA. *See* Middle cerebral artery

McLeod syndrome, 155–156
MD. *See* Movement disorder
MDS. *See* Movement Disorder Society
Medical Research Council (MRC), 169, 218
MERRF. *See* Mitochondrial epilepsy with ragged
    red fibers
Methicillin-resistant *Staphylococcus aureus*
    (MRSA), 285
MIBG SPECT. *See* Iodine-121-
    metaiodobenzylguanidine single-photon
    emission computed tomography
Middle cerebral artery (MCA), 276
Minimal cerebrospinal fluid, 235
Mini-mental state examination (MMSE), 98, 279
Mitochondrial epilepsy with ragged red fibers
    (MERRF), 257–258
MLPA. *See* Multiplex ligation-dependent probe
    amplification
MMSE. *See* Mini-mental state examination
Montreal Cognitive Assessment (MoCA), 162
Morvan syndrome (MVS), 139
Movement disorder (MD), 168–170, 229–231, 276
    contracted ankle, 170
    dystonic postures, 170
    Zolpidem's effect, 230
Movement Disorder Society (MDS), 176
MRC. *See* Medical Research Council
MRI. *See* Magnetic resonance imaging
MRSA. *See* Methicillin-resistant *Staphylococcus aureus*
MS. *See* Multiple sclerosis
MSA. *See* Multiple system atrophy
Multifocal dystonia, 215–216. *See also* Cervical
    dystonia; Dopa-responsive dystonia (DRD);
    Dystonia-improvement-dystonia (DID);
    DYT6 dystonia; Improvement-dystonia-
    improvement (IDI); Task-specific action
    dystonia
Multiple sclerosis (MS), 144–149
    MS plaque lesions, 148
    multiple MS plaques, 147
    periventricular white matter plaques, 145
    white matter MS plaque, 146
Multiple system atrophy (MSA), 89, 124, 301
Multiplex ligation-dependent probe amplification
    (MLPA), 47, 212
MVS. *See* Morvan syndrome
Myoclonic jerking, 257
Myoclonus syndrome, 285, 286
Myoglobinuria, 217

NAD. *See* Neuroaxonal dystrophy
NBIA. *See* Neurodegeneration with brain iron
    accumulation
NCC. *See* Neurocysticercosis
Nerve conduction studies (NCS), 218, 250
Neuroacanthocytosis syndromes, 241
Neuroaxonal dystrophy (NAD), 45
Neurocysticercosis (NCC), 57

Neurodegeneration with brain iron accumulation
  (NBIA), 43–48, 188, 253
  cerebellar atrophy, 45
  hypointensity of globus pallidus, 45
  NBIA genetic forms, 46–47
Neuroleptic malignant syndrome
  (NMS), 24–26, 50–52
Neuromuscular junction (NMJ), 219
Neuromyotonia (NMT), 139
Neuronal ceroid lipofuscinosis, 44
Neuropsychiatric symptoms, 35
New variant Creutzfeldt-Jakob disease (nvCJD),
  175–177. *See also* Sporadic Creutzfeldt-Jakob
  disease (sCJD)
Niemann-Pick disease type C (NPC), 68, 80, 81
NMDA. *See* Anti-*N*-methyl ᴅ-aspartate
NMJ. *See* Neuromuscular junction
NMR. *See* Nuclear magnetic resonance
NMS. *See* Neuroleptic malignant syndrome
NMT. *See* Neuromyotonia
Nonparaneoplastic limbic encephalitis, 137–139
Normal pressure hydrocephalus (NPH), 63
NPC. *See* Niemann-Pick disease type C
NPH. *See* Normal pressure hydrocephalus
Nuclear magnetic resonance (NMR), 107
nvCJD. *See* New variant Creutzfeldt-Jakob disease

OMD. *See* Oromandibular dystonia
Organic from psychogenic tic disorders, 272–274
Oromandibular dystonia (OMD), 202
Osteopetrosis, 115–118

Pantothenate kinase-associated neurodegeneration
  (PKAN), 44, 184–186, 252–254
Paraneoplastic disorder (PND), 80–82. *See also*
  Progressive supranuclear palsy (PSP)
Paraneoplastic syndrome, 138, 241, 285–286
Paraphilia, 8
PARK 2. *See* Autosomal recessive juvenile onset
  Parkinson's disease
Parkin parkinsonism. *See* Autosomal recessive
  juvenile onset Parkinson's disease (PARK 2)
Parkinsonian disorders. *See* Parkinson's
  disease (PD)
Parkinsonian manifestations, malignant, 26
Parkinsonian syndrome. *See* Parkinsonism
Parkinsonism, 40–42. *See also* Chorea;
  Huntington's disease (HD); Parkinson's
  disease (PD); Sydenham's chorea (SC)
  acute onset, 54–56
  asymmetric, 88–90
  atypical, 74–75
  reversible unilateral, 101–102
  reversible, 57–59
Parkinson's disease (PD), 2. *See also* Parkinsonism;
  Tremors
  acute onset parkinsonism, 54–56
  atypical parkinsonism, 74–75

  catatonia, 51, 52
  clinical trial, 16–17
  DBS surgery side effects, 27–28
  DDS, 10–12
  de novo parkinsonism vs. depression, 33–34
  dopamine dysregulation cases, 31–32
  DRD, 66–69
  dystonia, 2–6
  FOG, 18–19
  hallucinations and REM behavior disorder, 13–15
  HD, 60–61
  hypophonia and parkinsonism, 40–42
  ICDs in, 7–8
  impulse control disorders, 20–22
  lessons from extended family, 29–30
  NBIA, 44–48
  NMS, 25–26, 50–52
  PSP phenotype, 71–72
  reversible parkinsonism, 57–59
  VaP, 62–64
  warning from RBD, 35–36
Paroxysmal dystonic choreoathetosis (PDC), 276
Paroxysmal kinesigenic choreoathetosis
  (PKC), 276
Partial thromboplastin time (PTT), 152
PCR. *See* Polymerase chain reaction
PD. *See* Parkinson's disease
PDC. *See* Paroxysmal dystonic choreoathetosis
PEG. *See* Percutaneous endoscopic gastrostomy
PEP. *See* Postencephalitic parkinsonism
Percutaneous endoscopic gastrostomy
  (PEG), 174, 285
Periodic slow wave complex (PSWC), 107, 109
PET. *See* Positron emission tomography;
  Prolonged exercise test
Phospholipase A2 VI-associated
  neurodegeneration (PLAN), 44, 45
PKAN. *See* Pantothenate kinase-associated
  neurodegeneration
PKC. *See* Paroxysmal kinesigenic choreoathetosis
PLAN. *See* Phospholipase A2 VI-associated
  neurodegeneration
PND. *See* Paraneoplastic disorder
Polymerase chain reaction (PCR), 99, 107, 166
  CGG repeat analysis of FMR1 gene, 125
  to detect deletion mutations, 213
Polysomnography (PSG), 35
Positron emission tomography (PET), 41
Postencephalitic parkinsonism (PEP), 80, 81
Premutation carriers, 124
Prion protein (PRNP; PrP), 78, 108
Progressive supranuclear palsy (PSP), 70–72, 77,
  80, 84–87, 98, 230. *See also* Paraneoplastic
  disorder (PND); Supranuclear gaze palsy
  clinical variants, 85
  differential diagnosis, 80, 81
  no-no head tremor, 84, 85
  PSP-like syndromes, 85

Progressive supranuclear palsy-corticobasal syndrome (PSP-CBS), 85
Progressive supranuclear palsy-parkinsonism (PSP-P), 85
Progressive supranuclear palsy-progressive nonfluent aphasia (PSP-PNFA), 85
Progressive supranuclear palsy-pure akinesia with gait freezing (PSP-PAGF), 85
Prolonged exercise test (PET), 218
Pseudo-psychogenic movement disorder, 148
PSG. See Polysomnography
PSP. See Progressive supranuclear palsy
PSP CBS. See Progressive supranuclear palsy-corticobasal syndrome
PSP-P. See Progressive supranuclear palsy-parkinsonism
PSP-PAGF. See Progressive supranuclear palsy-pure akinesia with gait freezing
PSP-PNFA. See Progressive supranuclear palsy-progressive nonfluent aphasia
PSWC. See Periodic slow wave complex
Psychogenic bizarre-gait pigeonhole, 290–291
Psychogenic gait disorders, 259–261
Psychogenic movement disorder, 145, 148, 292–293
  bizarre exorcist-like movements, 295–297
  psychogenic bizarre-gait pigeonhole, 290–291
PTT. See Partial thromboplastin time
Punding, 21

Rapidly developing dementia (RDD), 109
Rapid-onset dystonia parkinsonism (RDP), 208
REM sleep behavior disorder (RBD), 13–15, 35–36, 70
Renal tubular acidosis (RTA), 117
Retrocollis, 207, 208
Right upper extremity (RUE), 70

Satoyoshi syndrome, 217–221
  painful muscle spasms, 218
  posturing of hands and feet, 218
SC. See Sydenham's chorea
SCA. See Spinocerebellar ataxia; Spinocerebellar atrophy
Schizophrenia, 240–242. See also Catatonia
sCJD. See Sporadic Creutzfeldt-Jakob disease
SD. See Spasmodic dysphonia
Segawa disease. See Dopa-responsive dystonia (DRD)
Selective serotonergic reuptake inhibitor (SSRI), 34
Senataxin (SETX), 250
Serum glutamic pyruvic transaminase (SGPT), 168
SET. See Short exercise test
SETX. See Senataxin
SFEMG. See Single-fiber electromyography
SGPT. See Serum glutamic pyruvic transaminase
Short-duration response, 2
Short exercise test (SET), 218

SIADH. See Syndrome of inappropriate antidiuretic hormone
Single-fiber electromyography (SFEMG), 218
Single nucleotide polymorphism (SNP), 167
Single-photon emission computed tomography (SPECT), 19, 71, 102
SLE. See Systemic lupus erythematosus
SN. See Substantia nigra
SNGP. See Supranuclear gaze palsy
SNP. See Single nucleotide polymorphism
Spasmodic dysphonia (SD), 201–202
SPECT. See Single-photon emission computed tomography
Spinocerebellar ataxia (SCA), 207–209, 230. See also Ataxia
  type 1, 250
  type 2, 300–302
  type 3, 75
  type 12, 131–132
  type 19, 123
Spinocerebellar atrophy (SCA), 188
Sporadic Creutzfeldt-Jakob disease (sCJD), 77–78. See also New variant Creutzfeldt-Jakob disease (nvCJD)
SPS. See Stiff person syndrome
SSRI. See Selective serotonergic reuptake inhibitor
STA MCA. See Superficial temporal artery–middle cerebral artery
Steatorrhea, 242
Stereotactic surgery, 96
Stereotypies, hereditary, 268–270. See also Catatonia
Stiff person syndrome (SPS), 248
STN. See Subthalamic nucleus
STN DBS surgery. See Subthalamic nucleus-deep brain stimulation surgery
Substantia nigra (SN), 36
Subthalamic nucleus (STN), 27, 91, 143
Subthalamic nucleus-deep brain stimulation surgery (STN-DBS surgery), 27–28
Superficial temporal artery–middle cerebral artery (STA-MCA), 277
Supranuclear gaze palsy (SNGP), 80
Supranuclear gaze palsy, 98–99. See also Progressive supranuclear palsy (PSP)
Sydenham's chorea (SC), 160–161. See also Chorea; Huntington's disease (HD)
Syndrome of inappropriate antidiuretic hormone (SIADH), 98
Systemic lupus erythematosus (SLE), 152

Task-specific action dystonia, 222–223. See also Cervical dystonia; Dopa-responsive dystonia (DRD); Dystonia-improvement-dystonia (DID); DYT6 dystonia; Improvement-dystonia-improvement (IDI); Multifocal dystonia
TB. See Tuberculosis

TCD. *See* Transcranial duplex sonography
TDPD. *See* Tremor dominant Parkinson disease
Thyroid-stimulating hormone (TSH), 244, 255
Thyroid transcription factor 1 (TITF-1), 244
Tics. *See also* Gilles de la Tourette syndrome
  HD, 264–265
  hereditary stereotypies, 268–270
  LTG for involuntary movements, 266–267
  organic from psychogenic tic disorders,
    272–274
TITF-1. *See* Thyroid transcription factor 1
Torsion dystonia, 200
Torticollis, 232, 233
Transcranial duplex sonography (TCD), 276–277
Tremor dominant Parkinson disease
  (TDPD), 91–93
Tremors. *See also* Parkinson's disease (PD);
  Parkinsonism
  disabling postural and resting tremor, 140–143
  DYT6 dystonia, 134–135
  FXTAS, 122–126, 127–130
  multiple sclerosis, 144–149
  nonparaneoplastic limbic encephalitis, 137–139
  SCA 12, 131–132
TSH. *See* Thyroid-stimulating hormone
Tuberculosis (TB), 91

UK Parkinson's Disease Society Brain Bank
  criteria (UK PDSBBC), 70

Unified Parkinson's Disease Rating Scale
  (UPDRS), 24
University of Nebraska Medical Center
  (UNMC), 29
University of Tennessee, 166

Vascular parkinsonism (VaP), 62–64. *See also*
  Parkinsonism
  gait assessments, 64
  NPH dichotomy vs., 64
Venereal Disease Research Laboratory (VDRL),
  247, 260
Ventralis intermedius thalamotomy
  (Vim thalamotomy), 91, 143
Ventralis oralis posterior (VOP), 96
Ventriculoperitoneal shunt (VPS), 57, 63
Vertical supranuclear gaze palsy (VSGP), 77, 78
Voltage-gated potassium channel
  (VGKC), 138, 139

Wechsler Adult Intelligence Scale-Revised
  (WAIS-R), 188
Wilson's disease (WD), 44, 204–205. *See also*
  Kayser-Fleischer ring; Parkinsonism

Zona incerta lesion (ZI lesion), 91
Zoophilia, 8

42925546R00190

Made in the USA
Lexington, KY
10 July 2015